T0318356

Japanese Kampo Medicines for the Treatment of Common Diseases: Focus on Inflammation

Japanese Kampo Medicines for the Treatment of Common Diseases: Focus on Inflammation

Somasundaram Arumugam

Kenichi Watanabe

Department of Clinical Pharmacology
Niigata University of Pharmacy and Applied Life Sciences
Niigata, Japan

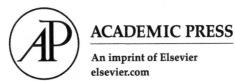

ACADEMIC PRESS

An imprint of Elsevier
elsevier.com

Academic Press is an imprint of Elsevier
125 London Wall, London EC2Y 5AS, United Kingdom
525 B Street, Suite 1800, San Diego, CA 92101-4495, United States
50 Hampshire Street, 5th Floor, Cambridge, MA 02139, United States
The Boulevard, Langford Lane, Kidlington, Oxford OX5 1GB, United Kingdom

Notices
Knowledge and best practice in this field are constantly changing. As new research and experience broaden our
understanding, changes in research methods, professional practices, or medical treatment may become necessary.

Practitioners and researchers must always rely on their own experience and knowledge in evaluating and using any
information, methods, compounds, or experiments described herein. In using such information or methods they
should be mindful of their own safety and the safety of others, including parties for whom they have a professional
responsibility.

To the fullest extent of the law, neither the Publisher nor the authors, contributors, or editors, assume any liability
for any injury and/or damage to persons or property as a matter of products liability, negligence or otherwise, or
from any use or operation of any methods, products, instructions, or ideas contained in the material herein.

Library of Congress Cataloging-in-Publication Data
A catalog record for this book is available from the Library of Congress

British Library Cataloguing-in-Publication Data
A catalogue record for this book is available from the British Library

ISBN: 978-0-12-809398-6

For information on all Academic Press publications visit our website at
https://www.elsevier.com/books-and-journals

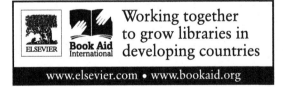
Working together
to grow libraries in
developing countries

www.elsevier.com • www.bookaid.org

Publisher: Mica Haley
Acquisition Editor: Kristine Jones
Editorial Project Manager: Tracy Tufaga
Production Project Manager: Edward Taylor
Designer: Mark Rogers

Typeset by TNQ Books and Journals

Contents

Biographies

Somasundaram Arumugam, MPharm, PhD

Reader, Department of Clinical Pharmacology

Niigata University of Pharmacy and Applied Life Sciences

Niigata, Japan

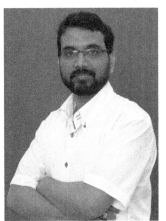

Dr. Somasundaram Arumugam is a Reader in the Department of Clinical Pharmacology at Niigata University of Pharmacy and Applied Life Sciences. Dr. Arumugam received the Japanese Circulation Society Young Investigator Award for International Students in 2014. He received the Young Investigator Award at the 6th International Congress on Cardiovascular Diseases in 2011. He is an Editorial Board Member of *International Journal of Innovative Pharmaceutical Sciences and Research*. He is serving as an expert reviewer in various journals and has more than 50 scientific publications to his credit.

Kenichi Watanabe, PhD

Professor of Clinical Pharmacology

Niigata University of Pharmacy and Applied Life Sciences

Niigata, Japan

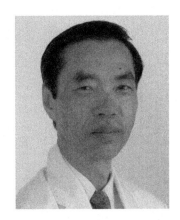

Prof./Dr. Kenichi Watanabe received his PhD in Medical Sciences at Niigata University and PhD in Pharmaceutical Sciences at Shizuoka Prefectural University. Currently, he is working as a Clinical Pharmacologist and Cardiologist at Niigata University of Pharmacy and Applied Life Sciences, Niigata, Japan. His research has focused on heart diseases, diabetes mellitus, hypertension, inflammation, Kampo traditional Japanese medicine, and metabolic syndrome. Based on this research and fellow-ship training, he has received several awards and honors, such as the Best Paper Award from the Society of Experimental Biology and Medicine. Dr. Watanabe is serving as an editorial member of several reputed journals as well as an expert reviewer. He has over 500 scientific publications to his credit.

List of Contributors

Shanish Antony   Government Medical College, Kottayam, India

Somasundaram Arumugam   Niigata University of Pharmacy and Applied Life Sciences, Niigata, Japan

Sahana S. Babu   Houston Methodist Research Institute, Houston, TX, United States

Vijayasree V. Giridharan   The University of Texas Health Science Center at Houston (UTHealth), Houston, TX, United States

Meilei Harima   Niigata University of Pharmacy and Applied Life Sciences, Niigata, Japan

Darukeshwara Joladarashi   Houston Methodist Research Institute, Houston, TX, United States

Geetha Kandasamy   KMCH College of Pharmacy, Coimbatore, Tamilnadu, India

Vengadeshprabhu Karuppagounder   Niigata University of Pharmacy and Applied Life Sciences, Niigata, Japan

Akihiko Komuro   Niigata University of Pharmacy and Applied Life Sciences, Niigata, Japan

Tetsuya Konishi   NUPALS Liaison R/D Promotion Division, Niigata, Japan; Changchun University of Chinese Medicine, Changchun, China; HALD Food Function Research Institute, Niigata, Japan

Prasanna Krishnamurthy   Houston Methodist Research Institute, Houston, TX, United States

K.T. Manisenthil Kumar   KMCH College of Pharmacy, Coimbatore, Tamilnadu, India

Arunkumar Nagalingam   KMCH College of Pharmacy, Coimbatore, Tamilnadu, India

Mayumi Nomoto   Niigata University of Pharmacy and Applied Life Sciences, Niigata, Japan

J. Quedevo   The University of Texas Health Science Center at Houston (UTHealth), Houston, TX, United States; The University of Texas Graduate School of Biomedical Sciences at Houston, Houston, TX, United States; University of Southern Santa Catarina (UNESC), Criciúma, SC, Brazil

V. Ravichandiran   National Institute of Pharmaceutical Education and Research, Kolkata, India

Hirohito Sone   Niigata University Graduate School of Medical and Dental Sciences, Niigata, Japan

Remya Sreedhar   Niigata University of Pharmacy and Applied Life Sciences, Niigata, Japan

Takao Sunaga   Niigata Kido Clinic, Niigata, Japan

Hiroshi Suzuki   Niigata University of Pharmacy and Applied Life Sciences, Niigata, Japan; Niigata University Graduate School of Medical and Dental Sciences, Niigata, Japan

Kenji Suzuki   Niigata University Graduate School of Medical and Dental Sciences, Niigata, Japan

Rajarajan A. Thandavarayan   Houston Methodist Research Institute, Houston, TX, United States

Alex Thomas   International Institute of Biotechnology and Toxicology, Kancheepuram, Tamilnadu, India

Murugan Veerapandian   National Institute of Pharmaceutical Education and Research, Kolkata, India

Kenichi Watanabe   Niigata University of Pharmacy and Applied Life Sciences, Niigata, Japan

CHAPTER 1

Introduction to Japanese Kampo Medicines

Remya Sreedhar, Kenichi Watanabe, Somasundaram Arumugam
Niigata University of Pharmacy and Applied Life Sciences, Niigata, Japan

Introduction

Traditional medicines or herbal medicines are known to have played an important role in providing first-line and basic health services for patients having numerous disease conditions from the very beginning of human history. This traditional medicine system (TMS) has different names in different cultures, like traditional Chinese medicine (TCM; China), Ayurveda (India), Japanese Kampo medicine (Japan), etc. According to the World Health Organization (WHO), traditional medicine includes a diversity of health practices, approaches, knowledge, and beliefs and incorporates plant, animal, and/or mineral-based medicines; spiritual therapies; manual techniques; and exercises, which are applied singly or in combination to maintain well-being and to treat or prevent illness. The National Center for Complementary and Alternative Medicine established at the National Institutes of Health in the United States in October 1998 recategorized traditional medicine as complementary and alternative medicine.

Natural products and related structures are essential sources of new pharmaceuticals, because of the immense variety of functionally relevant secondary metabolites of plant or microbial species. Owing to the great development of chemical and pharmacological screening methods over the past several years, natural products and related structures continue to be extremely important elements of pharmacopoeias. Moreover the increased scientific significance and commercial potential of TMSs attract international attention and global market demands (Mehta et al., 2015; Ngo et al., 2013; Yu et al., 2006). In recent years, an increasing number of people are choosing herbal medicines or products, either alone or in combination with others, to improve their health. According to the WHO, 75% of the world's population uses herbs for basic health care needs. Nowadays, many practitioners of conventional medicine do not hesitate to recommend herbs, herbal products, or complementary or alternative medicine therapy to their patients for the effective treatment of diseases (Pan et al., 2014).

Japanese Kampo Medicine

Kampo medicines are Japanese herbal medicines of traditional Chinese origin, but adapted to the Japanese culture. TCM is a complete system of healing that developed in China about

Japanese Kampo Medicines for the Treatment of Common Diseases: Focus on Inflammation. http://dx.doi.org/10.1016/B978-0-12-809398-6.00001-9

3000 years ago and reached a modified form about 2000 years ago. It includes herbal medicine, acupuncture, moxibustion, and massage, among other techniques. In recent decades, it has developed a popularity in China and, as a complementary medicine, throughout the world. TCM has been adopted in modified form in Far East countries like Japan and Korea. The methods and theories of diagnosis and treatment in TCM and Kampo differ from those of Western medicine. Western medicine follows the disease-based diagnosis, whereas TCM and Kampo follow a patient-based diagnosis (Yu et al., 2006).

History of Kampo Medicine

Traditional Japanese medicine has been used for 1500 years and includes Kampo, acupuncture, and acupressure (Shiatsu). The word Kampo (also written as Kanpo) refers to the herbal system used in China that developed during the Han Dynasty. Today the word is also used to describe a unique system of Japanese herbal medicine. Kampo is widely practiced in Japan, where it is fully integrated into the modern health care system (Watanabe et al., 2011). During the 5th and 6th centuries TCM was brought to Japan through the Korean Peninsula. Although Japanese practitioners initially followed TCM, later Japan started to modify the Chinese medicine mainly because the materials were unique to China and needed to be adjusted to conditions in Japan. During the Meiji Restoration, the focus was changed to Western countries and Western medicine was adopted, especially German medicine. As a consequence, Kampo medicine lost its importance and was almost forgotten. However, after the Second World War, the first modern Kampo specialists carried on the tradition from the Edo period. Kampo products, mainly herbal extracts, have been included in the Japanese National Health Insurance Drug List since 1971. A total of 148 Kampo herbal medicines are covered under the national health insurance system as of this writing (Ishibashi et al., 2005; Watanabe et al., 2011; Yu et al., 2006).

Therapeutic Policy of Kampo Medicine

The therapeutic policies underlying Kampo medicine are based on the physical constitution and current symptoms of each patient. Kampo therapy is referred to as "tailor-made medicine" and has properties similar to "mind and body" or psychosomatic medicine (Ushiroyama, 2013). Kampo medicine uses a treatment formulation corresponding to "Sho," which is based on the patient's symptoms at a given moment. The concept of Sho comes from the "Zheng" concept of TCM, but is simpler because of the simplified Kampo theory.

Sho is recognized in terms of:

1. Qi (well-being, energy, illness, vigor), blood, and water;
2. the eight principles (indicating the eight fundamental concepts of Yin–Yang, interior–exterior, cold–heat, and deficiency–excess);

3. the five parenchymatous viscera (all living and nonliving things in this world are composed of these five elements; in human beings, the five elements are allocated to five organs, liver, heart, spleen, lung, and kidney, which are in balanced interaction with one another);

4. six stages of disease (taiyang, shaoyang, yangming, taiyin, shaoyin, and jueyin).

Kampo physicians take the advantage of both Kampo and Western medicine diagnostic tools in most cases. The Kampo therapy consists of talking with the patient, an audio-olfactorial investigation, investigation of the tongue and skin, and palpation of the forearm and abdomen. Then the physician diagnoses the disease pattern and assigns it to a corresponding therapy (Efferth et al., 2007; Ishibashi et al., 2005; Terasawa, 1994; Yu et al., 2006).

Clinical Applications of Kampo Medicine

There is no separate license for the use of traditional medicine in Japan, because the Meiji government adopted a single license system for medical practitioners. Therefore, only Western physicians are allowed to prescribe Kampo drugs, and currently more than 70% of Japanese physicians are using Kampo medicine in their daily practice together with high-tech medical treatments such as organ transplantation and robotic operation (Iwase et al., 2012). Even though 148 Kampo formulas are listed under the Japanese insurance program, Kampo practitioners are also able to use decoctions, selecting several herbs from among 243 kinds available under the insurance system.

Research

Both basic and clinical research on Kampo medicine is actively pursued. In the clinical field, the main effort is on the application of Kampo in modern medicine. Numerous research studies are published every year and some of them are discussed in later sections. In clinical research, the studies are carried out according to the patient's condition based on the traditional logic of Kampo therapy.

Kampo Medicine for Gastrointestinal Tract Disorders

Kampo medicines are usually prescribed as a combination of several herbs, indicating that the combination of multiple herbs may be crucial for effective antiinflammatory activity. Kampo medicines are used mainly for the treatment of inflammation associated with the gastrointestinal tract. Numerous reports have suggested the use of Kampo medicines such as saireito, tokishakuyakusan, jumihaidokuto, hangeshashinto, etc., in cases of inflammatory bowel disorders (Endo et al., 2009; Fujisawa et al., 2005; Kawashima et al., 2004; Oikawa et al., 2012; Sreedhar et al., 2015a; Sreedhar et al., 2015b).

Kampo Medicines for Skin Diseases

Atopic dermatitis (AD), a common skin disease accompanied by intense itching and relapsing eczema, is caused by immune imbalances and skin-barrier disruption. Current treatment options for AD include topical corticosteroids and oral antiallergy drugs. Traditional Kampo medicine has a long history of playing a role in the prevention and treatment of AD. Some of the Kampo medicines and their formulations used for the treatment of AD are listed in Table 1.1 (Chino et al., 2010; Funakushi et al., 2011; Gao et al., 2005; Jiang et al., 2009; Kobayashi et al., 2003; Yamashita et al., 2013; Yanagihara et al., 2013). In addition to this, Kampo medicines such as byakkokakeishito, shoseiryuto, byakkokaninjinto, etc., are widely used for the treatment of skin allergies (Makino et al., 2014; Sakaguchi et al., 1996; Tatsumi et al., 2001).

Table 1.1: Some Commonly Used Kampo Formulas for Atopic Dermatitis

Kampo Medicine	Component
Juzentaihoto	Astragali radix
	Cinnamomi cortex
	Rehmanniae radix
	Paeoniae radix
	Cnidii rhizoma
	Atractylodis lanceae rhizoma
	Angelicae radix
	Panacis ginseng radix
	Poria
	Glycyrrhizae radix
Yokukansan	Atractylodis lanceae rhizoma
	Poria
	Cnidii rhizoma
	Angelicae radix
	Bupleuri radix
	Glycyrrhizae radix
	Uncariae cum uncis ramulus
Hochuekkito	Astragali radix
	Atractylodis lanceae radix
	Panacis ginseng radix
	Angelicae radix
	Bupleuri radix
	Zizyphi fructus
	Aurantii nobilis pericarpium
	Glycyrrhizae radix
	Cimicifugae rhizoma
	Zingiberis rhizoma
Orengedokuto	Coptidis rhizoma
	Scutellariae radix
	Phellodendri cortex
	Gardeniae fructus

Kampo Medicines for Eye Diseases

Kampo medicines have been used to treat a variety of ocular disease conditions such as dry eye, blurred vision, decreased visual acuity, and visual field defects. Oral administration of orenge-dokuto and kakkonto decreased aqueous flare elevation after small-incision cataract surgery. Tokishakuyakusan significantly increases ocular blood flow and can be used, either alone or in combination with topical medications such as tafluprost, as an effective strategy to improve fundus circulation in glaucoma patients, especially in patients with normal tension glaucoma. Oral administration of goshajinkigan improved ocular surface disorders in patients with type 1 diabetes mellitus (Hayasaka et al., 2012; Ikeda et al., 2001; Takayama et al., 2014).

Kampo Medicines for Respiratory Tract Disorders

Many diseases of the respiratory tract are treated with Kampo medicine in daily practice. Because the spread of steroid inhalants has fundamentally changed the basic Western medical therapy of asthma, Kampo preparations are now used less frequently than in the past. But owing to the adverse effects produced by the long-term use of bronchodilators or steroids, there is a strong demand for Kampo preparations. Various clinical studies are also going on to investigate the efficacy of Kampo formulations for the treatment of respiratory tract diseases. Reports have suggested that bakumondoto, a Kampo formulation, effectively suppresses cough in elderly patients with chronic obstructive pulmonary disease. In addition to this, bakumondoto could be useful and safe for the treatment of postinfectious prolonged cough. Saibokuto is effective for the treatment of asthma and it also has an antiinflammatory effect on bronchial eosinophilic infiltration (Irifune et al., 2011; Kamei et al., 2003; Mukaida et al., 2011; Urata et al., 2002).

Kampo Medicines for Liver Diseases

Hepatitis C virus (HCV) infection frequently causes hepatitis, which is linked to the development of liver cirrhosis and hepatocellular carcinoma. Most physicians who practice Kampo medicine in Japan have observed that Kampo medicine can be as effective as interferon therapy in the treatment of chronic hepatitis. An assessment of clinical treatment with ninjin-yoeito for chronic hepatitis showed an inhibitory effect on HCV infection and protective effect on immunological hepatopathy. Nonalcoholic steatohepatitis (NASH) is a multifactorial disease and has close correlations with other metabolic disorders. Although several Kampo formulations are used for other liver diseases, only a few studies have investigated their effects on NASH. Shosaikoto and juzentaihoto inhibited necroinflammation and fibrosis in the liver of a mouse model of NASH. Bofutsushosan, a well-known antiobesity medicine in Japan and other Asian countries, has been shown to reduce body weight and improve insulin resistance and hepatic steatosis (Cyong et al., 2000; Jadeja et al., 2014; Ono et al., 2014; Takahashi et al., 2014).

Kampo Medicines for Kidney Diseases

Kampo medicine has been used for the cure and prevention of urinary calculi for many years, but the effects and mechanism of this use of Kampo medicines are unclear. Gorinsan, which contains sanshishi and takusha, has been used for the treatment of urolithiasis. Oxidative stress and peritubular capillary injury are involved in the progression of chronic kidney diseases. Shichimotsukokato, a Kampo formulation, protected against nephrosclerosis and hypertension in chronic kidney diseases through the mechanism of antioxidative activity and maintenance of peritubular capillary networks. Several studies have also suggested the use of this Kampo formulation in cases of diabetic nephropathy and other kidney-related diseases (Goto et al., 2003; Mitsuma et al., 1999; Nishihata et al., 2013; Ono et al, 2013).

Kampo Medicine for Infectious Disease

Owing to the appearance of antibiotics and antibacterial agents, various vaccines, and fluid replacements, the application of Kampo medicine to the treatment of infectious diseases in modern Japan is now quite limited. However, many diseases are still treated with Kampo preparations either alone or in combination with modern medical therapies. For the common cold and the common cold syndrome, Kampo medicines are used as the first line choice. In Japan, there is a proverb stating "The cold is the origin of all diseases." Not only during the initial stages of common cold, but also with a whole group of similar conditions, attempts have been made to cure the emerging symptoms with Kampo medicine. *Streptococcus pyogenes* causes various serious diseases, including necrotizing fasciitis and streptococcal toxic shock syndrome, and a serious problem associated with therapy for this infection is attenuation of the antibiotic effect, especially penicillin treatment failure and macrolide resistance. Hainosankyuto is a traditional Kampo medicine used for the treatment of infectious purulent diseases in Japan. This drug increased survival rate after *S. pyogenes* infection and upregulated both bactericidal activity and macrophage phagocytic activity through modulation of inflammatory cytokines. Kakkonto is another traditional Kampo formulation that is used for the treatment of infectious diseases and is reported to have some efficacy against infection with herpes simplex virus type 1 (Hottenbacher et al., 2013; Minami et al., 2011; Nagasaka et al., 1995).

Kampo Medicine for Cancer Therapy

In this field, there are no Kampo prescriptions that are definitely effective; still, various studies are going on. However, Kampo medicines are used as adjunctive therapy following surgery for various malignant tumors or else in combination with chemotherapy or radiation therapy to provide relief for the suffering of the patients by preventing or alleviating the side effects of the Western medical therapies. Patients with cancer exhibit various symptoms induced by cancer itself and its therapy leading to fatigue. Restoration and maintenance of mental and physical energy are important for successful cancer treatment. Administration of Kampo along with Western medicine can restore the energy of patients. One of the characteristics of Kampo medicine is that Kampo diagnosis does not target the disease, but the patient with the disease. The appropriate use of Kampo formulas, such as "Ho-zai," formulas to vitalize fatigued patients (e.g., hochuekkito, juzentaihoto, ninjinyoeito), "Hojin-zai," formulas to restore energy (e.g., goshajinkigan), and "Kuoketsu-zai," formulas to resolve stagnant blood flow (e.g., keishibukuryogan, tokakujokito, tokishakuyakusan), is to administer them in combination. Consequently, basic autonomic functions, such as appetite, sleep, defecation, and urination, are normalized and the nutritional and mental conditions are restored. These favorable changes in the patient's condition allow completion of the standard cancer therapy course, resulting in an improved outcome of cancer therapy and successful treatment (Inoue and Hoshino, 2015; Nagata, 2015; Okumi and Koyama, 2014; Watanabe, 2015; Yamakawa et al., 2013b). Daikenchuto is a Kampo formulation that exhibits a higher antitumor effect in gastric, breast, esophageal, and colon cancer cells. Juzentaihoto shows immunoaugmentation effects and increased regulatory activities in T cells in advanced pancreatic cancer patients. Goshajinkigan is used for the treatment of several neurological symptoms and useful in preventing neuropathy in breast cancer patients treated with docetaxel (Abe et al., 2013; Gao et al., 2012; Ikemoto et al., 2014; Nagata et al., 2016).

Current Usage of Kampo and Applications in Western Medicine

According to a survey by the journal *Nikkei Medical*, more than 70% of physicians in Japan prescribe Kampo drugs today (Yamakawa et al., 2013a). The Japan Society for Oriental Medicine is the biggest society for Kampo medicine and has 8600 members and 2600 certified board members. Kampo education for medical students was incorporated into the "model core curriculum" by the Japanese Ministry of Education, Culture, Sports, Science, and Technology (Ishibashi et al., 2005). The availability of modern ready-to-use spray-dried granular extracts of the original Kampo formulas is directly related to the increased use of Kampo medicine. They have increasingly replaced the traditional decoctions of the crude drugs, even though they are also covered by the national insurance system. In addition to the simpler administration, industrial production has enabled several other advantages. There are over 15 pharmaceutical companies in Japan that are manufacturing Kampo extracts with government approval. Their manufacture is governed by pharmaceutical affairs law and strictly controlled by other government regulations, including good manufacturing practice (GMP) and good laboratory practice. GMP for pharmaceutical products includes reduction of human errors to a minimum, prevention of contamination of the drugs, and establishment of a system to guarantee high quality. As a result the products are assured of quality and safety at the highest level. Today extract preparations make up 95% of the Japanese Kampo market (Watanabe et al., 2011).

In Western countries, for example the United States, mainly TCM is receiving increasing interest. The practitioners practice herbal therapy often in combination with acupuncture, which is often a mixture of Chinese, Japanese, and Korean acupuncture styles. Kampo drugs are available only over the counter, meeting Japanese GMP criteria. Several Japanese pharmaceutical companies have started clinical trials in the United States and several drugs have already been registered as investigational new drugs by the Food and Drug Administration. In Europe, especially in Germany, there is a long tradition of herbal medicine, and there is a growing interest in Chinese phytotherapy and Japanese Kampo (Watanabe et al., 2011).

Conclusion

Kampo is a holistic and individualized treatment option with a long tradition, and future research is required to take this into account. Looking back through its history, the time has come for Kampo medicine to be approached from a fresh global perspective. Sustained clinical and basic research is required for the expanded integration of Kampo medicine into Western medicine. Also, the future establishment of Kampo education in Japanese medical schools requires fostering instructors knowledgeable in and responsible for Kampo education and the development of Kampo therapy integrated with Western medicine.

References

Abe, H., Kawai, Y., Mori, T., Tomida, K., Kubota, Y., Umeda, T., Tani, T., 2013. The Kampo medicine Goshajinkigan prevents neuropathy in breast cancer patients treated with docetaxel. Asian Pac. J. Cancer Prev. 14 (11), 6351–6356.

Chino, A., Okamoto, H., Hirasaki, Y., Terasawa, K., 2010. A case of atopic dermatitis successfully treated with juzentaihoto (Kampo). Altern. Ther. Health Med. 16 (1), 62–64.

Cyong, J.C., Ki, S.M., Iijima, K., Kobayashi, T., Furuya, M., 2000. Clinical and pharmacological studies on liver diseases treated with Kampo herbal medicine. Am. J. Chin. Med. 28 (3–4), 351–360. http://dx.doi.org/10.1142/S0192415X00000416.

Efferth, T., Miyachi, H., Bartsch, H., 2007. Pharmacogenomics of a traditional Japanese herbal medicine (Kampo) for cancer therapy. Cancer genom. proteom. 4 (2), 81–91.

Endo, M., Oikawa, T., Hoshino, T., Hatori, T., Matsumoto, T., Hanawa, T., 2009. Suppression of murine colitis by Kampo medicines, with special reference to the efficacy of saireito. J. Tradit. Med. 26 (3), 110–121. http://dx.doi.org/10.11339/jtm.26.110.

Fujisawa, M., Oguchi, K., Yamaura, T., Suzuki, M., Cyong, J.C., 2005. Protective effect of hawthorn fruit on murine experimental colitis. Am. J. Chin. Med. 33 (2), 167–180. http://dx.doi.org/10.1142/S0192415X05002849.

Funakushi, N., Yamaguchi, T., Jiang, J., Imamura, S., Kuhara, T., Suto, H., Ikeda, S., 2011. Ameliorating effect of Yokukansan on the development of atopic dermatitis-like lesions and scratching behavior in socially isolated NC/Nga mice. Arch. Dermatol. Res. 303 (9), 659–667. http://dx.doi.org/10.1007/s00403-011-1137-9.

Gao, J.J., Song, P.P., Qi, F.H., Kokudo, N., Qu, X.J., Tang, W., 2012. Evidence-based research on traditional Japanese medicine, Kampo, in treatment of gastrointestinal cancer in Japan. Drug Discov. Ther. 6 (1), 1–8.

Gao, X.K., Fuseda, K., Shibata, T., Tanaka, H., Inagaki, N., Nagai, H., 2005. Kampo medicines for mite antigen-induced allergic dermatitis in NC/Nga mice. Evid. Based Complement. Altern. Med. 2 (2), 191–199. http://dx.doi.org/10.1093/ecam/neh077.

Goto, H., Shimada, Y., Tanikawa, K., Sato, S., Hikiami, H., Sekiya, N., Terasawa, K., 2003. Clinical evaluation of the effect of daio (rhei rhizoma) on the progression of diabetic nephropathy with overt proteinuria. Am. J. Chin. Med. 31 (2), 267–275. http://dx.doi.org/10.1142/S0192415X03000850.

Hayasaka, S., Kodama, T., Ohira, A., 2012. Traditional Japanese herbal (kampo) medicines and treatment of ocular diseases: a review. Am. J. Chin. Med. 40 (5), 887–904. http://dx.doi.org/10.1142/S0192415X12500668.

Hottenbacher, L., Weisshuhn, T.E., Watanabe, K., Seki, T., Ostermann, J., Witt, C.M., 2013. Opinions on Kampo and reasons for using it—results from a cross-sectional survey in three Japanese clinics. BMC Complement. Altern. Med. 13, 108. http://dx.doi.org/10.1186/1472-6882-13-108.

Ikeda, N., Hayasaka, S., Nagaki, Y., Hayasaka, Y., Kadoi, C., Matsumoto, M., 2001. Effects of traditional Sino-Japanese herbal medicines on aqueous flare elevation after small-incision cataract surgery. J. Ocul. Pharmacol. Ther. 17 (1), 59–65. http://dx.doi.org/10.1089/108076801750125694.

Ikemoto, T., Shimada, M., Iwahashi, S., Saito, Y., Kanamoto, M., Mori, H., Utsunomiya, T., 2014. Changes of immunological parameters with administration of Japanese Kampo medicine (Juzen-Taihoto/TJ-48) in patients with advanced pancreatic cancer. Int. J. Clin. Oncol. 19 (1), 81–86. http://dx.doi.org/10.1007/s10147-013-0529-6.

Inoue, M., Hoshino, E., 2015. Symptoms of cancer patients and kampo formulas effective for them. Gan To Kagaku Ryoho 42 (13), 2418–2422.

Irifune, K., Hamada, H., Ito, R., Katayama, H., Watanabe, A., Kato, A., Higaki, J., 2011. Antitussive effect of bakumondoto a fixed kampo medicine (six herbal components) for treatment of post-infectious prolonged cough: controlled clinical pilot study with 19 patients. Phytomedicine 18 (8–9), 630–633. http://dx.doi.org/10.1016/j.phymed.2011.02.017.

Ishibashi, A., Kosato, H., Ohno, S., Sakaguchi, H., Yamada, T., Matsuda, K., 2005. General introduction to kampo. Introd. Kampo, Jpn. Tradit. Med. 2–13.

Iwase, S., Yamaguchi, T., Miyaji, T., Terawaki, K., Inui, A., Uezono, Y., 2012. The clinical use of Kampo medicines (traditional Japanese herbal treatments) for controlling cancer patients' symptoms in Japan: a national cross-sectional survey. BMC Complement. Altern. Med. 12, 222. http://dx.doi.org/10.1186/1472-6882-12-222.

Jadeja, R., Devkar, R.V., Nammi, S., 2014. Herbal medicines for the treatment of nonalcoholic steatohepatitis: current scenario and future prospects. Evid. Based Complement. Altern. Med. 2014, 648308. http://dx.doi.org/10.1155/2014/648308.

Jiang, J., Yamaguchi, T., Funakushi, N., Kuhara, T., Fan, P.S., Ueki, R., Ogawa, H., 2009. Oral administration of Yokukansan inhibits the development of atopic dermatitis-like lesions in isolated NC/Nga mice. J. Dermatol. Sci. 56 (1), 37–42. http://dx.doi.org/10.1016/j.jdermsci.2009.07.003.

Kamei, J., Nakamura, R., Ichiki, H., Kubo, M., 2003. Antitussive principles of Glycyrrhizae radix, a main component of the Kampo preparations Bakumondo-to (Mai-men-dong-tang). Eur. J. Pharmacol. 469 (1–3), 159–163.

Kawashima, K., Nomura, A., Makino, T., Saito, K., Kano, Y., 2004. Pharmacological properties of traditional medicine (XXIX): effect of Hange-shashin-to and the combinations of its herbal constituents on rat experimental colitis. Biol. Pharm. Bull. 27 (10), 1599–1603.

Kobayashi, H., Mizuno, N., Kutsuna, H., Teramae, H., Ueoku, S., Onoyama, J., Ishii, M., 2003. Hochu-ekki-to suppresses development of dermatitis and elevation of serum IgE level in NC/Nga mice. Drugs Exp. Clin. Res. 29 (2), 81–84.

Makino, T., Shiraki, Y., Mizukami, H., 2014. Interaction of gypsum and the rhizome of Anemarrhena asphodeloides plays an important role in anti-allergic effects of byakkokakeishito in mice. J. Nat. Med. 68 (3), 505–512. http://dx.doi.org/10.1007/s11418-014-0827-y.

Mehta, P., Shah, R., Lohidasan, S., Mahadik, K.R., 2015. Pharmacokinetic profile of phytoconstituent(s) isolated from medicinal plants—A comprehensive review. J. Tradit Complement. Med. 5 (4), 207–227. http://dx.doi.org/10.1016/j.jtcme.2014.11.041.

Minami, M., Ichikawa, M., Hata, N., Hasegawa, T., 2011. Protective effect of hainosankyuto, a traditional Japanese medicine, on *Streptococcus pyogenes* infection in murine model. PLoS One 6 (7), e22188. http://dx.doi.org/10.1371/journal.pone.0022188.

Mitsuma, T., Yokozawa, T., Oura, H., Terasawa, K., Narita, M., 1999. Clinical evaluation of kampo medication, mainly with wen-pi-tang, on the progression of chronic renal failure. Nihon Jinzo Gakkai Shi 41 (8), 769–777.

Mukaida, K., Hattori, N., Kondo, K., Morita, N., Murakami, I., Haruta, Y., Kohno, N., 2011. A pilot study of the multiherb Kampo medicine bakumondoto for cough in patients with chronic obstructive pulmonary disease. Phytomedicine 18 (8–9), 625–629. http://dx.doi.org/10.1016/j.phymed.2010.11.006.

Nagasaka, K., Kurokawa, M., Imakita, M., Terasawa, K., Shiraki, K., 1995. Efficacy of kakkon-to, a traditional herb medicine, in herpes simplex virus type 1 infection in mice. J. Med. Virol. 46 (1), 28–34.

Nagata, N., 2015. Current status of Japanese traditional medicine 'kampo' in chemotherapy. Gan To Kagaku Ryoho 42 (13), 2423–2429.

Nagata, T., Toume, K., Long, L.X., Hirano, K., Watanabe, T., Sekine, S., Tsukada, K., 2016. Anticancer effect of a Kampo preparation Daikenchuto. J. Nat. Med. http://dx.doi.org/10.1007/s11418-016-0989-x.

Ngo, L.T., Okogun, J.I., Folk, W.R., 2013. 21st century natural product research and drug development and traditional medicines. Nat. Prod. Rep. 30 (4), 584–592. http://dx.doi.org/10.1039/c3np20120a.

Nishihata, M., Kohjimoto, Y., Hara, I., 2013. Effect of Kampo extracts on urinary stone formation: an experimental investigation. Int. J. Urol. 20 (10), 1032–1036. http://dx.doi.org/10.1111/iju.12098.

Oikawa, T., Ito, G., Hanawa, T., 2012. Kampo therapy for inflammatory bowel diseases. Nihon Rinsho 70 (Suppl. 1), 365–369.

Okumi, H., Koyama, A., 2014. Kampo medicine for palliative care in Japan. Biopsychosoc. Med. 8 (1), 6. http://dx.doi.org/10.1186/1751-0759-8-6.

Ono, M., Ogasawara, M., Hirose, A., Mogami, S., Ootake, N., Aritake, K., Oben, J.A., 2014. Bofutsushosan, a Japanese herbal (Kampo) medicine, attenuates progression of nonalcoholic steatohepatitis in mice. J. Gastroenterol. 49 (6), 1065–1073. http://dx.doi.org/10.1007/s00535-013-0852-8.

Ono, T., Kamikado, K., Morimoto, T., 2013. Protective effects of Shichimotsu-koka-To on irreversible Thy-1 nephritis. Biol. Pharm. Bull. 36 (1), 41–47.

Pan, S.Y., Litscher, G., Gao, S.H., Zhou, S.F., Yu, Z.L., Chen, H.Q., Ko, K.M., 2014. Historical perspective of traditional indigenous medical practices: the current renaissance and conservation of herbal resources. Evid. Based Complement. Altern. Med. 2014, 525340. http://dx.doi.org/10.1155/2014/525340.

Sakaguchi, M., Iizuka, A., Yuzurihara, M., Ishige, A., Komatsu, Y., Matsumiya, T., Takeda, H., 1996. Pharmacological characteristics of Sho-seiryu-to, an antiallergic Kampo medicine without effects on histamine H1 receptors and muscarinic cholinergic system in the brain. Methods Find Exp. Clin. Pharmacol. 18 (1), 41–47.

Sreedhar, R., Arumugam, S., Karuppagounder, V., Thandavarayan, R.A., Giridharan, V.V., Pitchaimani, V., Watanabe, K., 2015a. Jumihaidokuto effectively inhibits colon inflammation and apoptosis in mice with acute colitis. Int. Immunopharmacol. 29 (2), 957–963. http://dx.doi.org/10.1016/j.intimp.2015.10.009.

Sreedhar, R., Arumugam, S., Thandavarayan, R.A., Giridharan, V.V., Karuppagounder, V., Pitchaimani, V., Watanabe, K., 2015b. Toki-shakuyaku-san, a Japanese kampo medicine, reduces colon inflammation in a mouse model of acute colitis. Int. Immunopharmacol. 29 (2), 869–875. http://dx.doi.org/10.1016/j.intimp.2015.08.029.

Takahashi, Y., Soejima, Y., Kumagai, A., Watanabe, M., Uozaki, H., Fukusato, T., 2014. Inhibitory effects of Japanese herbal medicines sho-saiko-to and juzen-taiho-to on nonalcoholic steatohepatitis in mice. PLoS One 9 (1), e87279. http://dx.doi.org/10.1371/journal.pone.0087279.

Takayama, S., Shiga, Y., Kokubun, T., Konno, H., Himori, N., Ryu, M., Nakazawa, T., 2014. The traditional kampo medicine tokishakuyakusan increases ocular blood flow in healthy subjects. Evid. Based Complement. Altern. Med. 2014, 586857. http://dx.doi.org/10.1155/2014/586857.

Tatsumi, T., Yamada, T., Nagai, H., Terasawa, K., Tani, T., Nunome, S., Saiki, I., 2001. A Kampo formulation: Byakko-ka-ninjin-to (Bai-Hu-Jia-Ren-Sheng-Tang) inhibits IgE-mediated triphasic skin reaction in mice: the role of its constituents in expression of the efficacy. Biol. Pharm. Bull. 24 (3), 284–290.

Terasawa, H., 1994. Diagnosis and treatment of respiratory emergencies. Nihon Kyobu Shikkan Gakkai Zasshi 32, 39–43.

Urata, Y., Yoshida, S., Irie, Y., Tanigawa, T., Amayasu, H., Nakabayashi, M., Akahori, K., 2002. Treatment of asthma patients with herbal medicine TJ-96: a randomized controlled trial. Respir. Med. 96 (6), 469–474.

Ushiroyama, T., 2013. The role of traditional Japanese medicine (Kampo) in the practice of psychosomatic medicine: the usefulness of Kampo in the treatment of the stress-related symptoms of women, especially those with peri-menopausal disorder. Biopsychosoc. Med. 7 (1), 16. http://dx.doi.org/10.1186/1751-0759-7-16.

Watanabe, K., 2015. Kampo therapy for patients with cancer—the role of kampo medicine in team therapy. Gan To Kagaku Ryoho 42 (13), 2414–2417.

Watanabe, K., Matsuura, K., Gao, P., Hottenbacher, L., Tokunaga, H., Nishimura, K., Witt, C.M., 2011. Traditional Japanese kampo medicine: clinical research between modernity and traditional medicine—the state of research and methodological suggestions for the future. Evid. Based Complement. Altern. Med. 2011, 513842. http://dx.doi.org/10.1093/ecam/neq067.

Yamakawa, J., Moriya, J., Takeuchi, K., Nakatou, M., Motoo, Y., Kobayashi, J., 2013a. Significance of Kampo, Japanese traditional medicine, in the treatment of obesity: basic and clinical evidence. Evid. Based Complement. Altern. Med. 2013, 943075. http://dx.doi.org/10.1155/2013/943075.

Yamakawa, J., Motoo, Y., Moriya, J., Ogawa, M., Uenishi, H., Akazawa, S., Kobayashi, J., 2013b. Role of Kampo medicine in integrative cancer therapy. Evid. Based Complement. Altern. Med. 2013, 570848. http://dx.doi.org/10.1155/2013/570848.

Yamashita, H., Tanaka, H., Inagaki, N., 2013. Treatment of the chronic itch of atopic dermatitis using standard drugs and kampo medicines. Biol. Pharm. Bull. 36 (8), 1253–1257.

Yanagihara, S., Kobayashi, H., Tamiya, H., Tsuruta, D., Okano, Y., Takahashi, K., Ishii, M., 2013. Protective effect of hochuekkito, a Kampo prescription, against ultraviolet B irradiation-induced skin damage in hairless mice. J. Dermatol. 40 (3), 201–206. http://dx.doi.org/10.1111/1346-8138.12050.

Yu, F., Takahashi, T., Moriya, J., Kawaura, K., Yamakawa, J., Kusaka, K., Kanda, T., 2006. Traditional Chinese medicine and Kampo: a review from the distant past for the future. J. Int. Med. Res. 34 (3), 231–239.

CHAPTER 2

Kampo Medicine for Human Homeostasis

Takao Sunaga[1], Kenichi Watanabe[2]
[1]*Niigata Kido Clinic, Niigata, Japan;* [2]*Niigata University of Pharmacy and Applied Life Sciences, Niigata, Japan*

Three Roots of Eastern Traditional Medicine

There are three major roots of Eastern traditional medicine, Ayurveda, Yunani (Unani), and Chinese. Ayurveda is a system of medicine with historical roots in the Indian subcontinent. Globalized and modernized practices derived from Ayurvedic traditions are a type of complementary or alternative medicine. Ayurvedic therapies are varied and have evolved over more than 2 millennia. Therapies are typically based on complex herbal compounds (Patwardhan et al., 2005), whereas treatises have introduced mineral and metal substances. Second, Yunani or Unani is the term for Perso-Arabic traditional medicine as practiced in Mughal India and in the Muslim culture in southern Asia and modern day central Asia. The term is derived from Arabic "Greek," as the Perso-Arabic system of medicine was in turn based on the teachings of the Greek physicians Hippocrates and Galen. The Hellenistic origin of Yunani medicine is still visible in its being based on the classical four humors, phlegm (balgham), blood (dam), yellow bile (ṣafra), and black bile (sauda) (Secretion et al., 1998), but it has also been influenced by the Indian and Chinese traditional systems. Third, traditional Chinese medicine is a style of traditional Asian medicine informed by modern medicine but built on a foundation of more than 2500 years of Chinese medical practice that includes various forms of herbal medicine, acupuncture, massage, exercise, and dietary therapy (Tabish, 2008). It is primarily used as a complementary alternative medicine approach. Traditional Chinese medicine is widely used in China and is becoming increasingly prevalent in Europe and North America.

Kampo Medicine

There are several terminologies used for dealing with Kampo medicine, such as Kampo formula, Kampo prescription, Kampo extract, Kampo product, crude drug product, Wakan-yaku, herbal medicine, complementary and alternative medicine, Oriental medicine, traditional Japanese medicine, traditional Chinese medicine, traditional Korean medicine, etc. In this chapter, we use the word "Kampo medicine," which means traditional Japanese medicine in general.

Kampo medicine, often known simply as Kampo or Kanpo, is the study of traditional Chinese medicine in Japan following its introduction, by way of Korea, beginning in the 6th century. Since then, the Japanese have created their own unique system of diagnosis and therapy. The term Kampo itself incorporates two characters: "Kam" or "Kan," an adjectival modifier for things Chinese, and "Po" or "Pho," denoting method or prescription. Thus, Kampo means modified Chinese-style medicine. The term appeared during the late Edo period to draw a line against the growing influence of Western medicine, which was called Rampo (Dutch-style medicine) by its adherents. Kampo medicine is widely practiced in Japan and is fully integrated into the modern health care system. Kampo is based on traditional Chinese medicine but adapted to Japanese culture.

Sho: The Patient's Constitution

Japanese traditional medicine uses most of the Chinese therapies, including acupuncture and moxibustion, but Kampo in its present-day sense is primarily concerned with the study of herbs. The term "Sho" refers to the particular pathological status of a patient evaluated by the Kampo diagnosis and is patterned according to the patient's constitution, symptoms, etc. A Kampo medicine should be used after confirmation that it is suitable for the identified Sho of the patient.

The Five Elements

Kampo medicine is based on the rationalization of certain concepts of the universe, and all known facts are related to and incorporated into these theories. Everything started with "Ki; Chi," divided into light and heavy, "Ki; Chi," which gave birth to heaven and earth and then "In; Yin" and "Yo; Yang." From these two forces there arose five elements, which in turn form the basis of all matters related to life, including the philosophic concepts concerned in medical practice (Kohn, 1997).

The "Five Elements" (also known as Wu Xing, Pinyin, Five Phases, Five Agents, Five Movements, Five Processes, Five Steps, Five Stages, and Five Planets) is the short form for the five types of Qi (Chi) that dominate at different times (Fig. 2.1). It is a fivefold conceptual scheme that many traditional Kampo and Chinese fields use to explain a wide array of phenomena, from cosmic cycles to the interactions between internal organs, and from the succession of political regimes to the properties of medicinal drugs. The five phases are wood, fire, earth, metal, and water (Fig. 2.2). This order of presentation is known as the mutual generation sequence. In the order of mutual overcoming, they are wood, earth, water, fire, and metal (Sallmann, 2006). The Doctrine of Five Phases describes two cycles, a generating or creation cycle, also known as mother–son, and an overcoming or destruction cycle, also known as grandfather–nephew, of interactions between the phases. Within Kampo and Chinese medicine the effects of these two main relations are further elaborated.

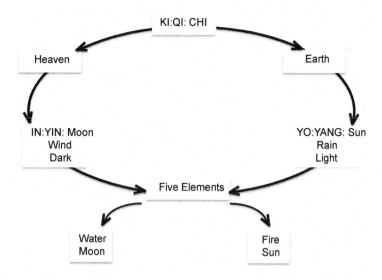

Figure 2.1: **The five elements (wood, fire, metal, earth, and water).**
Theory of the origin of the universe as conceptualized by Kampo medicine. Various organs are interrelated according to the five element theory.

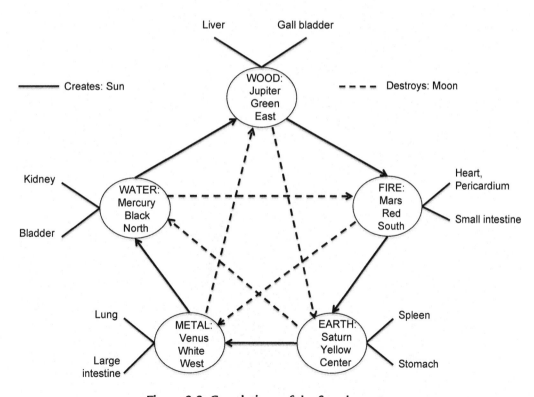

Figure 2.2: **Correlations of the five elements.**
The five elements and five note scales make the following correlations: movement, planet, color, and Arctic direction. Also, there is a strong relationship between the five elements and the body organs.

Creation (generation; straight line in Fig. 2.2): the common memory jobs, which help to remind us of the order of the phases, are wood feeds fire, fire creates earth, earth bears metal, metal enriches water (water with minerals is better than pure water), and water nourishes wood. Other common words for this cycle include begets, engenders, and mothers.

Destruction (overcoming; dotted line in Fig. 2.2): wood parts earth, earth dams water, water extinguishes fire, fire melts metal, and metal chops wood. This cycle might also use the words controls, restrains, and fathers.

The System of Five Phases was used for describing interactions and relationships between phenomena. After it came to maturity in the 2nd or 1st century BCE during the Han dynasty, this device was employed in many fields of early Chinese thought, including seemingly disparate fields such as geomancy or feng shui, astrology, traditional Chinese medicine, music, military strategy, and martial arts. The system is still used as a reference in some forms of complementary and alternative medicine and martial arts.

Yin (In) and Yang (Yo)

In Kampo philosophy, Yin (In) and Yang (Yo) describe how opposite or contrary forces are actually complementary, interconnected, and interdependent in the natural world, and how they give rise to each other as they interrelate to one another (Fig. 2.3). Many tangible dualities (such as light and dark, fire and water, expanding and contracting) are thought of as physical manifestations of the duality symbolized by Yin (In) and Yang (Yo). This duality lies at the origins of many branches of classical Japanese science and philosophy, as well as being a primary guideline of traditional Japanese and Chinese medicine and a central principle of various forms of Japanese martial arts and exercise. A term has been coined: dualistic monism or dialectical monism. Yin (In) and Yang (Yo) can be thought of as complementary (rather

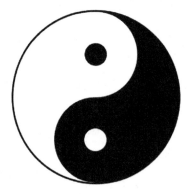

Figure 2.3: Yin (In) and Yang (Yo).
Many tangible dualities (such as light and dark, fire and water, expanding and contracting) are thought of as physical manifestations of the duality symbolized by Yin (In) and Yang (Yo).

than opposing) forces that interact to form a dynamic system in which the whole is greater than the assembled parts. Everything has both Yin (In) and Yang (Yo) aspects (for instance shadow cannot exist without light). Either of the two major aspects may manifest more strongly in a particular object, depending on the criterion of the observation. The symbol for "Yin (In) and Yang (Yo)" shows a balance between two opposites with a portion of the opposite element in each section (Cheng, 2000; Hu and Liu, 2012).

Yin (In) and Yang (Yo) are semantically complex words. The following provides translation equivalents.

Yin (In), shady side (of a mountain)

1. (in Japanese and Chinese philosophy) negative/passive/female principle in nature
2. surname Bound morpheme
3. the moon
4. shaded orientation
5. covert, concealed, hidden, negative
6. north side of a hill
7. south bank of a river

Yang (Yo), sunny side (of a mountain)

1. (in Japanese and Chinese philosophy) positive/active/male principle in nature
2. the sun
3. in relief
4. open, overt
5. south side of a hill
6. north bank of a river

Dropping a stone in a calm pool of water will simultaneously raise waves and create lower troughs between them, and this alternation of high and low points in the water will radiate outward until the movement dissipates and the pool is calm once more. Yin and Yang thus are always opposite and equal qualities. Further, whenever one quality reaches its peak, it will naturally begin to transform into the opposite quality: for example, grain that reaches its full height in summer [fully Yang (Yo)] will produce seeds and die back in winter [fully Yin (In)] in an endless cycle.

Yin is the black side with the white dot in it, and Yang is the white side with the black dot in it. The relationship between Yin (In) and Yang (Yo) is often described in terms of sunlight playing over a mountain and a valley. Yin (literally the "shady place" or "north slope") is the dark area occluded by the mountain's bulk, and Yang (Yo) (literally the "sunny place" or "south slope") is the brightly lit portion. As the sun moves across the sky, Yin (In) and Yang (Yo) gradually trade places with each other, revealing what was obscured and obscuring what was revealed.

Yin (In) is characterized as slow, soft, yielding, diffuse, cold, wet, and passive, and is associated with water, earth, the moon, femininity, and nighttime. Yang (Yo), by contrast, is fast, hard, solid, focused, hot, dry, and active, and is associated with fire, sky, the sun, masculinity, and daytime. Yin (In) and Yang (Yo) apply to the human body. In traditional Japanese medicine good health is directly related to the balance between the Yin (In) and the Yang (Yo) qualities within oneself. If Yin (In) and Yang (Yo) become unbalanced, one of the qualities is considered deficient or has vacuity.

How to Use Kampo Medicine: An Example Using Kakkonto

The use of Kampo medicine applies to both chronic diseases (including cancers, cerebrovascular diseases, heart diseases, hyperlipidemia, hypertension, diabetes mellitus, osteoporosis, etc.) and acute diseases (acute bronchitis, influenza, norovirus lumbago, herpes zoster, etc.) in Japan currently (Yasui, 2008).

Almost all Japanese doctors use Kampo medicine for patients with many kinds of diseases (JSOM and SBE, 2002). For example, the ethical use of kakkonto extract granules is indicated for the relief of the following symptoms of those patients with comparatively strong constitution: headache, fever, rigor, shoulder stiffness without spontaneous sweating, common cold, the initial stages of febrile diseases, inflammatory diseases (conjunctivitis, keratitis, otitis media, tonsillitis, mastitis, and lymphadenitis), neuralgia in the upper body, and urticaria. The usual adult dose is 7.5 g/day orally in two or three divided doses before or between meals. The dosage may be adjusted according to the patient's age, body weight, and symptoms.

Precaution and Careful Administration

Kakkonto should be administered with care to the following patients:

1. patients in a period of weakness after disease or with greatly declined constitution (adverse reactions are likely to occur, and the symptoms may be aggravated);
2. patients with an extremely weak gastrointestinal tract (anorexia, epigastric distress, nausea, vomiting, etc., may occur);
3. patients with anorexia, nausea, or vomiting (these symptoms may be aggravated);
4. patients showing a remarkable tendency for sweating (excess sweating and/or generalized weakness may occur);
5. patients with cardiovascular disorders, including angina pectoris, myocardial infarction, etc., or those with a history of such disorders;
6. patients with severe hypertension;
7. patients with severe renal dysfunction;
8. patients with dysuria;
9. patients with hyperthyroidism.

For (5)–(9), these diseases and symptoms may be aggravated.

Important Precautions

1. When kakkonto is used, the patient's Sho (constitution/symptoms) should be taken into account. The patient's progress should be carefully monitored, and if no improvement in symptoms/findings is observed, continuous treatment should be avoided.
2. Because kakkonto contains *Glycyrrhiza*, careful attention should be paid to the serum potassium level, blood pressure, etc., and if any abnormality is observed, administration should be discontinued.
3. When kakkonto is coadministered with other Kampo preparations, attention should be paid to the duplication of the contained crude drugs.

Drug Interactions

There are precautions for coadministration. Kakkonto should be administered with care when coadministered with the following drugs: (1) preparations containing ephedra herb; (2) preparations containing ephedrine-related compounds; (3) monoamine oxidase inhibitors; (4) thyroid preparations, thyroxine, liothyronine; (5) catecholamine preparations, epinephrine, isoprenaline; and (6) xanthine preparations, theophylline, diprophylline.

Adverse Reactions

Kakkonto has not been investigated (drug use investigations, etc.) for the incidence of adverse reactions. Therefore, the incidence of adverse reactions is not known.

Clinically Significant Adverse Reactions

1. Pseudoaldosteronism: Pseudoaldosteronism such as hypokalemia, increased blood pressure, retention of sodium/body fluid, edema, increased body weight, etc., may occur. The patient should be carefully monitored (measurement of serum potassium level, etc.), and if any abnormality is observed, administration should be discontinued and appropriate measures such as administration of potassium preparations should be taken.
2. Myopathy: Myopathy may occur as a result of hypokalemia. The patient should be carefully monitored, and if any abnormality such as weakness, convulsion/paralysis of limbs, etc., is observed, administration should be discontinued and appropriate measures such as administration of potassium preparations should be taken.
3. Hepatic dysfunction and jaundice: Hepatic dysfunction and/or jaundice with elevation of aspartate transaminase (AST, GOT), alanine transaminase (ALT, GPT), alkaline phosphatase (Al-P), and gamma glutamyl transpeptidase (γ-GTP) or other symptoms may occur. The patient should be carefully monitored for abnormal findings. Administration should be discontinued and appropriate therapeutic measures should be taken, if abnormalities are observed.

Other Adverse Reactions

Rash, redness, pruritus, insomnia, excess sweating, tachycardia, palpitation, generalized weakness, mental excitation, anorexia, epigastric distress, nausea, vomiting, urination disorder, and others. If such symptoms are observed, administration should be discontinued.

Use in the Elderly

Because elderly patients often have reduced physiological function, careful supervision and measures such as reducing the dose are recommended.

Use During Pregnancy, Delivery, or Lactation

The safety of kakkonto in pregnant women has not been established. Therefore, kakkonto should be used in pregnant women or women who may possibly be pregnant only if the expected therapeutic benefits outweigh the possible risks associated with treatment.

Pediatric Use

The safety of kakkonto in children has not been established (insufficient clinical data).

Other Precautions

Eczema, dermatitis, etc., may be aggravated.

Conclusion

Kampo medicine, Japanese traditional medicine, is useful for the maintenance of human homeostasis. *Homo sapiens* need a healthy body and a healthy mind. This means that in humans the ideal balance creates a microcosmic "utopia." Evidence of Kampo medicine treatment for almost all diseases has been reported and will be reported. "Understanding the past and predicting the future" should be one of the best therapeutic strategies in all diseases.

References

Cheng, J.T., 2000. Review: drug therapy in Chinese traditional medicine. J. Clin. Pharmacol. 40 (5), 445–450. Retrieved from: http://www.ncbi.nlm.nih.gov/pubmed/10806595.

Hu, J., Liu, B., 2012. The basic theory, diagnostic, and therapeutic system of traditional Chinese medicine and the challenges they bring to statistics. Stat. Med. 31 (7), 602–605. http://dx.doi.org/10.1002/sim.4409.

JSOM, SBE, 2002. Guide Kampo Traditional Medicine (In Japanese). Nankodo, Tokyo, Japan.

Kohn, L., 1997. Ying and Yang: the natural dimension of evil. In: Cohen, R.S., Tauber, A.I. (Eds.), Philosophies of Nature: The Human Dimension. Kluwer Academic Publishers, New York, pp. 91–106.

Patwardhan, B., Warude, D., Pushpangadan, P., Bhatt, N., 2005. Ayurveda and traditional Chinese medicine: a comparative overview. Evid. Based Complement. Altern. Med. 2 (4), 465–473. http://dx.doi.org/10.1093/ecam/neh140.

Sallmann, R., 2006. An Introduction to Wu Xing: The Five Phases, Also Called the Five Elements. Retrieved from: http://www.fengshui-harmony.net/fengshui-basics/89-five-elements-five-phases-feng-shui.

Secretion, F., Conjur, G.S., Attitude, S.P., 1998. Interviews with the dead. Using meta-life qualitative analysis to validate Hippocrates' theory of humours. CMAJ 159 (12), 1472–1473. Retrieved from: http://www.ncbi.nlm.nih.gov/pubmed/9875254.

Tabish, S.A., 2008. Complementary and alternative healthcare: is it evidence-based? Int. J. Health Sci. (Qassim) 2 (1), V–IX. Retrieved from: http://www.ncbi.nlm.nih.gov/pubmed/21475465.

Yasui, H., 2008. Kampo Traditional Medicine for Medical Students (In Japanese). Orient Arts and Sciences, Tokyo, Japan.

CHAPTER 3

General Mechanisms of Immunity and Inflammation

Remya Sreedhar, Kenichi Watanabe, Somasundaram Arumugam
Niigata University of Pharmacy and Applied Life Sciences, Niigata, Japan

Introduction

Inflammation is a local or systemic tissue reaction caused by external or internal stimuli with the objective of removing the noxa (injurious agent), inhibiting its further dissemination, and eventually repairing damaged tissue (Wilting et al., 2009). It is an acute cellular/tissue process and most commonly occurs upon exposure to pathogens and irritants or tissue injury. Under normal circumstances it is self-limiting, but upon persistent exposure to the inflammatory stimuli, it will lead to chronic inflammatory diseases (Ferrero-Miliani et al., 2007). There are several local reactions behind the pathogenesis of inflammation, which broadly include increased blood flow, vasodilation, cellular infiltration and edema, release of inflammatory mediators, increased sensitivity to pain, and activation of complement, coagulation, and fibrinolytic systems (Kumar et al., 2004). Here we will discuss various inflammatory stimuli, the biochemical processes and mediators involved in inflammation, and the identification of suitable targets for the treatment of chronic inflammatory diseases.

Definition of Inflammation

According to Cornelius Celsus, a Roman encyclopedist of ancient times, inflammation can be defined as "redness and swelling with heat and pain," and Rudolf Virchow later added "loss of function" to its signs. As per Ferrero-Miliani et al. (2007) inflammation can be explained as "part of the non-specific immune response that occurs in reaction to any type of bodily injury and that the cardinal signs of inflammation can be explained by increased blood flow, elevated cellular metabolism, vasodilatation, release of soluble mediators, extravasation of fluids and cellular influx."

Inflammatory Stimuli

Inflammation can be stimulated by a variety of causative agents, including bacterial/viral pathogens; foreign objects/matter entering into the tissue, such as sharp objects, metal parts, etc.; cells activated by local tissue injury; chemical agents such as alcohol; radiation; and autoimmunity. All these stimuli can activate acute inflammation, which is self-limiting upon removal of the causative agent. But with chronic exposure, it can turn into a chronic inflammatory disease. Skin is the mechanical and immunological barrier that protects our body from the environment. Any damage to this barrier causes the invasion of inflammation-causative agents into the body thereby stimulating the innate immune system, which typically initiates skin immune responses, while cells and cytokines of the adaptive immune system perpetuate the inflammation (Yazdi et al., 2016).

Immune System

Our body is provided with a protective self-defense against infection called the immune system, which can be broadly divided into the innate immune system, which is also called the nonspecific/inborn immune system, and the adaptive or acquired immune system. The innate immune system is present in our body evolutionarily, whereas the adaptive immune system is developed against any specific pathogen upon exposure to it, and its memory is stored in the form of B and T lymphocytes.

The innate immune system, which is essential for the prevention of microbial invasion, consists of genetically programmed defense mechanisms against the molecular components present especially in microorganisms (Jedynak et al., 2012). Innate immunity includes several defensive mechanisms such as anatomic or physical barriers, physiological barriers, phagocytosis, and inflammation (Toskala, 2014). It comprises cells that provide immediate protection against invading microbes or infectious agents by identifying specific disease-associated molecular patterns (DAMPs) present in the foreign pathogens via pattern-recognition receptors (PRRs) and releasing inflammatory mediators, causing swelling/inflammation to prevent further spread of the infection. Interferon (IFN)-β, soluble E-selectin, and soluble intercellular adhesion molecule-1 can activate the innate immune system via activation of Toll-like receptor (TLR)-3 (Lee et al., 2007). The innate immune system senses cytosolic double-stranded DNA (dsDNA) and bacterial cyclic dinucleotides and initiates signaling via the adaptor STING (stimulator of IFN genes), whereby Bruton's tyrosine kinase phosphorylates DEAD-box helicase 41 and activates its binding of dsDNA and STING to initiate a type I IFN response (Lee et al., 2015).

The innate immune system cannot provide long-lasting protection against infection and thereby stimulates the adaptive immune system. As an example, UV irradiation can cause aberrant induction of apoptosis in keratinocytes and contribute to the appearance of excessive apoptotic cells in the skin of cutaneous lupus erythematosus (CLE) patients and, if not cleared by phagocytes, they may undergo secondary necrosis and release proinflammatory compounds and potential autoantigens, which may contribute to the inflammatory micromilieu that leads to the formation of skin lesions. In addition to UV-mediated induction of apoptosis, the molecular and cellular factors that may cause the abnormal long-lasting photoreactivity in CLE include mediators of inflammation, such as cytokines and chemokines. In particular, IFNs are important players in the early activation of the immune system and have a specific role in the immunological interface between the innate and the adaptive immune systems. The fact that treatment with recombinant type I IFNs (α and β) can induce not only systemic organ manifestations but also LE-like skin lesions provides additional evidence for a pathogenic role of these IFNs in the disease (Kuhn et al., 2014). Deficiency of IFN-γ signaling alone had no effect on survival in mice, highlighting the importance of type I IFN in protection against infection, whereas the adaptive immune system is relatively unimportant in acute infections (Seymour et al., 2013). The adaptive immune response is activated in an antigen-specific way to eliminate the antigen and induce lasting protection. Hypersensitivity reactions occur when an exaggerated adaptive immune response is activated (Toskala, 2014).

Mechanisms of Adaptive Immune Function

Most of the cells in our body contain functional major histocompatibility complex (MHC) molecules, and among these cells, dendritic cells (DCs) and B lymphocytes are considered professional antigen-presenting cells (APCs). DCs engulf exogenous pathogens and present their antigens as a complex with type II MHCs to activate CD4$^+$ T helper (Th) cells in the lymph nodes, whereas the endogenous antigens are presented via a type I MHC to activate CD8$^+$ cytotoxic T cells. Once activated, cytotoxic T cells form effector cells to attack and destroy the affected/antigen-containing cells via either burst/lysis or apoptosis, but the Th cells cannot destroy the APCs; instead they release cytokines and activate cytotoxic T cells. There are two types of Th cells in our body, Th1 and Th2. Th1 cells produce IFN-γ to activate cell-mediated immunity against intracellular pathogens, whereas Th2 cells produce interleukins (IL)-4 and IL-5 to counter extracellular pathogens. Most of the activated T cells die and undergo phagocytosis by macrophages, whereas a few remain as memory cells and are activated upon further infection (Janeway et al., 2001). Apart from these, another class of regulatory T cells is also present in our immune system to control its aberrant activation against autoantigens, thereby preventing autoimmune diseases (Janeway et al., 2004).

Cytokines and Chemokines

Cytokines are involved in virtually every facet of immunity and inflammation, including innate immunity, antigen presentation, bone marrow differentiation, cellular recruitment and activation, and adhesion molecule expression (Borish and Steinke, 2003). The cytokines predominantly produced by monocytes include tumor necrosis factor (TNF) and several IL molecules known as IL-1, IL-6, IL-8, IL-12, IL-15, IL-18, and IL-23, which are involved in the innate immune system.

Immune responses directed against virus-infected and neoplastic cells are primarily mediated by CD8+ cytotoxic lymphocytes and natural killer cells. Cytokines that activate cytotoxic immunity include IL-2, IL-4, IL-5, IL-6, IL-7, IL-10, IL-12, and IL-15, as well as IL-11 and, most importantly, TNFα, TNFβ, and the IFNs (Borish and Steinke, 2003). A list of currently identified cytokines is presented in Table 3.1.

Chemokines are a group of small molecules that can induce chemotaxis in neutrophils, monocytes, lymphocytes, eosinophils, fibroblasts, and keratinocytes. The inflammatory chemokines recruit and activate leukocytes to mount an immune response and initiate wound healing. A few chemokines have a homeostatic or housekeeping function, involved in adaptive immune responses including lymphocyte trafficking, hematopoiesis, antigen sampling in secondary lymphoid tissue, and immune surveillance (Borish and Steinke, 2003). Chemokines may not regulate all stages of lymphocyte migration during inflammation, and paradigms describing their trafficking may need to account for the role of prostaglandin 2 (Ahmed et al., 2011). Currently, 19 different chemokine receptors have been discovered and separated into four subfamilies: C, CC, CXC, and CX3C. In humans, the CXC subfamily currently contains 7 chemokine receptors and 15 ligands. CXCR2 is a promising potential therapeutic target, because brain-penetrant inhibitors and a CXCR2 antagonist have provided

Table 3.1: List of Cytokines and Chemokines

Family	Name	Produced By	Function
Cytokines	IL-2	Th0 (naïve) lymphocytes	Promote regulatory T cells
	IFN-γ, TNFα, TNFβ, GM-CSF, IL-2, -3, -10, and -13	Th1 lymphocytes	Cell-mediated immunity
	IL-4, -5, -9, and -25, TNFα, GM-CSF, IL-2, -3, -10, and -13	Th2 lymphocytes	Allergic immune responses
	TGF-β and IL-10	Th3 lymphocytes	Immunosuppression
Chemokines	**CC family**		
	CCL1–5, 7, 8, 11, 13, 17, 20, 22, 24, 26, and 28		Inflammation
	CCL17–22, 25, 27, and 28		Homeostasis
	CCL6, 9, 10, 12, 14–16, 23		Unknown
	C family		
	XCL1 and XCL2		Unknown
	CXC family		
	CXCL1–3, 8–11, and 16		Inflammation
	CXCL13 and 14		Homeostasis
	CXCL4–7, 12, and 15		Unknown
	CX3C family		
	CX3CL1		Inflammation

GM-CSF, granulocyte macrophage-colony stimulating factor; *IFN*, interferon; *IL*, interleukin; *TGF*, transforming growth factor; *Th*, T helper; *TNF*, tumor necrosis factor.

promising results in various clinical trials for Alzheimer's disease and chronic obstructive pulmonary disease, respectively. The mechanisms of CXCR2 in various disease models and environments have not been totally defined yet, so vigilance should be exercised because of the complex biological role CXCR2 carries out (Veenstra and Ransohoff, 2012). A list of identified chemokines along with their roles is presented in Table 3.1.

Immunoglobulins

B lymphocytes produce specific antibodies, also called immunoglobulins, into the circulation against antigens present in pathogens. Unlike T cells (which recognize MHC), B cells detect the antigen in its native form. Upon activation B cells are modified into effector cells called plasma cells, secreting antibodies targeted against the pathogenic antigen and making them targets for phagocytes. There are five classes of immunoglobulins, IgA, IgD, IgE, IgG, and IgM, each of them recognizing unique antigens (Janeway et al., 2001).

Signaling Processes in Inflammation and Immunity

Innate immune cells recognize pathogen invasion or cell damage with intracellular or surface-expressed PRRs, which detect, either directly or indirectly, pathogen-associated molecular patterns (PAMPs), such as microbial nucleic acids, lipoproteins, and carbohydrates, or DAMPs released from injured cells. Activated PRRs then oligomerize and assemble large multisubunit complexes that initiate signaling cascades that trigger the release of factors that promote recruitment of leukocytes to the region (Newton and Dixit, 2012).

Members of the TLR family are major PRRs in cells and they recognize distinct PAMPs and play a critical role in innate immune responses. They participate in the first line of defense against invading pathogens and play a significant role in inflammation, immune cell regulation, survival, and proliferation. Signaling by TLRs involves five adaptor proteins known as myeloid differentiation 88 (MyD88), MyD88-adapter-like, Toll/IL-1 receptor (TIR) domain-containing adapter-inducing IFN-β (TRIF), TLR4 adapter (TRAM), and sterile α- and armadillo-motif-containing protein (O'Neill and Bowie, 2007). The activation of the TLR signaling pathway originates from the cytoplasmic TIR domain-containing adaptor, MyD88, which recruits IL-1 receptor-associated kinase-4 (IRAK-4) to TLRs through interaction of the death domains of both molecules. TNF receptor-associated factor (TRAF)-6 activates and associates with IRAK-1, thereby activating the IκB kinase (IKK) complex and leading to activation of mitogen-activated protein kinases (MAPKs) (JNK, p38 MAPK) and nuclear factor (NF)-κB. Activation of MyD88-independent pathways occurs via TRIF and TRAF3, leading to recruitment of IKKε/TBK1, phosphorylation of IFN-regulatory factor 3, and expression of IFN-β. TIR domain-containing adaptors such as TIR-associated protein, TRIF, and TRAM regulate TLR-mediated signaling pathways by providing specificity for individual TLR signaling cascades. TRAF3 plays a critical role in the regulation of both MyD88-dependent and

TRIF-dependent signaling via TRAF3 degradation, which activates MyD88-dependent signaling and suppresses TRIF-dependent signaling (Barton and Kagan, 2009; Blasius and Beutler, 2010; O'Neill and Bowie, 2007).

Activated p38 MAPK acts on two levels of the antiviral IFN response. Initially the kinase regulates IFN induction and, at a later stage, p38 controls IFN signaling and thereby expression of IFN-stimulated genes. Thus, inhibition of p38 MAPK may be an antiviral strategy that protects mice from lethal influenza by suppressing excessive cytokine expression (Borgeling et al., 2014).

IFN-γ induces the loss of intestinal epithelial barrier function and disruption of tight-junction proteins, by upregulation of hypoxia-inducible factor-1α expression through the NF-κB pathway (Yang et al., 2014). NF-κB transcription factors are evolutionarily conserved, coordinating regulators of immune and inflammatory responses (Tornatore et al., 2012). NF-κB can modulate Notch-1 signaling and both pathways operate synergistically for the production of proinflammatory cytokines (Cao et al., 2011).

NF-κB family members regulate the expression of cytokines, inducible nitric oxide synthase, and cyclooxygenase 2 (Shi et al., 2015). Aberrant NF-κB action is found to play a crucial role in several diseases, making it an intensively studied target for drug interventions. However, given its pleiotropic functions in inflammation and immunity, a more targeted modulation of its activity, at a cell-type-specific or disease-stage-specific level, could provide safer therapeutic solutions (Xanthoulea et al., 2005). Induction of the heat shock response (HSR) before a proinflammatory signal inhibits NF-κB activation and NF-κB-dependent proinflammatory gene expression, via inhibition of IKK activation and increased de novo expression of the IκBα gene, thereby providing a potential mechanism through which the HSR can modulate cellular proinflammatory signaling (Malhotra and Wong, 2002).

Transforming growth factor (TGF)-β is considered the main fibrogenic cytokine; however, in some pathological settings TGF-β also has antiinflammatory properties (Rodrigues-Diez et al., 2015). Impairment of TGF-β signaling enhances TNFα/NF-κB activity (Al-Mulla et al., 2011). For example, IL-15 causes impairment of TGF-β-mediated signaling, thereby promoting and sustaining intestinal inflammation in celiac disease, suggesting that IL-15 is a meaningful therapeutic target in inflammatory diseases associated with irreducible elevation of IL-15 (Benahmed et al., 2007).

IFN-γ has a dual role as a pro- or antiinflammatory cytokine (Mata-Espinosa and Hernandez-Pando, 2008). Subsequent to viral infection, secreted IFNs bind and activate the type I IFN receptor, thereby leading to the activation of IFN-stimulated gene factor 3, which translocates to the nucleus and induces the transcription of hundreds of effector molecules, called IFN-inducible genes, to establish an antiviral state (Uematsu and Akira, 2007). Thus, type I IFNs mediate both innate immune responses and the subsequent development of adaptive immunity to viruses. Suppression of IFN signaling by FOXA3 provides a plausible mechanism that may serve to limit ongoing Th1 inflammation during the resolution of acute viral infection; however, inhibition of innate immunity by FOXA3 may contribute to susceptibility to viral infections associated with chronic lung disorders accompanied by chronic goblet cell metaplasia (Chen et al., 2014).

Conclusion

Understanding the complexity of the early response to infection with respect to the innate immune response is required for the future development of drugs that will effectively control infectious diseases (Jedynak et al., 2012). Although inflammation is a tissue-protective phenomenon, it affects organ functions where the cells are postmitotic, such as the spinal cord (Popovich and Jones, 2003). Thus, limiting its severity by targeting any of the mediators is essential to maintain or bring back the normal function of the organ. Although various antiinflammatory agents are currently available, research is still progressing to identify effective therapeutic agents against inflammation. In this regard, natural medicine offers a major source of antiinflammatory agents with potential benefits and the fewest side effects.

References

Ahmed, S.R., McGettrick, H.M., Yates, C.M., Buckley, C.D., Ratcliffe, M.J., Nash, G.B., Rainger, G.E., 2011. Prostaglandin D2 regulates CD4+ memory T cell trafficking across blood vascular endothelium and primes these cells for clearance across lymphatic endothelium. J. Immunol. 187 (3), 1432–1439. http://dx.doi.org/10.4049/jimmunol.1100299.

Al-Mulla, F., Leibovich, S.J., Francis, I.M., Bitar, M.S., 2011. Impaired TGF-beta signaling and a defect in resolution of inflammation contribute to delayed wound healing in a female rat model of type 2 diabetes. Mol. Biosyst. 7 (11), 3006–3020. http://dx.doi.org/10.1039/c0mb00317d.

Barton, G.M., Kagan, J.C., 2009. A cell biological view of Toll-like receptor function: regulation through compartmentalization. Nat. Rev. Immunol. 9 (8), 535–542. http://dx.doi.org/10.1038/nri2587.

Benahmed, M., Meresse, B., Arnulf, B., Barbe, U., Mention, J.J., Verkarre, V., Cerf-Bensussan, N., 2007. Inhibition of TGF-beta signaling by IL-15: a new role for IL-15 in the loss of immune homeostasis in celiac disease. Gastroenterology 132 (3), 994–1008. http://dx.doi.org/10.1053/j.gastro.2006.12.025.

Blasius, A.L., Beutler, B., 2010. Intracellular toll-like receptors. Immunity 32 (3), 305–315. http://dx.doi.org/10.1016/j.immuni.2010.03.012.

Borgeling, Y., Schmolke, M., Viemann, D., Nordhoff, C., Roth, J., Ludwig, S., 2014. Inhibition of p38 mitogen-activated protein kinase impairs influenza virus-induced primary and secondary host gene responses and protects mice from lethal H5N1 infection. J. Biol. Chem. 289 (1), 13–27. http://dx.doi.org/10.1074/jbc.M113.469239.

Borish, L.C., Steinke, J.W., 2003. 2. Cytokines and chemokines. J. Allergy Clin. Immunol. 111 (2 Suppl), S460–S475. Retrieved from: http://www.ncbi.nlm.nih.gov/pubmed/12592293.

Cao, Q., Kaur, C., Wu, C.Y., Lu, J., Ling, E.A., 2011. Nuclear factor-kappa beta regulates Notch signaling in production of proinflammatory cytokines and nitric oxide in murine BV-2 microglial cells. Neuroscience 192, 140–154. http://dx.doi.org/10.1016/j.neuroscience.2011.06.060.

Chen, G., Korfhagen, T.R., Karp, C.L., Impey, S., Xu, Y., Randell, S.H., Whitsett, J.A., 2014. Foxa3 induces goblet cell metaplasia and inhibits innate antiviral immunity. Am. J. Respir. Crit. Care Med. 189 (3), 301–313. http://dx.doi.org/10.1164/rccm.201306-1181OC.

Ferrero-Miliani, L., Nielsen, O.H., Andersen, P.S., Girardin, S.E., 2007. Chronic inflammation: importance of NOD2 and NALP3 in interleukin-1beta generation. Clin. Exp. Immunol. 147 (2), 227–235. http://dx.doi.org/10.1111/j.1365-2249.2006.03261.x.

Janeway Jr., C.A., Travers, P., Walport, M., Shlomchik, M.J., 2001. Immunobiology, fifth ed. Garland Science, New York.

Janeway, C.A., Travers, P., Walport, M., Shlomchik, M.J., 2004. Immunobiology. Garland Science, New York.

Jedynak, M., Siemiatkowski, A., Rygasiewicz, K., 2012. Molecular basics of sepsis development. Anaesthesiol. Intensive Ther. 44 (4), 221–225. Retrieved from: http://www.ncbi.nlm.nih.gov/pubmed/23348491.

Kuhn, A., Wenzel, J., Weyd, H., 2014. Photosensitivity, apoptosis, and cytokines in the pathogenesis of lupus erythematosus: a critical review. Clin. Rev. Allergy Immunol. 47 (2), 148–162. http://dx.doi.org/10.1007/s12016-013-8403-x.

Kumar, R., Clermont, G., Vodovotz, Y., Chow, C.C., 2004. The dynamics of acute inflammation. J. Theor. Biol. 230 (2), 145–155. http://dx.doi.org/10.1016/j.jtbi.2004.04.044.

Lee, K.G., Kim, S.S., Kui, L., Voon, D.C., Mauduit, M., Bist, P., Lam, K.P., 2015. Bruton's tyrosine kinase phosphorylates DDX41 and activates its binding of dsDNA and STING to initiate type 1 interferon response. Cell Rep. 10 (7), 1055–1065. http://dx.doi.org/10.1016/j.celrep.2015.01.039.

Lee, M.T., Hooper, L.C., Kump, L., Hayashi, K., Nussenblatt, R., Hooks, J.J., Detrick, B., 2007. Interferon-beta and adhesion molecules (E-selectin and s-intraclular adhesion molecule-1) are detected in sera from patients with retinal vasculitis and are induced in retinal vascular endothelial cells by Toll-like receptor 3 signalling. Clin. Exp. Immunol. 147 (1), 71–80. http://dx.doi.org/10.1111/j.1365-2249.2006.03253.x.

Malhotra, V., Wong, H.R., 2002. Interactions between the heat shock response and the nuclear factor-kappa B signaling pathway. Crit. Care Med. 30 (Suppl. 1), S89–S95. Retrieved from: http://www.ncbi.nlm.nih.gov/pubmed/11782566.

Mata-Espinosa, D.A., Hernandez-Pando, R., 2008. Gamma interferon: basics aspects, clinic significance and terapeutic uses. Rev. Invest. Clin. 60 (5), 421–431. Retrieved from: http://www.ncbi.nlm.nih.gov/pubmed/19227440.

Newton, K., Dixit, V.M., 2012. Signaling in innate immunity and inflammation. Cold Spring Harb. Perspect. Biol. 4 (3). http://dx.doi.org/10.1101/cshperspect.a006049.

O'Neill, L.A., Bowie, A.G., 2007. The family of five: TIR-domain-containing adaptors in Toll-like receptor signalling. Nat. Rev. Immunol. 7 (5), 353–364. http://dx.doi.org/10.1038/nri2079.

Popovich, P.G., Jones, T.B., 2003. Manipulating neuroinflammatory reactions in the injured spinal cord: back to basics. Trends Pharmacol. Sci. 24 (1), 13–17. Retrieved from: http://www.ncbi.nlm.nih.gov/pubmed/12498725.

Rodrigues-Diez, R., Rayego-Mateos, S., Orejudo, M., Aroeira, L.S., Selgas, R., Ortiz, A., Ruiz-Ortega, M., 2015. TGF-Beta blockade increases renal inflammation caused by the C-Terminal module of the CCN2. Mediat. Inflamm. 2015, 506041. http://dx.doi.org/10.1155/2015/506041.

Seymour, R.L., Rossi, S.L., Bergren, N.A., Plante, K.S., Weaver, S.C., 2013. The role of innate versus adaptive immune responses in a mouse model of O'nyong-nyong virus infection. Am. J. Trop. Med. Hyg. 88 (6), 1170–1179. http://dx.doi.org/10.4269/ajtmh.12-0674.

Shi, G., Li, D., Fu, J., Sun, Y., Li, Y., Qu, R., Li, D., 2015. Upregulation of cyclooxygenase-2 is associated with activation of the alternative nuclear factor kappa B signaling pathway in colonic adenocarcinoma. Am. J. Transl. Res. 7 (9), 1612–1620. Retrieved from: http://www.ncbi.nlm.nih.gov/pubmed/26550460.

Tornatore, L., Thotakura, A.K., Bennett, J., Moretti, M., Franzoso, G., 2012. The nuclear factor kappa B signaling pathway: integrating metabolism with inflammation. Trends Cell Biol. 22 (11), 557–566. http://dx.doi.org/10.1016/j.tcb.2012.08.001.

Toskala, E., 2014. Immunology. Int. Forum Allergy Rhinol. 4 (Suppl. 2), S21–S27. http://dx.doi.org/10.1002/alr.21380.

Uematsu, S., Akira, S., 2007. Toll-like receptors and Type I interferons. J. Biol. Chem. 282 (21), 15319–15323. http://dx.doi.org/10.1074/jbc.R700009200.

Veenstra, M., Ransohoff, R.M., 2012. Chemokine receptor CXCR2: physiology regulator and neuroinflammation controller? J. Neuroimmunol. 246 (1–2), 1–9. http://dx.doi.org/10.1016/j.jneuroim.2012.02.016.

Wilting, J., Becker, J., Buttler, K., Weich, H.A., 2009. Lymphatics and inflammation. Curr. Med. Chem. 16 (34), 4581–4592. Retrieved from: http://www.ncbi.nlm.nih.gov/pubmed/19903150.

Xanthoulea, S., Curfs, D.M., Hofker, M.H., de Winther, M.P., 2005. Nuclear factor kappa B signaling in macrophage function and atherogenesis. Curr. Opin. Lipidol. 16 (5), 536–542. Retrieved from: http://www.ncbi.nlm.nih.gov/pubmed/16148538.

Yang, S., Yu, M., Sun, L., Xiao, W., Yang, X., Sun, L., Yang, H., 2014. Interferon-gamma-induced intestinal epithelial barrier dysfunction by NF-kappaB/HIF-1alpha pathway. J. Interferon. Cytokine Res. 34 (3), 195–203. http://dx.doi.org/10.1089/jir.2013.0044.

Yazdi, A.S., Rocken, M., Ghoreschi, K., 2016. Cutaneous immunology: basics and new concepts. Semin. Immunopathol. 38 (1), 3–10. http://dx.doi.org/10.1007/s00281-015-0545-x.

CHAPTER 4

Antioxidant Property Is the Basic Feature of Kampo Medicine

Tetsuya Konishi[1,2,3]

[1]*NUPALS Liaison R/D Promotion Division, Niigata, Japan;* [2]*Changchun University of Chinese Medicine, Changchun, China;* [3]*HALD Food Function Research Institute, Niigata, Japan*

Introduction

In a long-lived society, diseases like cancer, diabetes, and dementia are the major factors decreasing the quality of life. Because such diseases involve multiple pathogenic processes and pathological features, the Western medicine–based concept of a single molecule attacking a specific receptor responsible for the disease usually does not provide an effective treatment strategy. Thus preventive medicine is recognized as more important for suppressing these disorders, as is developing an alternate strategy for treating these diseases (Konishi, 2009). In this sense, a specific physiological condition named "mibyou," or subhealthy condition, is attracting much attention as the primary target of preventive medicine, because many of the aforementioned serious disorders develop from the mibyou condition (Uebaba et al., 2011).

In Oriental medicine, it is recognized that there is no clear boundary between health and diagnosed disease and the mibyou was defined as the state between them, and the endpoint diseases develop from this condition. It shows no clear specific symptom, but several abnormalities, such as coldness of hands and feet, stiffness of the shoulders, and abnormalities of autonomic nerve function, such as constipation. From the view of Western medicine, mibyou might be implicated as a complex pathological condition reflected in health check data such as high blood pressure, high plasma cholesterol level, and high blood sugar. Therefore, the strategy of Western medicine to remove a specific pathological target by a single drug is usually not effective for treating mibyou. Traditional Oriental medicines such as Kampo medicine, on the other hand, have an advantage by treating not only the diagnosed disease, like cancer or diabetes, as complementary and alternate medicines, but also the mibyou (Terasawa, 2004).

It is known that stressors induce physiological abnormalities, producing conditions similar to mibyou (Grippo and Johnson, 2009). At the same time, without distinction of physical and psychological stressors, an excess stressor causes so-called oxidative stress (Tomanek, 2015; Wang et al., 2007), in that overproduction of harmful chemical species such as reactive oxygen and nitrogen species (ROS and RNS) tends to damage important cellular molecules such as DNA, protein, and sugar, leading to cell death. Indeed, oxidative stress is associated with the pathogenesis and progression of various diseases (Rahman et al., 2012). It is, therefore, reasonable to postulate that oxidative stress is behind the pathogenesis of mibyou. This implies that the primary target of herbal medicines, including Kampo medicines, is oxidative stress (Konishi, 2009). This idea is supported by the fact that they are usually prescribed as a combination of several herbs, and the herbs are usually rich sources of antioxidant components such as polyphenols.

Oxidative Stress and Diseases

Molecular oxygen is an essential element for the life of aerobic organisms. The development of a metabolism called oxidative phosphorylation for effective ATP production was a paradigm for the organisms on the earth to gain enough energy for living. In this process molecular oxygen is the final acceptor of electrons extracted from low-entropy substrates being decomposed in the mitochondria to CO_2 and H_2O (Caprette, 1996).

During the process, partially reduced oxygen species named primary ROS are produced, such as superoxide radical, H_2O_2, and hydroxyl radical. They successively react with nearby cellular substrates to produce other reactive species such as peroxynitrite, hydroperoxy radicals, and alkoxyl radicals (Ozcan and Ogun, 2015). These species behave as toxic oxidants to react with and decompose or modify various physiologically important molecules, including lipids, DNA, sugars, and proteins. Thus, living systems have developed defense systems against ROS abuse at the early stage of development, such as the so-called antioxidant enzymes, like superoxide dismutase (SOD), catalase, and glutathione peroxidase (Gpx), and low-molecular-weight antioxidants, such as reduced glutathione and uric acid, to eliminate excess ROS and prevent cellular damage. In addition to these physiological defense systems, externally available antioxidant molecules such as polyphenols in the diet also participate in the antioxidant protection against tissue damage caused by ROS. ROS, on the other hand, play important roles as physiological signal molecules. ROS are thus two-faced, like Janus; they play a critical role in modulating cellular signaling via their redox properties, on one side, but are critical in the pathogenesis of many endpoint diseases on the other. When ROS production overcomes their elimination, cellular components tend to be damaged. Such condition is called oxidative stress and is associated with not only pathogenesis but also aggravation of many diseases (Uttara et al., 2009). Therefore, the control of oxidative stress is a basic strategy for preventing diseases, such as cancer, and also the effects of aging. Thus, how to manage or control oxidative stress is an emerging social concern for human health.

Oxidative Stress as the Target of Kampo Medicine

Currently the disease preventive functions of antioxidant ingredients in food are attracting much attention and discussion (WHO Technical Report Series No. 916). Kampo medicines are implicated as a model for food because they have been used not only for disease treatment but also in prevention. For example, "yakuzen," a pharmacologically active cuisine, is designed for health promotion and is one of the approaches of Kampo medicine to prevent disease and maintain health (Whang, 1981).

Kampo medicine, on the other hand, has such characteristics that the same prescription is often used to treat different pathological conditions and the same disorder is treated with different prescriptions, indicating that there are certain common or basic targets for such prescriptions. Because oxidative stress is one of the common pathologies associated with many diseases (Hybertson et al., 2011), it is inferred that oxidative stress is the primary target of Oriental medicine (Konishi, 2009).

This agrees with the fact that Kampo medicines are usually formulated with various substances, at least two, mainly originating from plants and with different properties and functions, whereas in folk medicine, a single herb is used for medication. The plants or herbs are well-known rich sources of antioxidant ingredients, such as polyphenols, having free radical scavenging properties, and a book of knowledge has accumulated on their physiological and pharmacological functions, such as cancer chemoprevention (Dashwood, 2007), protection against vascular endothelial injury (Vita, 2005), and neural protection (Bhullar and Rupasinghe, 2013). Therefore, herbal medicines like Kampo medicines are basically antioxidants, and thus antioxidant protection will be one of the underlying mechanisms of their functions.

Antioxidant Properties of Kampo Formulas and Herbal Components

As antioxidant activity is the basic factor of food function and also plays an important role in herbal medicine function, the antioxidant activity of many herbal resources and Kampo formulas has been studied and much information has accumulated. However, the term "antioxidant" comprises rather complex features; for example, there are several methods to evaluate antioxidant activity and the unit to show the potential, such as ferric-reducing antioxidant power (FRAP), radical scavenging potency, Trolox equivalent antioxidant capacity, and oxygen radical absorbance capacity (ORAC). Therefore, it is often difficult to make comparisons of the antioxidant activities of interest obtained by the many fragmented studies so far published. Some systematic surveys of series of foods and herbs using the same method and conditions are provided for the public as databases (Nishimura et al., 2011; Paur et al., 2011). For example, Carlsen et al. (2010) measured the FRAP activity of more than 3100 foods, beverages, spices, herbs, and supplements and some Kampo formulas provided worldwide (Carlsen et al., 2010). According to the data, traditional medicines and their component herbs formed a category of high antioxidant activity, although a large variation is present among them, such that the mean and median values are 91.7 and 14.2 mmol/100 g, respectively. Among them, goshuyutou is one of the Kampo formulas showing a high antioxidant potential, 132.6–706.3 mmol/100 g. The FRAP values of some Kampo formulas picked up from the database are given in Table 4.1.

Table 4.1: Antioxidant Activity of Some Kampo Formulas Measured by Ferric-Reducing Antioxidant Power

Kampo Formula	Antioxidant Content (mmol/100 g)
Goshuyuto	132.58
Hochuekkito	9.67
Juzentaihoto	14.2
Saikokeishito	21.4
Hangebyakujutsutemmato	5.15

Selected from NCBI bookshelf www.ncbi.nlm.gov/books/NBK92763/.

Table 4.2: Antioxidant Activity of Kampo Formulas Used for Mental and Gastrointestinal Symptoms

Kampo Formula	ORAC Unit (Formula/Day)
Kakkonto	3469
Kososan	3390
Yokukansankachimpihange	3151
Saikokeishikankyoto	3041
Orengedokuto	2771
Bukuryouingohangekobokuto	2518
Keishikashakuyakuto	3425
Ogikenchuto	2174
Keishikashakuyakuto	1797

Selected from Nishimura et al., 2011. EBCAM, Article ID 81263.

A series of Kampo formulas and component herbs was also systematically measured by the ORAC method. From the data provided by Nishimura et al. (2011), some formulas used frequently to treat symptoms related to psychological (upper four in the table) and gastrointestinal (lower three) disorders were selected, and their antioxidant activities in ORAC units compared with daily dose are shown in Table 4.2. All showed rather high ORAC values; however, there was no characteristic tendency between the formulas applied for mental or psychological dysfunctions and those for gastrointestinal symptoms. This also indicates that antioxidant property plays certain common roles in Kampo medicine.

The Brain Is a Primary Target of Antioxidant Kampo Medicines

The brain is fragile against oxidative stress, as it has high contents of oxidizable substrates, high opportunity for oxidant production through normal metabolism, and low levels of antioxidant enzymes (Konishi, 2009). Indeed, psychological stress induces oxidative stress in the midbrain in rodents as shown by our developed whisker cut model (Wang et al., 2007). Because brain stress is a pathogenic factor of mibyou, we studied the protective function of the Kampo formula shengmaisan against brain oxidative stress. Shengmaisan is a well-known formula, having been used clinically to treat heart failure in China, and comprises three herbs, *Panax ginseng*, *Ophiopogon japonicus*, and *Schisandra chinensis* (Ko, 2002). In the old Oriental medicine theory, the functions related to the brain overlap with the functions of the heart (Konishi, 2009). This formula successfully prevented cerebral oxidative injury in a forebrain ischemia–reperfusion rat model (Xuejiang et al., 1999) and also in a Parkinson's model induced by 1-methyl-4-phenyl-1,2,3,6-tetrahydropyridine (MPTP) (Giridharan et al., 2015b). The brain-protective function of shengmaisan was also demonstrated using a scopolamine-induced dementia model in rats (Giridharan et al., 2011). Further, several other Kampo medicine formulas were studied for their preventive effects on brain damage induced by ischemia–reperfusion and MPTP, such as reikeijutsukantou (Giridharan et al., 2015b), zokumeito (Motoshima et al., 2007), choutousan (Motoshima et al., 2007), and a Chinese Oriental medicine, qizhutang (Xuejiang et al., 2001). All of them inhibited brain oxidative damage and also the decline of functions such as kinesis and memory, although they all had different compositions of herbs. Further, their antioxidant protection activities in vivo were comparable even if their antioxidant properties were diverse, such that shengmaisan has a rather higher radical scavenging potential for hydroxyl radical than for superoxide radical, but other formulas showed rather strong activity toward superoxide radical. This indicated that the complex formulations with different antioxidant components are the beneficial backgrounds for their antioxidant functions, because each antioxidant molecule has a specific territory against different oxidant molecules under diverse cellular environments (Nakagawa et al., 2000).

Single Antioxidant Molecules Have Multiple Functions in a Formula

It is interesting to note that schisandrin B, a lignan component of *S. chinensis*, prevents brain damage as well as the complete formula shengmaisan in a cisplatin model system (Giridharan et al., 2012) and also prevents amyloid-β-induced brain dysfunction in an Alzheimer's disease model (Giridharan et al., 2015a). These observations provide some debate on the beneficial use of single antioxidant molecules or mixed formulas like Kampo medicine. The anti-cerebral oxidative damage activities of complete and incomplete formulas of shengmaisan and each of its component herbs were precisely examined both in vitro and in vivo (Ichikawa and Konishi, 2002; Ichikawa et al., 2003). The results revealed that the complete formula showed the strongest in vivo protective activity against oxidative damage, even if the in vitro antioxidant activities of some component herbs like *S. chinensis* and their incomplete formulas showed higher activity than complete shengmaisan. *Ophiopogon* did not show any thiobarbituric acid-reactive substance (TBARS) inhibition, but prevented Gpx activity loss the same as the complete formula. Among the antioxidant indexes examined, 2,2-diphenyl-1-picrylhydrazyl (DPPH) radical scavenging and crocin-quenching activities showed rather good correlation to the in vivo protective activities, followed by superoxide radical scavenging, although strong hydroxyl radical scavenging activity is a characteristic feature of the shengmaisan formula. It should be noted that there was some synergism among the component herbs of shengmaisan in terms of antioxidant enzyme induction, whereby a synergistic enhancement of SOD activity of *Schisandra* occurred both with *Ophiopogon* and with ginseng, but the activity of the complete mix of three component herbs was moderately adjusted. In the case of Gpx activity, no two-herb combination changed the activity, but the complete shengmaisan mix showed a markedly enhanced activity (Li et al., 2007).

Is an Herbal Mixture More Beneficial for Antioxidant Protection?

In addition to the differential reactivity of antioxidants with different ROS and RNS, the topical distribution and intracellular localization are determinants of their antioxidant function, and the factors directing to the target site or location are their chemical and physical properties. Moreover, not only direct scavenging of radicals but also redox modulation of cellular signals is a mechanism of antioxidant molecules (Hybertson et al., 2011). Therefore, it is easy to imagine that a Kampo formula, as a cocktail of many types of antioxidant ingredients that may concertedly work in the cell, is a more reasonable strategy for the integrative regulation of cellular homeostasis than a single antioxidant molecule. It is not, however, exceptional that a pharmacologically active single antioxidant molecule, such as schisandrin B, can produce multiple functionalities as discussed elsewhere (Konishi, 2014), but the effects will be restricted.

Conclusion and Remarks

Owing to the complexity of antioxidant action, it happens frequently that the antioxidant potential determined in vitro is not directly reflected in the damage-protective potential, in terms of inhibition of oxidative stress and physiological reactions such as antioxidant enzyme modulation, in vivo. The advantage of Kampo medicines containing several antioxidant ingredients will be obvious in the treatment of mibyou when we consider the complexity of antioxidant action and the role of oxidative stress in mibyou. Although synergism among the components was observed in enzyme induction activity, the in vitro antioxidant activity measured by DPPH was basically correlated to TBARS inhibition. This indicates that antioxidative protection is essentially involved behind the function of herbal mixtures like Kampo medicines. At present, the practical or clinical significance of the in vitro antioxidant activity data is yet limited; they will be reliable indexes of the quality of Kampo medicines together with chemotaxonomy. Further understanding of the concerted mechanisms of antioxidant and pharmacological actions is necessary for Kampo medicine.

References

Bhullar, K.S., Rupasinghe, H.P., 2013. Polyphenols: multipotent therapeutic agents in neurodegenerative diseases. Oxid. Med. Cell Longev. 2013, 891748. http://dx.doi.org/10.1155/2013/891748.

Caprette, D.R., 1996, 2005. Retrieved from: http://www.ruf.rice.edu/~bioslabs/studies/mitochondria/mitets.html.

Carlsen, M.H., Halvorsen, B.L., Holte, K., Bohn, S.K., Dragland, S., Sampson, L., et al., 2010. The total antioxidant content of more than 3100 foods, beverages, spices, herbs and supplements used worldwide. Nutr. J. 9, 3. http://dx.doi.org/10.1186/1475-2891-9-3.

Dashwood, R.H., 2007. Frontiers in polyphenols and cancer prevention. J. Nutr. 137 (Suppl. 1), 267S–269S. http://www.ncbi.nlm.nih.gov/pubmed/17182838.

Giridharan, V.V., Thandavarayan, R.A., Sato, S., Ko, K.M., Konishi, T., 2011. Prevention of scopolamine-induced memory deficits by schisandrin B, an antioxidant lignan from *Schisandra chinensis* in mice. Free Radic. Res. 45 (8), 950–958. http://dx.doi.org/10.3109/10715762.2011.571682.

Giridharan, V.V., Thandavarayan, R.A., Bhilwade, H.N., Ko, K.M., Watanabe, K., Konishi, T., 2012. Schisandrin B, attenuates cisplatin-induced oxidative stress, genotoxicity and neurotoxicity through modulating NF-kappaB pathway in mice. Free Radic. Res. 46 (1), 50–60. http://dx.doi.org/10.3109/10715762.2011.638291.

Giridharan, V.V., Thandavarayan, R.A., Arumugam, S., Mizuno, M., Nawa, H., Suzuki, K., et al., 2015a. Schisandrin B ameliorates ICV-infused amyloid beta induced oxidative stress and neuronal dysfunction through inhibiting RAGE/NF-kappaB/MAPK and up-regulating HSP/Beclin expression. PLoS One 10 (11), e0142483. http://dx.doi.org/10.1371/journal.pone.0142483.

Giridharan, V.V., Thandavarayan, R.A., Konishi, T., 2015b. Antioxidant formulae, shengmai san, and LingGuiZhuGanTang, prevent MPTP induced brain dysfunction and oxidative damage in mice. Evid. Based Complement. Alternat. Med. 2015, 584018. http://dx.doi.org/10.1155/2015/584018.

Grippo, A.J., Johnson, A.K., 2009. Stress, depression and cardiovascular dysregulation: a review of neuro-biological mechanisms and the integration of research from preclinical disease models. Stress 12 (1) , 1–21. http://dx.doi.org/10.1080/10253890802046281.

Hybertson, B.M., Gao, B., Bose, S.K., McCord, J.M., 2011. Oxidative stress in health and disease: the therapeutic potential of Nrf2 activation. Mol. Aspects Med. 32 (4–6), 234–246. http://dx.doi.org/10.1016/j.mam. 2011.10.006.

Ichikawa, H., Konishi, T., 2002. In vitro antioxidant potentials of traditional Chinese medicine, shengmai san and their relation to in vivo protective effect on cerebral oxidative damage in rats. Biol. Pharm. Bull. 25 (7), 898–903. http://dx.doi.org/10.1248/bpb.25.898.

Ichikawa, H., Wang, X., Konishi, T., 2003. Role of component herbs in antioxidant activity of shengmai san—a traditional Chinese medicine formula preventing cerebral oxidative damage in rat. Am. J. Chin. Med. 31 (4), 509–521. http://dx.doi.org/10.1142/S0192415X03001193.

Ko, R.K.M., 2002. Shengmai San. Taylor & Francis, London.

Konishi, T., 2009. Brain oxidative stress as basic target of antioxidant traditional oriental medicines. Neurochem. Res. 34 (4), 711–716. http://dx.doi.org/10.1007/s11064-008-9872-9.

Konishi, T., 2014. "Weak direct" and "Strong indirect" interactions are the mode of action of food factors. JFFHD 4, 254–263.

Li, Y., Gong, M., Konishi, T., 2007. Antioxidant synergism among component herbs of traditional Chinese medicine formula, shengmai san studied in vitro and in vivo. J. Health Sci. 53 (6), 692–699. http://dx.doi.org/10.1248/jhs.53.692.

Motoshima, T., Sato, S., Konishi, T., 2007. The effect of Zokumei-to in cerebral oxidative model in rats and mice. Pharmacometrics 72, 57–62.

Nakagawa, K., Kawagoe, M., Yoshimura, M., Arata, H., Minamikawa, T., Nakamura, M., Matsumoto, A., 2000. Differential effects of flavonoid quercetin on oxidative damages induced by hydrophilic and lipophilic radical generators in hepatic lysosomal fractions of mice. Eisei kagaku 46 (6), 509–512. http://dx.doi.org/10.1248/jhs.46.509.

Nishimura, K., Osawa, T., Watanabe, K., 2011. Evaluation of oxygen radical absorbance capacity in Kampo medicine. Evid. Based Complement. Alternat. Med. 2011, 812163. http://dx.doi.org/10.1093/ecam/nen082.

Ozcan, A., Ogun, M. (Eds.), 2015. Biochemistry of Reactive Oxygen and Nitrogen Species. InTech.

Paur, I., Carlsen, M.H., Halvorsen, B.L., Blomhoff, R., 2011. Antioxidants in herbs and spices. In: Benzie, I.F.F., Wachtel-Galor, S. (Eds.), Herbal Medicine: Biomolecular and Clinical Aspects. CRC Press/Taylor & Francis: NCBI Bookshelf.

Rahman, T., Hosen, I., Islam, M.M.T., Shekhar, H.U., 2012. Oxidative stress and human health. Adv. Biosci. Biotechnol. 03 (07), 23. http://dx.doi.org/10.4236/abb.2012.327123.

Terasawa, K., 2004. Evidence-based reconstruction of Kampo medicine: part I-is Kampo CAM? Evid. Based Complement. Alternat. Med. 1 (1), 11–16. http://dx.doi.org/10.1093/ecam/neh003.

Tomanek, L., 2015. Proteomic responses to environmentally induced oxidative stress. J. Exp. Biol. 218 (Pt 12), 1867–1879. http://dx.doi.org/10.1242/jeb.116475.

Uebaba, K., Xu, F., Ogawa, H., & Yatsuzuka, Y., 2011. Concept and Treatment of Mibyou, Presymptomatic State. www.inm.u-toyama.ac.jp/jp/nennpo/10np/10_sosetu.pdf.

Uttara, B., Singh, A.V., Zamboni, P., Mahajan, R.T., 2009. Oxidative stress and neurodegenerative diseases: a review of upstream and downstream antioxidant therapeutic options. Curr. Neuropharmacol. 7 (1), 65–74. http://dx.doi.org/10.2174/157015909787602823.

Vita, J.A., 2005. Polyphenols and cardiovascular disease: effects on endothelial and platelet function. Am. J. Clin. Nutr. 81 (Suppl. 1), 292S–297S. Retrieved from: http://www.ncbi.nlm.nih.gov/pubmed/15640493.

Wang, L., Muxin, G., Nishida, H., Shirakawa, C., Sato, S., Konishi, T., 2007. Psychological stress-induced oxidative stress as a model of sub-healthy condition and the effect of TCM. Evid. Based Complement. Alternat. Med. 4 (2), 195–202. http://dx.doi.org/10.1093/ecam/nel080.

Whang, J., 1981. Chinese traditional food therapy. J. Am. Diet. Assoc. 78 (1), 55–57. Retrieved from: http://www.ncbi.nlm.nih.gov/pubmed/7217561.

WHO Technical Report Series No 916 (TRS 916) Diet, Nutrition and the Prevention of Chronic Diseases: Report of the Joint WHO/FAO Expert Consultation, 2003.

Xuejiang, W., Magara, T., Konishi, T., 1999. Prevention and repair of cerebral ischemia-reperfusion injury by Chinese herbal medicine, shengmai san, in rats. Free Radic. Res. 31 (5), 449–455. Retrieved from: http://www.ncbi.nlm.nih.gov/pubmed/10547189.

Xuejiang, W., Ichikawa, H., Konishi, T., 2001. Antioxidant potential of qizhu tang, a Chinese herbal medicine, and the effect on cerebral oxidative damage after ischemia reperfusion in rats. Biol. Pharm. Bull. 24 (5), 558–563. Retrieved from: http://www.ncbi.nlm.nih.gov/pubmed/11379780.

CHAPTER 5

Japanese Kampo Medicines for Inflammatory Bowel Disease

Meilei Harima[1], Remya Sreedhar[1], Kenji Suzuki[2]

[1]Niigata University of Pharmacy and Applied Life Sciences, Niigata, Japan; [2]Niigata University Graduate School of Medical and Dental Sciences, Niigata City, Japan

Introduction

The Japanese traditional herbal medicine, Kampo, is a unique form of pharmacological therapy that originated in ancient China and was developed further in Japan (Watanabe et al., 2011). Kampo medicines have been used as prescription drugs for additional treatment of patients with unexplained physical symptoms such as nausea, abdominal pain, diarrhea, and constipation in the gastroenterology field in Japan. The therapeutic strategies of Kampo medicine, thus, largely depend on the experience of the individual doctor and supposedly lack basic and clinical evidence. Therefore, according to the definition of the National Center for Complementary and Alternative Medicine, such agents are regarded as complementary and alternative medicine, i.e., a group of diverse medical and health care systems, practices, and products that are not currently considered to be part of conventional medicine (Manabe et al., 2010). However, extensive evidence for the clinical efficacies or pharmacological mechanisms of Kampo medicines has gradually accumulated over past decades. In this chapter, we provide an overview of Kampo medicine for gastrointestinal (GI) disorders and then discuss its role in inflammatory bowel disease.

Kampo Medicines for Gastrointestinal Disorders

The Japanese traditional herbal medicines or Kampo medicines are standardized with regard to quality and quantity of their ingredients and have been approved by the Japanese Ministry of Health and Welfare. In contrast to herbal medicinal products from many other, less well regulated countries, Kampo medicines are primarily extract granules, and notably their pharmacologic actions have been studied and elucidated at the molecular level (Yuan et al., 2016). An emerging therapeutic target for Kampo medicines in clinical practice is GI functional disorders, in which conventional pharmacotherapy is either only partly effective or associated with adverse events. Extensive evidence for the clinical efficacy or pharmacological mechanisms of Kampo medicines has gradually accumulated over past decades; however, more multiple, randomized placebo-controlled trials (preferably international) using common endpoints are required to establish the Kampo medicines as evidence-based standardized medicines as opposed to experience-based alternative medicines (Oka et al., 2014; Tominaga and Arakawa, 2013).

Rikkunshito and daikenchuto are two major Kampo medicines used for GI disorders at present in Japan. There are other Kampo medicines used for these disorders; however, they lack evidence, or their efficacy and mechanism of pharmacologic action are elucidated incompletely. Therefore, we introduce the two major Kampo drugs, which have relatively firm evidence for their efficacy and mechanism of action.

The GI tract is divided into two parts: upper and lower. The upper GI tract is composed of the esophagus, stomach, and duodenum. The lower includes the small intestine, colon, and rectum. Rikkunshito is widely used for upper GI disorders; in contrast, daikenchuto is prescribed for patients with lower GI disorders.

Rikkunshito is prepared by compounding eight herbal medicines listed in the Japanese Pharmacopoeia, which include *Atractylodes lancea* rhizome, ginseng, *Pinellia* tuber, *Poria* sclerotium, jujube, *Citrus unshiu* peel, *Glycyrrhiza*, and ginger. It has been shown that oral administration of rikkunshito stimulates the secretion of ghrelin from the stomach. Ghrelin is an orexigenic hormone mainly secreted from the stomach, and it plays an important role in the motility of the stomach and duodenum. Rikkunshito is considered a complementary medicine for gastroesophageal reflux disorder and functional dyspepsia. It is also prescribed for patients with diverse GI disorders. Combination therapy with modern Western medicine and Japanese traditional medicine has also been used for various gastric disease conditions (Saegusa et al., 2015; Tominaga and Arakawa, 2015; Tominaga et al., 2015).

Daikenchuto, a mixture of herbal medicines such as processed ginger, ginseng, *Zanthoxylum* fruit, and maltose sugar, is mainly indicated for the relief of abdominal cold feeling and pain accompanied by abdominal flatulence. It has also been used to improve GI motility, postoperative adhesion, and paralytic ileus after abdominal surgery (Endo et al., 2014; Numata et al., 2014; Okada et al., 2013; Sato, 2014). Daikenchuto extract powder (Tsumura & Co., Tokyo, Japan) is manufactured as an aqueous extract containing 2.2% Japanese pepper, 5.6% processed ginger, 3.3% ginseng, and 88.9% maltose syrup powder. Daikenchuto exhibits antiinflammatory effects. It ameliorates microvascular dysfunction and inhibits mucosal injuries and adhesion of the colonic serosa. Daikenchuto induces the production of calcitonin gene-related peptide (CGRP), a neuropeptide produced by the sensory neurons of the gut. CGRP is an important mediator of microvascular vasodilation in the human body and it also has antiinflammatory and trophic actions in the gut (Kono et al., 2009). Daikenchuto is considered a complementary medicine for several GI disorders and is even prescribed in combination with Western medicine for postoperative bowel motility.

Inflammatory Bowel Disease

Inflammatory bowel disease (IBD), which comprises ulcerative colitis (UC) and Crohn's disease (CD), is characterized by chronically relapsing inflammation in the bowel of unknown etiology (Baumgart and Carding, 2007). IBD generally affects young people, and approximately 30% of patients with UC will undergo a colectomy in the course of their lifetime, whereas about 80% of all patients with CD require surgery at least once during the course of their disease (Yamamoto, 2005). Thus, IBD is a serious disease affecting the quality of life for a long period. The number of patients with IBD has been increasing in Asia as well as in the European and North American countries (Asakura et al., 2009).

The pathophysiology of the IBD is not yet clear, but it seems as if genetic, immune, environmental, inflammatory, neurological, and physiological factors have some role in the disease progression. CD includes discontinuous transmural inflammation involving the thickening of the bowel wall and inflammatory responses, and the location of the disease includes the entire GI tract, including small intestine, colon, esophagus, and stomach. UC is characterized by the impairment of the normal anatomy and physiology of the colon combined with the occurrence of extraintestinal manifestations and incidence of dysplasia and colorectal cancer (Sreedhar et al., 2016).

In recent years, the treatment for IBD has been greatly improved and established. The conventional treatment for IBD includes the use of aminosalicylates, corticosteroids, immunosuppressants, antibiotics, calcineurin inhibitors, and anti-tumor necrosis factor antibodies. However, unfortunately, many patients are not sufficiently helped by conventional therapy or suffer from relevant adverse events, including the risks of infection and malignancy. In addition, IBD requires lifelong treatment, such as induction and maintenance therapy, given the difficulty of predicting and controlling the frequency and severity of disease exacerbation.

Kampo Medicines for Inflammatory Bowel Disease

Treatment for IBD mainly focuses on the regulation of inflammatory cells and their secretion of various inflammatory mediators like proinflammatory cytokines, chemokines, etc., and also suppressing the inflammation and cell death associated with oxidative stress and endoplasmic reticulum stress. Maintenance of intestinal microbial dysbiosis, host genetics, and environmental factors also have important roles in IBD treatment. The incorporation of natural products into the therapeutic regimen is an attractive approach for improving disease treatment because of their generally low toxicity profiles and high patient compliance. Japanese Kampo medicines are highly standardized for their quality and widely used for the treatment of various diseases. Several Kampo medicines have been investigated using animal studies and clinical trials to evaluate their potential beneficial effects (Sreedhar et al., 2015b).

As previously described, daikenchuto is a Kampo that is widely used for various ailments in the GI tract. Daikenchuto has been reported to upregulate the adrenomedullin (ADM)/CGRP system, which is involved in intestinal vasodilation. Therefore, it ameliorates the microvascular dysfunction by the upregulation of ADM in CD (Kono et al., 2010, 2011). It may be effective in improving blood flow and reducing inflammatory changes by augmenting secretion of ADM from the intestinal mucosal epithelium, which supplements the decreased production of CGRP from damaged neuronal tissues in CD (Kono et al., 2009).

There are several studies in process at the time of this writing to investigate the efficacy of Kampo formulas in the treatment of IBD. Hangeshashinto is a Japanese Kampo formula that has been used to treat inflammatory ulcerative gut diseases. Crude herbal drugs include *Pinellia* tuber, *Scutellaria* root, ginseng, jujube, *Glycyrrhiza*, *Coptis* rhizome, and steamed ginger (Kawashima et al., 2004).

Tokishakuyakusan is a traditional Kampo medicine that improves blood circulation and is used to treat various gynecological disorders. This Kampo formulation is made from six different herbs, i.e., hoelen, *Cnidium* rhizome, *Angelica sinensis*, peony root, *Atractylodes* rhizome, and *Alisma* rhizome. Use of this Kampo formula in a murine acute colitis model showed attenuation of clinical symptoms of the disease and also alleviated the inflammatory mechanisms by reducing the inflammatory mediators and thereby downregulating endoplasmic reticulum stress and apoptotic signaling. It has been suggested that tokishakuyakusan may be a promising agent for the treatment of colitis, because it alleviates the disease progression and severity (Sreedhar et al., 2015b).

Jumihaidokuto is another Kampo formula, which is currently prescribed for skin inflammatory conditions like atopic dermatitis, acne vulgaris, and chronic eczema. It is composed of 10 medicinal herbs mixed together, i.e., *Platycodon* root, *Bupleurum* root, *Cnidium* rhizome, *Poria* sclerotium, *Quercus* bark, *Aralia* rhizome, *Saposhnikovia* root, *Glycyrrhiza*, *Schizonepeta* spike, and ginger. A dose of 1 g of jumihaidokuto per kilogram per day taken orally produced beneficial effects on dextran sulfate sodium-induced colitis in mice (Sreedhar et al., 2015a). One of the components of jumihaidokuto, *Platycodon* root, contains platyconic acid and platycodin D, which were reported to possess antiinflammatory activity. The polysaccharides isolated from the roots of *Bupleurum chinense* and four compounds, namely, falcarindiol, 6-hydroxy-7-methoxy dihydroligustilide, ligustilidiol, and senkyunolide H isolated from the extract of the rhizome of *Cnidium officinale*, showed antiinflammatory properties. Treatment with jumihaidokuto for acute colitis resulted in the attenuation of inflammatory cascades and thereby reduced oxidative stress, endoplasmic reticulum stress, and apoptosis, which strongly recommends the use of jumihaidokuto as a therapeutic option for IBD (Sreedhar et al., 2015a).

Conclusion

IBD is mainly associated with the infiltration of the inflammatory cascade into the intestinal wall and can be effectively suppressed by the use of various Kampo formulations that have antiinflammatory activity. The Japanese traditional herbal medicines or Kampo medicines are standardized with regard to quality and quantity of the ingredients. Kampo medicines have been used as prescription drugs for various disease conditions in the gastroenterology field in Japan. The incorporation of natural products into therapy can improve disease treatment because the toxicity profile is low for natural products. Therefore Kampo formulas can play an important role as an effective treatment option for IBD. There are very few reports of clinical trials available for Kampo medicines, and therefore future studies should focus on large clinical studies to confirm the therapeutic potential of Kampo medicines for IBD and other GI disorders.

References

Asakura, K., Nishiwaki, Y., Inoue, N., Hibi, T., Watanabe, M., Takebayashi, T., 2009. Prevalence of ulcerative colitis and Crohn's disease in Japan. J. Gastroenterol. 44 (7), 659–665. http://dx.doi.org/10.1007/s00535-009-0057-3.

Baumgart, D.C., Carding, S.R., 2007. Inflammatory bowel disease: cause and immunobiology. Lancet 369 (9573), 1627–1640. http://dx.doi.org/10.1016/s0140-6736(07)60750-8.

Endo, M., Hori, M., Ozaki, H., Oikawa, T., Hanawa, T., 2014. Daikenchuto, a traditional Japanese herbal medicine, ameliorates postoperative ileus by anti-inflammatory action through nicotinic acetylcholine receptors. J. Gastroenterol. 49 (6), 1026–1039. http://dx.doi.org/10.1007/s00535-013-0854-6.

Kawashima, K., Nomura, A., Makino, T., Saito, K., Kano, Y., 2004. Pharmacological properties of traditional medicine (XXIX): effect of Hange-shashin-to and the combinations of its herbal constituents on rat experimental colitis. Biol. Pharm. Bull. 27 (10), 1599–1603.

Kono, T., Kanematsu, T., Kitajima, M., 2009. Exodus of Kampo, traditional Japanese medicine, from the complementary and alternative medicines: is it time yet? Surgery 146 (5), 837–840. http://dx.doi.org/10.1016/j.surg.2009.06.012.

Kono, T., Kaneko, A., Hira, Y., Suzuki, T., Chisato, N., Ohtake, N., Watanabe, T., 2010. Anti-colitis and -adhesion effects of daikenchuto via endogenous adrenomedullin enhancement in Crohn's disease mouse model. J. Crohns Colitis 4 (2), 161–170. http://dx.doi.org/10.1016/j.crohns.2009.09.006.

Kono, T., Omiya, Y., Hira, Y., Kaneko, A., Chiba, S., Suzuki, T., Watanabe, T., 2011. Daikenchuto (TU-100) ameliorates colon microvascular dysfunction via endogenous adrenomedullin in Crohn's disease rat model. J. Gastroenterol. 46 (10), 1187–1196. http://dx.doi.org/10.1007/s00535-011-0438-2.

Manabe, N., Camilleri, M., Rao, A., Wong, B.S., Burton, D., Busciglio, I., Haruma, K., 2010. Effect of daikenchuto (TU-100) on gastrointestinal and colonic transit in humans. Am. J. Physiol. Gastrointest. Liver Physiol. 298 (6), G970–G975. http://dx.doi.org/10.1152/ajpgi.00043.2010.

Numata, T., Takayama, S., Tobita, M., Ishida, S., Katayose, D., Shinkawa, M., Yaegashi, N., 2014. Traditional Japanese medicine daikenchuto improves functional constipation in poststroke patients. Evid. Based Complement. Altern. Med. 2014, 231258. http://dx.doi.org/10.1155/2014/231258.

Oka, T., Okumi, H., Nishida, S., Ito, T., Morikiyo, S., Kimura, Y., Murakami, M., 2014. Effects of Kampo on functional gastrointestinal disorders. Biopsychosoc. Med. 8, 5. http://dx.doi.org/10.1186/1751-0759-8-5.

Okada, K., Kawai, M., Uesaka, K., Kodera, Y., Nagano, H., Murakami, Y., Investigators, J.-P., 2013. Effect of Daikenchuto (TJ-100) on postoperative bowel motility and on prevention of paralytic ileus after pancreaticoduodenectomy: a multicenter, randomized, placebo-controlled phase II trial (the Japan-PD study). Jpn. J. Clin. Oncol. 43 (4), 436–438. http://dx.doi.org/10.1093/jjco/hyt005.

Saegusa, Y., Hattori, T., Nahata, M., Yamada, C., Takeda, H., 2015. A new strategy using rikkunshito to treat Anorexia and gastrointestinal dysfunction. Evid. Based Complement. Altern. Med. 2015, 364260. http://dx.doi.org/10.1155/2015/364260.

Sato, Y., 2014. Improvement effect of Daikenchuto on morphine-induced constipation through gastrointestinal peptides. Nihon Yakurigaku Zasshi 143 (3), 120–125. Retrieved from: http://www.ncbi.nlm.nih.gov/pubmed/24614634.

Sreedhar, R., Arumugam, S., Karuppagounder, V., Thandavarayan, R.A., Giridharan, V.V., Pitchaimani, V., Watanabe, K., 2015a. Jumihaidokuto effectively inhibits colon inflammation and apoptosis in mice with acute colitis. Int. Immunopharmacol. 29 (2), 957–963. http://dx.doi.org/10.1016/j.intimp.2015.10.009.

Sreedhar, R., Arumugam, S., Thandavarayan, R.A., Giridharan, V.V., Karuppagounder, V., Pitchaimani, V., Watanabe, K., 2015b. Toki-shakuyaku-san, a Japanese Kampo medicine, reduces colon inflammation in a mouse model of acute colitis. Int. Immunopharmacol. 29 (2), 869–875. http://dx.doi.org/10.1016/j.intimp.2015.08.029.

Sreedhar, R., Arumugam, S., Thandavarayan, R.A., Karuppagounder, V., Watanabe, K., 2016. Curcumin as a therapeutic agent in the chemoprevention of inflammatory bowel disease. Drug Discov. Today 21 (5), 843–849. http://dx.doi.org/10.1016/j.drudis.2016.03.007.

Tominaga, K., Arakawa, T., 2013. Kampo medicines for gastrointestinal tract disorders: a review of basic science and clinical evidence and their future application. J. Gastroenterol. 48 (4), 452–462. http://dx.doi.org/10.1007/s00535-013-0788-z.

Tominaga, K., Arakawa, T., 2015. Clinical application of Kampo medicine (rikkunshito) for common and/or intractable symptoms of the gastrointestinal tract. Front Pharmacol. 6, 7. http://dx.doi.org/10.3389/fphar.2015.00007.

Tominaga, K., Tanigawa, T., Watanabe, T., Fujiwara, Y., Arakawa, T., 2015. Kampo medicine (rikkunshito). Nihon Rinsho 73 (7), 1179–1184. Retrieved from: http://www.ncbi.nlm.nih.gov/pubmed/26165077.

Watanabe, K., Matsuura, K., Gao, P., Hottenbacher, L., Tokunaga, H., Nishimura, K., Witt, C.M., 2011. Traditional Japanese Kampo medicine: clinical research between modernity and traditional medicine—the state of research and methodological suggestions for the future. Evid. Based Complement. Altern. Med.: eCAM 2011, 513842. http://dx.doi.org/10.1093/ecam/neq067.

Yamamoto, T., 2005. Factors affecting recurrence after surgery for Crohn's disease. World J. Gastroenterol. 11 (26), 3971–3979.

Yuan, H., Ma, Q., Ye, L., Piao, G., 2016. The traditional medicine and modern medicine from natural products. Molecules 21 (5). http://dx.doi.org/10.3390/molecules21050559.

CHAPTER 6

Significance of Japanese Kampo Medicine in Supportive Care of Heart Failure/Function

Darukeshwara Joladarashi, Rajarajan A. Thandavarayan, Prasanna Krishnamurthy

Houston Methodist Research Institute, Houston, TX, United States

Historical Background: Japanese Traditional Herbal Medicine (Kampo Medicine)

Overview

Ancient Chinese medicine serves as the origin for Kampo, which is a traditional Japanese medicine and was significantly developed during the Edo era (AD 1603–1868). It includes characteristics such as the use of abdominal diagnosis for therapeutic indications and formulations with smaller amounts of herbs compared with Chinese medicine. In 1967, four Kampo formulations were covered by the Japanese national health insurance, and since 1986, 148 Kampo formulations have been accepted for ethical use (Tsutani, 1993). From 1967 to 1986, the ethical Kampo product approval process was based on a "consensus-based monograph" written by the Federation of Pharmaceutical Manufacturers' Associations of Japan under the supervision of the Ministry of Health and Welfare [renamed the Ministry of Health, Labor, and Welfare (MHLW) in 2001], and not on clinical evidence. The indications on the label were based on symptoms, not traditional Kampo medicine theory or Western medicine diagnosis. A slight modification to these indications was made during the MHLW reevaluation of 1985–2014.

Kampo Herbal Formulas in Japan

Generally, Kampo formulations are extracts of herbal formulations and prepared as described in the classical Kampo literature (Motoo, 2008; Motoo et al., 2009, 2011). The struggle to implement randomized controlled trials (RCTs) of Kampo medicines has frequently been accredited to the usage of Kampo diagnosis. Because high-quality good manufacturing practice-based extracts of Kampo formulas for ethical use have been prescribed in RCTs, the reproducibility of RCT results has been very high. Kampo is used in a Western-style medical system in Japan; and the medical doctors who are educated in Western medicine, but have basic knowledge of Kampo, prescribe it. It is mandatory for doctors, not by law, but as professionals, to have a basic knowledge of the indications for each Kampo formulation when prescribing, along with the knowledge of Western medical diagnosis. In 2011, 52% of Japanese medical doctors prescribed Kampo formulations based on Western medicine, 32% on Western medicine considering Kampo diagnosis, 10% on both Western medicine and Kampo medicine, and 6% on Kampo diagnosis, according to a survey by the Japan Kampo Medicines Manufacturers Association.

Kampo Diagnosis

Physical examination results serve as the basis for Kampo diagnosis, chiefly the abdominal palpation result, which is particular for Kampo medicine. Japan teaches Kampo medicine in all its 80 medical schools and it is part of the model core curriculum for medical education as of 2001 set by the Association of Cooperative Researchers on Medical and Dental Education under the supervision of the Ministry of Education, Culture, Sports, Science, and Technology of Japan. Approximately 2150 Kampo experts (medical doctors) as of March 2011 have been certified by the Japan Society for Oriental Medicine (JSOM); these experts have passed an examination and have completed a training program. Certainly, ordinary physicians who are not Kampo medicine experts can prescribe Kampo drugs, and health insurance essentially covers the cost of prescribed drugs as named in Western medicine for that particular disease. Hence, Japanese doctors are allowed to prescribe Kampo formulations based on Western medical diagnosis. As it is not clear that this system is sufficient, evidence should be assembled from RCTs of Kampo medicines prescribed on the basis of Kampo diagnosis.

RCTs of Kampo medicines have been conducted in many clinical fields, like cardiology, gastroenterology, respirology, etc. The descriptions of Kampo products in the Japanese clinical practice guidelines have been investigated by the Committee for Evidence-Based Medicine of the JSOM, and the results of this investigation are presented (in "Clinical practice guidelines containing Kampo products in Japan," in Japanese) to the public on the website (http://www.jsom.or.jp/medical/ebm/cpg/index.html). Scrutiny of the results reveals that consumer packaged-goods developers have no adequate access to the evidence on Kampo.

In 2001, the first evidence-based study of Kampo treatment (EKAT project) was started, and in 2005, the first report was published. In 2005, an evidence report task force was established and in 2007, the EKAT project gained momentum. The EKAT 2010 (which was published in 2010) contained the structured abstracts of 345 RCTs of Kampo formulations, and has been linked to the Cochrane library (CENTRAL) as a specialized register (Wieland et al., 2013; EKAT, 2010). EKAT 2013 was made available in July 2014 and it covers all previous archived structured abstracts. Nevertheless, not all the articles on Kampo RCTs contain comments from a Kampo perspective. Additionally, studies of Kampo diagnosis used in each RCT are unresolved.

Heart Failure in Japan

According to the guidelines for the diagnosis and treatment of chronic heart failure (HF) of the American College of Cardiology/American Heart Association and the European Society of Cardiology, HF is defined as a multifaceted clinical disorder that can result from any structural or functional cardiac disorder that weakens the ability of the ventricle to fill with or eject blood (Hunt et al., 2005; Swedberg et al., 2005). Dyspnea and fatigue are the cardiac signs of HF, which may limit exercise tolerance, and fluid retention, which may lead to pulmonary congestion and peripheral edema (Hunt et al., 2005; Swedberg et al., 2005). Morbidity and mortality in industrialized countries are caused mainly by HF (Jessup and Brozena, 2003). It is also a growing public health problem, mainly because of the aging of the population and the increase in the prevalence of HF among the elderly (Massie and Shah, 1997).

Very limited information is available on the characteristics and outcome of patients with HF in Japan (Itoh et al., 1992; Koseki et al., 2003; Shiba et al., 2005). Tsutsui et al. (2001) have studied the comprehensive analysis of experimental characteristics, management, and outcome including mortality and HF-related readmission in Japan (Tsuchihashi et al., 2000, 2001; Tsutsui et al., 2001). They validated that HF patients were elderly; comprised a larger population of women, particularly at higher age; and had a higher incidence of overt HF despite a relatively normal ejection fraction (EF). In their study they found that as many as 35% of hospitalized patients with HF were readmitted within 1 year of hospital discharge. Earlier community-based studies also reported the same characteristics in the HF patient population (Kannel and Belanger, 1991; Cowie et al., 1999).

The Japanese cardiac registry of HF in cardiology (JCARECARD) was developed to provide a national prospective registry database describing the clinical characteristics, treatment, and outcomes of patients hospitalized because of worsening HF symptoms. It will also establish a framework for future initiatives to improve the outcomes of these patients. The prevalence of cardiovascular diseases in Japan remains low. The age-adjusted mortality from heart diseases has been declining recently. Shiba et al. have conducted a multicenter prospective cohort study of HF patients, named the Chronic HF Analysis and Registry, in the Tohoku district (CHART-1; $n = 1278$) since 2000. They report that the mortality rate of HF patients in Japan is high and is comparable with that seen in Western countries (Itoh et al., 1992; Koseki et al., 2003; Shiba et al., 2005).

It is estimated that there are 1.0 million patients with HF, and the number of outpatients with left-ventricular dysfunction is predicted to gradually increase to 1.3 million by 2030 in Japan. Trends in coronary heart disease (CHD) mortality and coronary risk factors have not been uniform and may vary by sex, age, and region. In the two largest metropolitan areas, Tokyo and Osaka, where 17% of the total Japanese population resides, the CHD mortality decline was small for men 30–49 years of age compared with those residing in the rest of Japan (Itoh et al., 1992; Koseki et al., 2003; Shiba et al., 2005).

Treatment for Heart Failure in Japan

From the CHART studies in Japan, it is clear that the use of renin–angiotensin system inhibitors and β-blockers in HF patients increased from 69.1% and 27.9%, respectively, in 2000–4 to 72.3% and 49.0% in 2006–10, whereas that of loop diuretics and digitalis decreased (Guo et al., 2013; Shiba and Shimokawa, 2008). In South Asian countries, it was reported that the most commonly used medications are β-blockers, angiotensin-converting enzyme (ACE) inhibitor/angiotensin receptor blocker, diuretics, and aldosterone antagonists (Cheung and Yung Cheung, 2014).

Although available data are limited, implantable cardioverter–defibrillators (ICDs) and/or cardiac resynchronization therapy are likely to be underused in Asian countries. In the CHART-2 study ($n = 10,219$), among 2778 patients with ischemic heart disease or dilated cardiomyopathy in New York Heart Association (NYHA) class II/III, 315 had a left-ventricular EF (LVEF) of ≤35% (Shiba and Shimokawa, 2008). Among them, according to the Japanese Circulation Society guidelines, 56 patients with a history of nonsustained ventricular tachycardia and the remaining 259 without it were considered to have class I and IIa recommendations for ICD implantation, respectively. However, the use of prophylactic ICD was only 30.4% and 6.6% in each group, respectively (Satake et al., 2015). It is also estimated that ICDs are underused, particularly in South Asia, partly because of limited accessibility and affordability (Pillai and Ganapathi, 2013). Although long-term mortality data are limited, Yoo et al. (2014) reported that 1-year mortality after discharge was 9.2% in HF patients with reduced LVEF in South Korea (Yoo et al., 2014). In the JCARECARD study, patients with serum uric acid ≥7.4 mg/dL had higher rates of all-cause death, cardiac death, rehospitalization, and all-cause death or rehospitalization due to worsening HF (Hamaguchi et al., 2011).

For treating HF patients at present, conventional therapeutic approaches are used, including ACE inhibitors, β-blockers, and diuretics. Although several of them have shown an important effectiveness, HF remains the leading cardiovascular disease with an increasing hospitalization burden and an ongoing drain on health care expenditure (Ramani et al., 2010). Therefore, it remains necessary to search for alternative and complementary treatments, of which traditional Japanese medicine takes a good proportion (Fu et al., 2011).

Kampo Medicine for Heart Failure Treatment

Distinctive herbal preparations are used in stable combinations to prepare the traditional Japanese pharmaceutical agents, Kampo medicines. Apart from Japan, these medicines are widely used in many parts of the world (Eisenberg et al., 1998; Stickel and Schuppan, 2007). Improving the natural resilience, strengthening the habitus, preventing disease, and adjusting the internal balance are used by Kampo medicines to place attention on and maintain basic health, thereby attracting worldwide attention (Zheng and Moritani, 2008). There is incomplete information on the cardiac effects of Kampo medicine in the literature, but from the available resources, this information is discussed in the following sections (Goldbeck-Wood, 1996; Inaki).

Mokuboito (Mu-Fang-Ji-Tang)

Mokuboito, a kind of Kampo formulation, has been used clinically for HF (Yakubu et al., 2002). It has been noted that mokuboito improves HF symptoms and reduces the rank of NYHA classification and the concentration of plasma brain natriuretic peptide (BNP) (Kasahara et al., 2002). Mokuboito mainly contains four herbal drugs: Cinnamomi cortex (Fukuda et al., 1995), *Sinomenium acutum*, gypsum, and Ginseng radix (Satoh, 2005). As every ingredient contains many chemical compounds, the resultant effect of mokuboito is shown as a net of the complex interactions among a lot of enclosed ingredients. Traditionally, mokuboito has been used for patients with symptoms like wheezing, dark complexion, and deep tight pulse.

In voltage-clamp experiments that used guinea pig cardiomyocytes, sinomenine (1 mmol/L) and tetrandrine (100 μmol/L) suppressed the concentration of ionic currents dose dependently (Satoh, 2013). Similarly, they also affected the action potential configurations. *S. acutum* (1 mg/mL) reduced the maximum rate of depolarization (V_{max}). Among the ingredients in *S. acutum*, tetrandrine (30 μmol/L) and sinomenine (300 μmol/L) also had comparable effects, but magnoflorine (1 mmol/L) had little or no effect. Sinomenine eliminated dysrhythmias that were induced by excess cellular Ca^{2+}. Even at critical administrations, these drugs exert active electropharmacological actions and cardioprotection. Satoh (2005) demonstrated that mokuboito and its constituents displayed cardiac electropharmacological actions and exerted conservative actions on cardiomyocytes. Their findings indicate that mokuboito, *S. acutum*, and sinomenine have effective pharmacological actions that improve chronic HF by recovering cardiac functions.

Chotosan (Diao-Teng-San)

Chotosan is used to treat brain and heart diseases effectively. In guinea pig ventricular cardiomyocytes, chotosan and its main constituent, Uncariae cum uncis ramulus, at 0.1–1 mg/mL inhibited the V_{max} and prolonged the action potential duration (APD) in a concentration-dependent manner. Chotosan decreased V_{max} by $15.4 \pm 3.0\%$ ($p < .05$) at 1 mg/mL, and prolonged 75% repolarization of APD by $1.2 \pm 0.3\%$ ($p > .05$) at 0.3 mg/mL. The APD prolongations were enhanced with an increase in the percentage repolarization from 50% repolarization to 90% repolarization. Washout recovered V_{max} to almost control values, but failed to shorten all the APDs (Satoh, 2013).

The main pharmacological action of chotosan would be vasodilatation, due to both endothelium-dependent and -independent actions. It has been found to be involved in complicated mechanisms for the inhibition of ion channels and protein kinase (PK) C activity, and also for nitric oxide release (Satoh, 2013).

Keisibukuryogan (Gui-Zhi-Fu-Ling-Wan) and Tokakujokito (Tao-He-Cheng-Qi-Tang)

Kampo formulations such as tokakujokito, keishibukuryogan, tokishakuyakusan (dang-gui-shao-tao-san), and kamishoyosan (jia-wei-xiao-yao-san) help in vasodilatation responsible for the modulation of endothelium-derived releasing factor, endothelium-derived hyperpolarizing factor, PKA, PKC, eicosanoids, phosphodiesterase, and K^+/Ca^{2+} channels, and further help in antioxidative action. In rat aorta, they produced marked vasodilatation by over 80–90% at 1 mg/mL of each formulation. These Kampo formulations improve vascular dysfunction that occurs with aging and can prevent the functional somatic syndrome (mibyo), which are clinically the disorders that present before the diagnosis of disease (Satoh, 2013).

Sinomenine

Sinomenine is one of the alkaloids extracted from the Chinese medical plant *S. acutum*. Sinomenine is known as one of the effective therapeutic drugs for HF and dysrhythmias, and may maintain cardiovascular functions by the modulation of cardiac ionic channels and blood vessels (Nishida and Satoh, 2007). Mokuboito, a Kampo formulation containing *S. acutum*, has been used for HF and improves HF symptoms and reduces NYHA class and plasma BNP concentration (Satoh, 2013).

Most recently, Satoh (2005) has demonstrated that sinomenine effectively modulates cardiac ionic channels. Sinomenine inhibits I_{Ca} and simultaneously produces an I_K decrease in cardiomyocytes, which results in APD prolongation. Modulation of Ca^{2+} channels induced by sinomenine is similarly exerted in vascular smooth muscle cells. The cardioprotective action of sinomenine on rat acute myocardial ischemia has also been demonstrated using reperfusion injury induced by ligating the rat left coronary artery for 15 min and reopening. Sinomenine can inhibit the incidence of arrhythmias and reduce intracellular Ca^{2+} concentration (Xie and Jin, 1993).

Sinomenine has multiple vasodilating mechanisms. The vasodilating agent is one of the great useful tools for HF and regulates pre- and afterloads of the cardiovascular system. Therefore, sinomenine-induced vasodilating actions may improve cardiac functions via the regulation of both pre- and afterloads in HF. In the future, therefore, sinomenine as a cardioprotective drug may be expected to have a respectable effectiveness for HF, mediated through the modulation of cardiac ion channels (including the regulation for dysrhythmias) and blood vessels.

Boiogito (TJ-20)

Boiogito, a traditional Japanese Kampo medicine, is prescribed as a remedy for arthritis, nephrosis, edema, hyperhidrosis, and obesity. In particular, it is effective for these diseases in patients with symptoms of fatigue, light complexion, and soft muscle. Boiogito is an extract composed of six herbal drugs including *Sinomenium* stem and *Astragalus* root. Sinomenine, an ingredient extracted from the *Sinomenium* stem, has demonstrated potential antiinflammatory activity (Gautam et al., 2014). Gautam et al. (2014) reported for the first time on the beneficial effects of Japanese Kampo medicine (TJ-20), in combination with conventional treatment, for chronic HF patients with renal insufficiency. The administration of TJ-20 significantly ameliorated renal function, decreased BNP levels, and improved NYHA functional class from baseline. They enrolled 26 patients with cardiorenal syndrome [18 men; mean age, 77 ± 8.4 years; mean serum BNP, 241.5 ± 196.6 pg/mL; mean estimated glomerular filtration rate (eGFR), 40.02 ± 10.54 mL/min 1.73 m^{-2}]. Treatment with TJ-20 was started at an average dose of 4.6 ± 1.5 g/day, which was increased to 5.2 ± 1.2 g/day at 3.5 months and to 5.9 ± 1.5 g/day at 9.4 months. TJ-20 treatment significantly increased mean eGFR (mL/min/1.73 m^2) to 44.60 ± 10.76 at 3.5 months ($p = .001$) and to 45.93 ± 11.57 at 9.4 months ($p = .0004$). In addition, the NYHA functional classification improved ($p = .019$), and serum BNP levels decreased significantly to 195.5 ± 145.7 pg/mL at 3.5 months ($p = .008$) and to 163.3 ± 130.2 pg/mL at 9.4 months ($p = .007$). The increase in eGFR had no correlation with the decrease in BNP level, indicating independent effects on both renal function and HF status. The addition of TJ-20, the Japanese Kampo boiogito, to standard HF treatment clearly demonstrated beneficial effects on the status of renal function and HF. The observations in the study of Gautam et al. (2014) suggest new strategies for utilizing traditional Japanese medicine in the management of cardiorenal syndrome (Gautam et al., 2014).

Sanoshashinto (TJ-113)

Sanoshashinto (code name TJ-113) is a Kampo medicine composed of three medicinal herbs (Scutellariae radix, Coptidis rhizoma, and Rhei rhizoma; volume ratio 1:1:1) and is used to treat climacteric disorder. Sakanashi et al. (2013) demonstrated for the first time that long-term oral treatment with a clinical dosage of TJ-113 markedly improved cardiac dysfunction and infarct size following reperfusion injury in ovariectomized rats through its inhibition of inducible nitric oxide synthase (iNOS) expression, suppression of peroxynitrite formation, and restoration of manganese-dependent superoxide dismutase activity (Sakanashi et al., 2013).

They have shown that long-term treatment with a clinical dosage of TJ-113 for 4 weeks markedly improved cardiac functional and morphological changes. Additionally, it improved the oxidative changes by reducing myocardial iNOS expression and peroxynitrite levels with restored antioxidant activity. Importantly, those beneficial actions of TJ-113 were significantly inhibited by the estrogen receptor antagonist fulvestrant, and the phytoestrogen emodin, a

TJ-113 ingredient, mimicked the actions of TJ-113, suggesting involvement of emodin in the effects of TJ-113. The results of Sakanashi et al. (2013) provide the first evidence that long-term treatment with TJ-113 protects the heart against reperfusion injury in a climacteric rat model (Sakanashi et al., 2013).

Tokishakuyakusan (TJ-23)

Tokishakuyakusan, a Japanese traditional herbal medicine, has a long history in Asia for the treatment of neurodegenerative, immune, and airway diseases. Aberle et al. (2003) examined the effect of TJ-23 on ventricular contractile function at the single cardiomyocyte level (Aberle et al., 2003). Ventricular cardiomyocytes from adult rat hearts were stimulated to contract at 0.5 Hz, and their mechanical properties were evaluated using an IonOptix Myocam system. Contractile properties analyzed included peak shortening (PS), time to PS (TPS), time to 90% relengthening (TR90), and maximal velocity of shortening/relengthening (dL/dt). TJ-23 (108–105 mg/mL) exhibited significant augmentation of PS, with a maximal response of 27.2%. TJ-23 at 107–105 mg/mL also increased dL/dt, shortened TR90, but had no effect on TPS. Pretreatment with the Na^+–K^+ ATPase inhibitor ouabain (1 M), removal of extracellular sodium from the contractile buffer (which inhibits the Na^+/Ca^{2+} exchanger), or both concurrently abolished the positive effect of TJ-23 in cell shortening without inhibiting the baseline cell shortening (Aberle et al., 2003). The study of Aberle et al. (2003) demonstrates a direct cardiac enhancement of TJ-23 at the ventricular cardiomyocyte level, possibly through a Na^+–K^+ ATPase and/or a Na^+/Ca^{2+} exchanger-associated mechanism.

Cardiac Effects of Clinically Available Kampo Medicines

Sugiyama et al. (2002) studied the chronotropic and inotropic effects of 10 kinds of clinically available Kampo extracts [kakkonto (TJ-1), daisaikoto (TJ-8), boiogito (TJ-20), choreito (TJ-40), rokumigan (TJ-87), tsudosan (TJ-105), goshajinkigan (TJ-107), sanoshashinto (TJ-113), saireito (TJ-114), and inchingoreisan (TJ-117)] using canine isolated blood-perfused heart preparations. They found that intracoronary injections of TJ-1, TJ-20, TJ-105, and TJ-113 increased the sinoatrial rate and developed tension in papillary muscle in a dose-related manner, which was significantly attenuated by pretreatment of the preparations with the β-blocker propranolol. Meanwhile, the other extracts hardly affected these parameters. TJ-1, TJ-20, and TJ-113 increased the adenylate cyclase activity in a dose-related manner, but their potency was significantly less compared with that of an equivalent concentration of isoproterenol. Moreover, TJ-105 did not increase the adenylate cyclase activity. In their study the authors showed that TJ-1, TJ-20, TJ-105, and TJ-113 possess positive chronotropic and inotropic actions, which may be exerted through the direct stimulation of the β-adrenoceptor and/or norepinephrine release from the postganglionic nerve terminals in the heart (Sugiyama et al., 2002).

Another study conducted by Sugiyama and Hashimoto (1989) demonstrated that TJ-15, TJ-36, and TJ-119, out of 10 Kampo extracts, produced dose-dependent positive chronotropic and inotropic effects and the results indicated that these three drugs act as β-adrenoceptor agonists to produce clinically useful cardiac effects (Sugiyama and Hashimoto, 1989).

Conclusion

In summary, Japanese Kampo medicines have shown potent cardioprotective actions in various studies conducted by many investigators. The observations of many clinical studies suggest a novel strategic approach for utilizing traditional Japanese Kampo medicines in the supportive care of HF and for better heart function.

Acknowledgments

This work was supported, in part, by National Institutes of Health Grant 1R01HL116729 to Dr. Prasanna Krishnamurthy and American Heart Association Grant-in-Aid GRNT 25860041 to Dr. Prasanna Krishnamurthy.

References

Aberle II, N.S., Hiramatsu, M., Ren, J., 2003. Japanese herbal medicine Toki-shakuyaku-san (TJ-23) enhances cardiac contractile function in isolated ventricular cardiomyocytes. J. Pharmacol. Sci. 91, 197–201.

Cheung, T.T., Yung Cheung, B.M., 2014. Managing blood pressure control in Asian patients: safety and efficacy of losartan. Clin. Interv. Aging 9, 443–450.

Cowie, M.R., Wood, D.A., Coats, A.J., Thompson, S.G., Poole-Wilson, P.A., Suresh, V., et al., 1999. Incidence and aetiology of heart failure; a population-based study. Eur. Heart J. 20, 421–428.

Eisenberg, D.M., Davis, R.B., Ettner, S.L., Appel, S., Wilkey, S., Van Rompay, M., et al., 1998. Trends in alternative medicine use in the United States, 1990–7: results of a follow-up national survey. JAMA 280, 1569–1575.

EKAT, 2010. Website. Available: http://www.jsom.or.jp/medical/ebm/ere/pdf/EKATE2010.pdf.

Fu, S., Zhang, J., Menniti-Ippolito, F., et al., 2011. Huangqi injection (a traditional Chinese patent medicine) for chronic heart failure: a systematic review. PLoS One 6, 19604.

Fukuda, K., Kido, T., Miura, N., Yamamoto, M., Komatsu, Y., 1995. Increase in nitric oxide synthase and cyclic GMP in vascular smooth muscle cells by treatment with aqueous extracts of Astragali Radix, Ginseng Radix and Scutellariae Radix. J. Trad. Med. 12, 38–44.

Gautam, M., Atsushi, I., Tatsuya, S., Saeko, Y., Hirohiko, M., Takeshi, T., et al., 2014. The traditional Japanese medicine (kampo) Boiogito has a dual Benefit in cardiorenal syndrome: a Pilot observational study. Shinshu Med. J. 62, 89–97.

Goldbeck-Wood, S., 1996. Complementary medicine is booming worldwide. BMJ 313, 131–133.

Guo, Y., Lip, G.Y.H., Banerjee, A., 2013. Heart failure in East Asia. Curr. Cardiol. Rev. 112–122.

Hamaguchi, S., Furumoto, T., Tsuchihashi-Makaya, M., Goto, K., Goto, D., Yokota, T., Kinugawa, S., Yokoshiki, H., Takeshita, A., Tsutsui, H., JCARE-CARD Investigators, 2011. Hyperuricemia predicts adverse outcomes in patients with heart failure. Int. J. Cardiol. 151, 143–147.

Hunt, S.A., Abraham, W.T., Chin, M.H., Feldman, A.M., Francis, G.S., Ganiats, T.G., et al., 2005. ACC/AHA 2005 guideline update for the diagnosis and management of chronic heart failure in the adult: a report of the American College of cardiology/American heart association task force on practice guidelines (writing committee to update the 2001 guidelines for the evaluation and management of heart failure): developed in collaboration with the American College of chest physicians and the international society for heart and Lung Transplantation: endorsed by the Heart Rhythm Society. Circulation 112, 154–235.

Inaki, K. Diseases and kampo. In: Sato, Y., Hanawa, T., Arai, M., Cyong, J., Fukuzawa, M., Mitani, K., Ogihara, Y., Sakiyama, T., Shimada, Y., Toriizuka, K., Ymamada, T. (Eds.) 2005, Introduction to Kampo, vol. 125. Elsevier, Japan.

Itoh, A., Saito, M., Haze, K., et al., 1992. Prognosis of patients with congestive heart failure: its determinants in various heart diseases in Japan. Intern. Med. 31, 304–309.

Japan Kampo Medicines Manufacturers Association, Actual Condition Survey on Prescription of Kampo Medicines–Summary Report– (in Japanese). Available: http://www.nikkankyo.org/aboutus/investigation/pdf/jittaichousa2011.pdf.

Jessup, M., Brozena, S., 2003. Heart failure. N. Engl. J. Med. 348, 2007–2018.

Kannel, W.B., Belanger, A.J., 1991. Epidemiology of heart failure. Am. Heart J. 121, 951–957.

Kasahara, Y., Goto, H., Shimada, Y., Sekiya, N., Yang, Q., Terasawa, K., 2002. Inhibitory effects of Cinnamomi cortex and cinnamaldehyde on oxygen-derived free radical-induced vasocontraction in isolated aorta of spontaneously hypertensive rats. J. Trad. Med. 19, 51–57.

Koseki, Y., Watanabe, J., Shinozaki, T., Sakuma, M., Komaru, T., Fukuchi, M., et al., 2003. Characteristics and 1-year prognosis of medically treated patients with chronic heart failure in Japan. Circ. J. 67, 431–436.

Massie, B.M., Shah, N.B., 1997. Evolving trends in the epidemiologic factors of heart failure: rationale for preventive strategies and comprehensive disease management. Am. Heart J. 133, 703–712.

Motoo, Y., Arai, I., Hyodo, I., Tsutani, K., 2009. Current status of Kampo (Japanese herbal) medicines in Japanese clinical practice guidelines. Complement. Ther. Med. 147–154.

Motoo, Y., Seki, T., Tsutani, K., 2011. Traditional Japanese medicine, Kampo: its history and current status. Chin. J. Integer. Med. 85–87.

Motoo, Y., 2008. Japanese herbal medicine in Western-style modern medical system. In: Watson, R.R., Preedy, V.R. (Eds.), Botanical Medicine in Clinical Practice. CAB International, New York, pp. 105–111.

Nishida, S., Satoh, H., 2007. Cardiovascular Pharmacology of sinomenine: the mechanical and electropharmacological actions. Drug Target Insights 2, 97–104.

Pillai, H.S., Ganapathi, S., 2013. Heart failure in South Asia. Curr. Cardiol. Rev. 102–111.

Ramani, G.V., Uber, P.A., Mehra, M.R., 2010. Chronic heart failure: contemporary diagnosis and management. Mayo Clin. Proc. 180–195.

Sakanashi, M., Matsuzaki, T., Noguchi, K., Nakasone, J., Sakanashi, M., Uchida, T., Kina-Tanada, M., Kubota, H., Arakaki, K., Tanimoto, A., Yanagihara, N., Sakanashi, M., Ohya, Y., Masuzaki, H., Ishiuchi, S., Sugahara, K., Tsutsui, M., 2013. Long-term treatment with san'o-shashin-to, a kampo medicine, markedly ameliorates cardiac ischemia-reperfusion injury in ovariectomized rats via the redox-dependent mechanism. Circ. J. 77, 1827–1837.

Satake, H., Fukuda, K., Sakata, Y., Miyata, S., Nakano, M., Kondo, M., Hasebe, Y., Segawa, M., Shimokawa, H., CHART-2 Investigators, 2015. Current status of primary prevention of sudden cardiac death with implantable cardioverter defibrillator in patients with chronic heart failure—a report from the CHART-2 Study. Circ. J. 381–390.

Satoh, H., 2005. Electropharmacological actions of the constituents of Sinomeni Caulis et Rhizome and Mokuboi-to in Guinea pig heart. Am. J. Chin. Med. 33, 967–979.

Satoh, H., 2013. Pharmacological characteristics of Kampo medicine as a mixture of constituents and ingredients. J. Integr. Med. 11, 11–16.

Shiba, N., Shimokawa, H., 2008. Chronic heart failure in Japan: implications of the CHART studies. Vasc. Health Risk Manag. 103–113.

Shiba, N., Watanabe, J., Shinozaki, T., Koseki, Y., Sakuma, M., Kagaya, Y., et al., 2005. Poor prognosis of Japanese patients with chronic heart failure following myocardial infarction—comparison with nonischemic cardiomyopathy. Circ. J. 69, 143–149.

Stickel, F., Schuppan, D., 2007. Herbal medicine in the treatment of liver diseases. Dig. Liver Dis. 39, 293–304.

Sugiyama, A., Hashimoto, K., 1989. Chronotropic and inotropic effects of Kampo extracts in the canine isolated, blood-perfused heart preparations. Jpn. J. Pharmacol. 51, 239–246.

Sugiyama, A., Takahara, A., Satoh, Y., Yoneyama, M., Saegusa, Y., Hashimoto, K., 2002. Cardiac effects of clinically available Kampo medicine assessed with canine isolated, blood-perfused heart preparations. Jpn. J. Pharmacol. 88, 307–313.

Swedberg, K., Cleland, J., Dargie, H., Drexler, H., Follath, F., Komajda, M., et al., 2005. Guidelines for the diagnosis and treatment of chronic heart failure: executive summary (update 2005): the task force for the diagnosis and treatment of chronic heart failure of the European society of cardiology. Eur. Heart J. 26, 1115–1140.

Tsuchihashi, M., Tsutsui, H., Kodama, K., Kasagi, F., Takeshita, A., 2000. Clinical characteristics and prognosis of hospitalized patients with congestive heart failure–a study in Fukuoka. Jpn. Circ. J. 64, 953–959.

Tsuchihashi, M., Tsutsui, H., Kodama, K., Kasagi, F., Setoguchi, S., Mohr, M., et al., 2001. Medical and socioenvironmental predictors of hospital readmission in patients with congestive heart failure. Am. Heart J. 142, E7.

Tsutani, K., 1993. The evaluation of herbal medicines: an East Asian perspective. In: Lewith, G.T., Aldridge, D. (Eds.), Clinical Research Methodology for Complementary Therapies. Hodder & Stoughton, London, pp. 365–393.

Tsutsui, H., Tsuchihashi, M., Takeshita, A., 2001. Mortality and readmission of hospitalized patients with congestive heart failure and preserved versus depressed systolic function. Am. J. Cardiol. 88, 530–533.

Wieland, L.S., Manheimer, E., Sampson, M., Barnabas, J.P., Bouter, L.M., et al., 2013. Bibliometric and content analysis of the Cochrane Complementary Medicine Field specialized register of controlled trials. Syst. Rev. 2, 51.

Xie, S.X., Jin, Q.Q., 1993. Prevention of sinomenine on isolated rat myocardial reperfusion injury. Zhongguo Yao Li Xue Bao (Suppl.), S12–S15.

Yakubu, S., Kinoshita, Y., Arakawa, Y., Takahashi, M., Kitanaka, S., 2002. Clinical evaluation of Moku-boi-to (Mu-Fang-Yi-Tang): a Japanese and Chinese traditional medicine for heart failure. J. Trad. Med. 19, 159–163.

Yoo, B.-S., Oh, J., Hong, B.-K., Shin, D.-H., Bae, J.-H., Yang, D.H., Shim, W.-J., Kim, H-seop, Kim, Su-H., Choi, J.-O., Chun, W.-J., Go, C.-W., Kang, H.-J., Baek, S.H., Cho, J-hyun, Hong, S.-K., Shin, J.-H., Oh, S.-K., Pyun, W.-B., Kwan, J., Hong, Y.-J., Jeong, J.-O., Kang, S.-M., Choi, D.-J., On behalf of the SUGAR Study, 2014. SUrvey of guideline Adherence for treatment of systolic heart failure in real world (SUGAR): a Multi-Center, Retrospective, observational study. PLoS One 9(1), e86596.

Zheng, A., Moritani, T., 2008. Effect of the combination of ginseng, oriental bezoar and glycyrrhiza on autonomic nervous activity as evaluated by power spectral analysis of HRV and cardiac depolarization-repolarization process. J. Nutr. Sci. Vitaminol. (Tokyo) 54, 148–153.

CHAPTER 7

Kampo Medicine for Hypertension and Related Disorders

Sahana S. Babu, Rajarajan A. Thandavarayan, Prasanna Krishnamurthy

Houston Methodist Research Institute, Houston, TX, United States

Background

Kampo medicine, the Japanese herbal medicine, has reemerged as an individualized treatment system with a long tradition, in which the overall condition of the patient and his or her constitut1ion are of real importance (Watanabe et al., 2011). Kampo has a holistic therapeutic approach, as the mind and body are seen as one entity. The therapeutic aim is to relieve symptoms and to restore harmony in bodily functions. The treatment regime is based on symptoms, in contrast to Western medicine, which seeks to target the sick parts of the body to identify and remove the cause of a sickness (Motoo et al., 2011). The basic concept underlying Kampo medicine is the methodology referred to as "matching of pattern and formula," which was emphasized by the physician Todo Yoshimasu. This methodology follows the principle that an appropriate treatment could be administered if a set pattern could be identified (Watanabe et al., 2011; Yakubo et al., 2014). Kampo medical treatments have transformed over time, with Kampo and Western/European medicines being combined in the 18th century by the Japanese surgeon Dr. Seishu Hanaoka, using Kampo mainly for internal medicine and European medicine for surgery (Yakubo et al., 2014).

Principally, Kampo medicine consists of formulas that are mixtures of the crude extracts of several herbs, each of which contains multiple components (Hayasaka et al., 2012). Thus, Kampo medicines are composed of not only one drug, but are used in combination with several other medicines depending on each symptom. These herbal medicines are efficacious for treating several human diseases such as hypertension, ocular disorders associated with type 1 diabetes mellitus, cancer, and primary dysmenorrhea (Arakawa et al., 2006; Hayasaka et al., 2012; Takeda et al., 2012; Terauchi et al., 2011).

Hypertension

Hypertension is a major predisposing factor for vascular dysfunction that leads to increased cardiovascular risk (Wojtowicz et al., 2010). In addition to others, we have characterized several molecular signaling pathways (such as mechanotransduction by zyxin) that lead to

59

hypertension-induced abnormal vascular remodeling, as a potential contributor to altered heart function (Beech, 2013; Ghosh et al., 2015; Krishnamurthy et al., 2010; Suresh Babu et al., 2012). High blood pressure also contributes to cerebrovascular disease, which in turn determines neurobiologic alterations (such as β-amyloid accumulation) resulting in neuro-pathologic damage and vascular dementia (Paglieri et al., 2008). Despite novel inventions in molecular research, hypertension-associated disorders remain as the major cause of death worldwide. Hypertension-associated disorders include aneurysms, eye damage, chronic kidney disease, peripheral artery disease, stroke, heart attack, heart failure, and cognitive decline such as memory loss, difficulty finding words, shoulder stiffness, headache, and dizziness (Lackland and Weber, 2015; Novak and Hajjar, 2010). Loss of cognitive function is one the most devastating manifestations of hypertension-induced vascular disease, contribut-ing significantly to increased mortality (Gasecki et al., 2013). In addition, the remedial measures for hypertension and related disorders are still under investigation.

Kampo Medicine Used in Hypertension

Kampo has been used for the purpose of relieving hypertension-related symptoms such as headache, dizziness, rush of blood to the head, shoulder stiffness, and tinnitus. Such Kampo medicines include shichimotsukokato (SKT), orengedokuto, keishibukuryogan, the Apiaceae family including *Angelica sinensis* and *Apium graveolens*, baicalin from *Scutellaria baicalensis,* and saikokaryukotsuboreito (Fig. 7.1 and Table 7.1).

Shichimotsukokato

SKT is a Kampo formula comprising *Astragalus* root, *Phellodendron* bark, *Rehmannia* root, peony root, *Cnidium* rhizome, Japanese *Angelica* root, and *Uncaria* hook. SKT is prescribed to hypertensive patients with a sensation of a rush of blood to the head, shoulder stiffness, tinnitus, and dull headache (Bai et al., 2012). SKT administration has been shown by several studies to have antihypertensive effects (Bai et al., 2012; Hiwara et al., 1994; Ma et al., 2016; Ono et al., 2013). Antihypertensive effects of SKT in nephrectomized Wistar rats were mediated by the dimethylaminohydrolase–dimethylarginine–nitric oxide pathway (Bai et al., 2012). SKT lowered systolic blood pressure in experimental animal models of hypertension (spontaneously hypertensive rats—SHRs) and displayed renoprotective effects in this animal model by decreasing urinary albumin excretion. Antialbuminuric effects of SKT were associ-ated with the amelioration of the loss of the critical podocyte proteins and components of the endocytic machinery that mediates the reabsorption of albumin in the renal proximal tubules of SHRs. A notable loss of chloride channel 5 (ClC-5) in the proximal renal tubules occurred in the SHR control group. Thus, the mechanism of SKT in reducing urinary albumin excre-tion is mediated at least partly by prevention of the loss of ClC-5 in the renal cortex of SHRs (Ma et al., 2016).

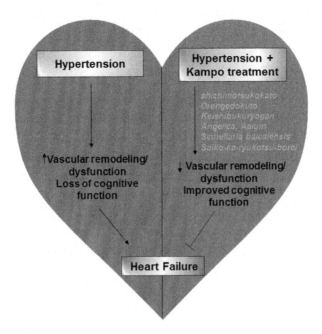

Figure 7.1: Schematic Representation of Kampo Medicines Used in Hypertension.
Hypertension or increased blood pressure leads to increased vascular remodeling and loss of cognitive function, leading to heart failure. Our hypothesis that the use of Kampo medicine could reduce hypertension-induced vascular remodeling and improve cognitive function, which restores heart function.

Table 7.1: Kampo Medicines Used in Hypertension

Kampo Medicine	Composition	Effect on Hypertensive Symptoms
Shichimotsukokato	*Astragalus* root, *Phellodendron* bark, *Rehmannia* root, peony root, *Cnidium* rhizome, Japanese *Angelica* root, and *Uncaria* hook	Reduces sensation of a rush of blood to the head, shoulder stiffness, tinnitus, and dull headache
Tsumura orengedokuto extract	Four herbal drugs	Reduces blood pressure, stress, or hyperactivation of the sympathetic nervous system, such as anger, stress, anxiety, and fear
Keishibukuryogan	*Cinnamomum cassia* Blume, *Paeonia lactiflora* Pallas, *Paeonia suffruticosa* Andrews, *Prunus persica* Batsch, and *Poria cocos* Wolf	Improves subjective sleep disturbances, alleviates perspiration Reduces systolic/diastolic pressure and heart rate
Apiaceae family, *Angelica sinensis*	Root, ferulic acid, and Z-ligustilide	Decreases pulmonary arterial pressure and increases cardiac output
Apiaceae family, *Apium graveolens*	Seed/celery	Displays vasorelaxant activity with antihypertensive effect
Baicalin	Flavonoid compound from the dry roots of *Scutellaria baicalensis* Georgi	Represses the elevation of right-ventricular systolic pressure Attenuates the pulmonary vascular structure remodeling of pulmonary arterioles induced by chronic hypoxia
Saikokaryukotsuboreito	Herbal kampo formula	Decreases oxidative stress

Orengedokuto

Tsumura's orengedokuto extract, a Kampo medicine in granular form containing four herbal drugs, was administered to hypertensive patients, and an improvement in accessory symptoms of hypertension was observed (Arakawa et al., 2006; Motoo et al., 2014). Furthermore, orengedokuto reduced spontaneous platelet activation in patients after oral administration (Kimura et al., 2006). These studies targeted the symptoms related to stress or hyperactivation of the sympathetic nervous system, such as anger, stress, anxiety, and fear. In this multicenter double-blind clinical trial, blood pressure tended to decrease in response to treatment. However, a significant improvement in accessory symptoms was observed. Orengedokuto extract showed more efficacy compared with benzodiazepine anxiolytics in this study of essential hypertension (Arakawa et al., 2006).

Keishibukuryogan

Keishibukuryogan (KBG) is one of the Kampo medicines, composed of five medicinal plants, *Cinnamomum cassia* Blume (Cinnamomi cortex), *Paeonia lactiflora* Pallas (Paeoniae radix), *Paeonia suffruticosa* Andrews (Moutan cortex), *Prunus persica* Batsch (Persicae semen), and *Poria cocos* Wolf (hoelen) (Nozaki et al., 2006). KBG has been widely administered to patients with blood stagnation to improve blood circulation (Yoshihisa et al., 2010). Terauchi et al. (2011) showed that patients who received KBG treatment over a period of 5 months showed improved subjective sleep disturbances, alleviated perspiration, and reduced systolic/diastolic pressure and heart rate (Terauchi et al., 2011). KBG has also been reported to have a beneficial effect on vascular endothelial function in patients with metabolic syndrome-related factors assessed by reactive hyperemia peripheral arterial tonometry (Nagata et al., 2012). Mechanistically, KBG protects vascular function by causing a significant decrease in vaso-contraction induced by free radicals and contractive prostanoids and a further decrease in serum NO_2^-/NO_3^- and blood viscosity (Goto et al., 2004).

Apiaceae: Angelica sinensis and Apium graveolens

Several extracts from the family Apiaceae, including *A. sinensis* and *A. graveolens*, are used commonly in Kampo medicine (Jorge et al., 2013). *Angelica* species of herbs, known as toki in Japanese, are usually a root containing ferulic acid and Z-ligustilide and used as a substitute for the crude drug toki in Kampo medicine (Zhao et al., 2003). Hypertensive patients were treated with 25% *A. sinensis* to investigate changes in hemodynamics, pulmonary function, and blood gas. The study showed that mean pulmonary arterial pressure was decreased and cardiac output was increased significantly in the patients (Xu et al., 1992). The extracts obtained from *A. graveolens*, a celery used commonly in Kampo medicine, has a vasorelaxant activity with an antihypertensive effect (Jorge et al., 2013). In addition, a study that investigated the effects of various *A. graveolens* seed extracts on blood pressure in normotensive and deoxycorticosterone acetate–induced hypertensive rats confirmed that these extracts have antihypertensive properties, which appear to be attributable to the actions of active hydrophobic constituents such as *n*-butylphthalide, and can be considered as antihypertensive agents in the chronic treatment of elevated blood pressure (Moghadam et al., 2013).

Scutellaria baicalensis *(Baicalin)*

Baicalin, a flavonoid Kampo compound purified from the dry roots of *S. baicalensis* Georgi, has been shown to possess the potential to be used as a novel drug in the treatment of pulmonary arterial hypertension (PAH) pathology (Huang et al., 2014). PAH is a cardiovascular disease characterized by enhanced pulmonary artery smooth muscle cell (SMC) proliferation and suppressed apoptosis (Zhang et al., 2014). An in vitro study showed that baicalin antagonizes hypoxia-inducible factor-α and aryl hydrocarbon receptor expression and subsequently decreases SMC proliferation and the phenotypic switch (Huang et al., 2014). In addition, baicalin reversed the hypoxia-induced reduction of p27 and increased AKT/protein kinase B phosphorylation both in vivo and in vitro (Zhang et al., 2014). In vivo, baicalin repressed the elevation of right-ventricular systolic pressure and attenuated the pulmonary vascular structure remodeling of pulmonary arterioles induced by chronic hypoxia and, thus, effectively attenuated hypoxic pulmonary hypertension (Zhang et al., 2014).

Saikokaryukotsuboreito

Saikokaryukotsuboreito (SKRBT) is a Japanese Kampo medicine used clinically for the treatment of hypertension, atherosclerosis, and hyperlipidemia (Hattori et al., 2010; Wei et al., 1997). SKRBT has been shown to be a feasible herbal medicine that protects against cardiovascular diseases through an increase in endothelial progenitor cell (EPC) function along with antioxidative effects (Iijima et al., 2013). EPCs are known to repair vascular injuries and the treatment with SKRBT reduced serum interleukin-6 level and increased EPC colony numbers significantly with a decrease in oxidative stress and without affecting blood pressure in SHRs (Iijima et al., 2013). Thus, SKRBT may affect the link between chronic inflammation and cardiovascular disease.

Clinical Application

The clinical efficacy of Kampo medicine has been tested in the treatment of several disorders. It improves accessory symptoms of hypertension, cancer treatment, and primary dysmenorrhea (Oya et al., 2008; Takeda et al., 2012; Terauchi et al., 2011). The clinical use of Kampo was made more appealing as a form of treatment by the "matching of pattern and formula" methodology according to some studies (Watanabe et al., 2011; Yakubo et al., 2014).

Kampo can be used in combination with Western medicine to avoid the adverse side effects of certain drugs (Arai et al., 2014; Yamakawa et al., 2013). For instance, the retrospective analysis by Arai et al. at the Pain Center of Aichi Medical University Hospital showed that two-thirds of the chronic pain patients experienced further pain improvement with the use of Kampo medicine combined with Western medicine. Steroids used as antiinflammatory drugs are helpful in treating inflammatory conditions but lead to the development of serious side effects that can harm the central nervous system and could lead to increased risk of cardiovascular diseases like heart failure and often limit their long-term use (Kallinich, 2015). Thus, considering the requirement for nonsteroidal antiinflammatory drugs, Kampo medicines can be introduced into clinical studies to reduce the severity of the condition (Oya et al., 2008).

Several Kampo medicines described in this chapter have been used in patients at clinically relevant doses. Patients treated with KBG showed improved subjective sleep disturbances and reduced systolic/diastolic pressure and heart rate (Terauchi et al., 2011). Kimura et al. demonstrated the inhibitory activity of orengedokuto on both platelet aggregation and platelet activation at a clinically relevant dose (Kimura et al., 2006). Administration of *A. sinensis* decreased pulmonary arterial pressure significantly in hypertensive patients (Xu et al., 1992). Baicalin drug has the potential to treat PAH pathology (Huang et al., 2014). SKRBT's beneficial effect against cytokines has been used to treat patients with hypogonadism-related symptoms (Tsujimura et al., 2011). Thus, Kampo medicine could be used to improve hypertension-associated symptoms (Fig. 7.1).

Kampo in Health Care

The study by Watanabe et al. (2011) that tested Kampo formulas reported that 148 formulas can be prescribed within the health insurance system and are listed on the Japanese insurance program (Watanabe et al., 2011; Yakubo et al., 2014). Kampo medicine has government-regulated prescription drugs and has been used under Japan's national health insurance scheme for 46 years (Katayama et al., 2013). In addition, the World Health Organization has set out to create an international classification of traditional Kampo medicines and plans to incorporate it into the International Statistical Classification of Diseases and Related Health Problems (Katayama et al., 2013; Watanabe et al., 2012).

Conclusion

Kampo is a holistic and individualized treatment with a long tradition, and future research is necessary to standardize Kampo diagnosis, which would help physicians to integrate Kampo medicine into their practice. The clinical efficacy of most Kampo medicines discussed in this chapter has been tested and thus, they could be used as a novel therapeutic approach based on traditional herbs to address hypertension and associated disorders.

References

Arai, Y.C., Yasui, H., Isai, H., Kawai, T., Nishihara, M., Sato, J., et al., 2014. The review of innovative integration of Kampo medicine and Western medicine as personalized medicine at the first multidisciplinary pain center in Japan. EPMA J. 5 (1), 10. http://dx.doi.org/10.1186/1878-5085-5-10.

Arakawa, K., Saruta, T., Abe, K., Iimura, O., Ishii, M., Ogihara, T., et al., 2006. Improvement of accessory symptoms of hypertension by TSUMURA Orengedokuto Extract, a four herbal drugs containing Kampo-Medicine Granules for ethical use: a double-blind, placebo-controlled study. Phytomedicine 13 (1–2), 1–10. http://dx.doi.org/10.1016/j.phymed.2004.02.012.

Bai, F., Makino, T., Ono, T., Mizukami, H., 2012. Anti-hypertensive effects of shichimotsukokato in 5/6 nephrectomized Wistar rats mediated by the DDAH-ADMA-NO pathway. J. Nat. Med. 66 (4), 583–590. http://dx.doi.org/10.1007/s11418-011-0625-8.

Beech, D.J., 2013. Characteristics of transient receptor potential canonical calcium-permeable channels and their relevance to vascular physiology and disease. Circ. J. 77 (3), 570–579. Retrieved from: http://www.ncbi.nlm.nih.gov/pubmed/23412755.

Gasecki, D., Kwarciany, M., Nyka, W., Narkiewicz, K., 2013. Hypertension, brain damage and cognitive decline. Curr. Hypertens. Rep. 15 (6), 547–558. http://dx.doi.org/10.1007/s11906-013-0398-4.

Ghosh, S., Kollar, B., Nahar, T., Suresh Babu, S., Wojtowicz, A., Sticht, C., et al., 2015. Loss of the mechanotransducer zyxin promotes a synthetic phenotype of vascular smooth muscle cells. J. Am. Heart Assoc. 4 (6), e001712. http://dx.doi.org/10.1161/JAHA.114.001712.

Goto, H., Shimada, Y., Sekiya, N., Yang, Q., Kogure, T., Mantani, N., et al., 2004. Effects of Keishi-bukuryo-gan on vascular function and hemorheological factors in spontaneously diabetic (WBN/kob) rats. Phytomedicine 11 (2–3), 188–195. http://dx.doi.org/10.1078/0944-7113-00336.

Hattori, T., Fei, W., Kizawa, T., Nishida, S., Yoshikawa, H., Kishida, Y., 2010. The fixed herbal drug composition "Saikokaryukotsuboreito" prevents bone loss with an association of serum IL-6 reductions in ovariectomized mice model. Phytomedicine 17 (3–4), 170–177. http://dx.doi.org/10.1016/j.phymed.2009.12.004.

Hayasaka, S., Kodama, T., Ohira, A., 2012. Traditional Japanese herbal (kampo) medicines and treatment of ocular diseases: a review. Am. J. Chin. Med. 40 (5), 887–904. http://dx.doi.org/10.1142/S0192415X12500668.

Hiwara, N., Uehara, Y., Takada, S., Kawabata, Y., Ohshima, N., Nagata, T., et al., 1994. Antihypertensive property and renal protection by shichimotsu-koka-to extract in salt-induced hypertension in Dahl strain rats. Am. J. Chin. Med. 22 (1), 51–62. http://dx.doi.org/10.1142/S0192415X94000073.

Huang, S., Chen, P., Shui, X., He, Y., Wang, H., Zheng, J., et al., 2014. Baicalin attenuates transforming growth factor-beta1-induced human pulmonary artery smooth muscle cell proliferation and phenotypic switch by inhibiting hypoxia inducible factor-1alpha and aryl hydrocarbon receptor expression. J. Pharm. Pharmacol. 66 (10), 1469–1477. http://dx.doi.org/10.1111/jphp.12273.

Iijima, H., Daikonya, A., Takamatsu, S., Kanno, A., Magariyama, K., Yoshikawa, K., et al., 2013. Effects of the herbal medicine composition "Saiko-ka-ryukotsu-borei-To" on the function of endothelial progenitor cells in hypertensive rats. Phytomedicine 20 (3–4), 196–201. http://dx.doi.org/10.1016/j.phymed.2012.10.014.

Jorge, V.G., Angel, J.R., Adrian, T.S., Francisco, A.C., Anuar, S.G., Samuel, E.S., et al., 2013. Vasorelaxant activity of extracts obtained from Apium graveolens: possible source for vasorelaxant molecules isolation with potential antihypertensive effect. Asian Pac. J. Trop. Biomed. 3 (10), 776–779. http://dx.doi.org/10.1016/S2221-1691(13)60154-9.

Kallinich, T., 2015. Regulating against the dysregulation: new treatment options in autoinflammation. Semin. Immunopathol. 37 (4), 429–437. http://dx.doi.org/10.1007/s00281-015-0501-9.

Katayama, K., Yoshino, T., Munakata, K., Yamaguchi, R., Imoto, S., Miyano, S., Watanabe, K., 2013. Prescription of kampo drugs in the Japanese health care insurance program. Evid. Based Complement. Alternat. Med. 2013, 576973. http://dx.doi.org/10.1155/2013/576973.

Kimura, Y., Shimizu, M., Kohara, S., Yoshii, F., Sato, H., Shinohara, Y., 2006. Antiplatelet effects of a kampo medicine, Orengedokuto. J. Stroke Cerebrovasc. Dis. 15 (6), 277–282. http://dx.doi.org/10.1016/j.jstrokecerebrovasdis.2006.09.002.

Krishnamurthy, P., Lambers, E., Verma, S., Thorne, T., Qin, G., Losordo, D.W., Kishore, R., 2010. Myocardial knockdown of mRNA-stabilizing protein HuR attenuates post-MI inflammatory response and left ventricular dysfunction in IL-10-null mice. FASEB J. 24 (7), 2484–2494. http://dx.doi.org/10.1096/fj.09-149815.

Lackland, D.T., Weber, M.A., 2015. Global burden of cardiovascular disease and stroke: hypertension at the core. Can. J. Cardiol. 31 (5), 569–571. http://dx.doi.org/10.1016/j.cjca.2015.01.009.

Ma, Y., Fujimoto, M., Watari, H., Kimura, M., Shimada, Y., 2016. The renoprotective effect of shichimotsukokato on hypertension-induced renal dysfunction in spontaneously hypertensive rats. J. Nat. Med. 70 (2), 152–162. http://dx.doi.org/10.1007/s11418-015-0945-1.

Moghadam, M.H., Imenshahidi, M., Mohajeri, S.A., 2013. Antihypertensive effect of celery seed on rat blood pressure in chronic administration. J. Med. Food 16 (6), 558–563. http://dx.doi.org/10.1089/jmf.2012.2664.

Motoo, Y., Seki, T., Tsutani, K., 2011. Traditional Japanese medicine, Kampo: its history and current status. Chin. J. Integr. Med. 17 (2), 85–87. http://dx.doi.org/10.1007/s11655-011-0653-y.

Motoo, Y., Arai, I., Tsutani, K., 2014. Use of kampo diagnosis in randomized controlled trials of kampo products in Japan: a systematic review. PLoS One 9 (8), e104422. http://dx.doi.org/10.1371/journal.pone.0104422.

Nagata, Y., Goto, H., Hikiami, H., Nogami, T., Fujimoto, M., Shibahara, N., Shimada, Y., 2012. Effect of keishibukuryogan on endothelial function in patients with at least one component of the diagnostic criteria for metabolic syndrome: a controlled clinical trial with crossover design. Evid. Based Complement. Alternat. Med. 2012, 359282. http://dx.doi.org/10.1155/2012/359282.

Novak, V., Hajjar, I., 2010. The relationship between blood pressure and cognitive function. Nat. Rev. Cardiol. 7 (12), 686–698. http://dx.doi.org/10.1038/nrcardio.2010.161.

Nozaki, K., Hikiami, H., Goto, H., Nakagawa, T., Shibahara, N., Shimada, Y., 2006. Keishibukuryogan (gui-zhi-fu-ling-wan), a Kampo formula, decreases disease activity and soluble vascular adhesion molecule-1 in patients with rheumatoid arthritis. Evid. Based Complement. Alternat. Med. 3 (3), 359–364. http://dx.doi.org/10.1093/ecam/nel025.

Ono, T., Kamikado, K., Morimoto, T., 2013. Protective effects of Shichimotsu-koka-To on irreversible Thy-1 nephritis. Biol. Pharm. Bull. 36 (1), 41–47. Retrieved from: http://www.ncbi.nlm.nih.gov/pubmed/23131611.

Oya, A., Oikawa, T., Nakai, A., Takeshita, T., Hanawa, T., 2008. Clinical efficacy of Kampo medicine (Japanese traditional herbal medicine) in the treatment of primary dysmenorrhea. J. Obstet. Gynaecol. Res. 34 (5), 898–908. http://dx.doi.org/10.1111/j.1447-0756.2008.00847.x.

Paglieri, C., Bisbocci, D., Caserta, M., Rabbia, F., Bertello, C., Canade, A., Veglio, F., 2008. Hypertension and cognitive function. Clin. Exp. Hypertens. 30 (8), 701–710. http://dx.doi.org/10.1080/10641960802563584.

Suresh Babu, S., Wojtowicz, A., Freichel, M., Birnbaumer, L., Hecker, M., Cattaruzza, M., 2012. Mechanism of stretch-induced activation of the mechanotransducer zyxin in vascular cells. Sci. Signal. 5 (254), ra91. http://dx.doi.org/10.1126/scisignal.2003173.

Takeda, T., Yamaguchi, T., Yaegashi, N., 2012. Perceptions and attitudes of Japanese gynecologic cancer patients to Kampo (Japanese herbal) medicines. Int. J. Clin. Oncol. 17 (2), 143–149. http://dx.doi.org/10.1007/s10147-011-0271-x.

Terauchi, M., Hiramitsu, S., Akiyoshi, M., Owa, Y., Kato, K., Obayashi, S., et al., 2011. Effects of three Kampo formulae: Tokishakuyakusan (TJ-23), Kamishoyosan (TJ-24), and Keishibukuryogan (TJ-25) on Japanese peri- and postmenopausal women with sleep disturbances. Arch. Gynecol. Obstet. 284 (4), 913–921. http://dx.doi.org/10.1007/s00404-010-1779-4.

Tsujimura, A., Miyagawa, Y., Okuda, H., Yamamoto, K., Fukuhara, S., Nakayama, J., et al., 2011. Change in cytokine levels after administration of saikokaryuukotsuboreito or testosterone in patients with symptoms of late-onset hypogonadism. Aging Male 14 (1), 76–81. http://dx.doi.org/10.3109/13685538.2010.502268.

Watanabe, K., Matsuura, K., Gao, P., Hottenbacher, L., Tokunaga, H., Nishimura, K., et al., 2011. Traditional Japanese kampo medicine: clinical research between Modernity and traditional medicine—the state of research and Methodological Suggestions for the future. Evid. Based Complement. Alternat. Med. 2011, 513842. http://dx.doi.org/10.1093/ecam/neq067.

Watanabe, K., Zhang, X., Choi, S.H., 2012. Asian medicine: a way to compare data. Nature 482 (7384), 162. http://dx.doi.org/10.1038/482162e.

Wei, M.J., Shintani, F., Kanba, S., Yagi, G., Asai, M., Kato, R., Nakaki, T., 1997. Endothelium-dependent and -independent vasoactive actions of a Japanese kampo medicine, Saiko-ka-ryukotsu-borei-to. Biomed. Pharmacother. 51 (1), 38–43. Retrieved from: http://www.ncbi.nlm.nih.gov/pubmed/9084728.

Wojtowicz, A., Babu, S.S., Li, L., Gretz, N., Hecker, M., Cattaruzza, M., 2010. Zyxin mediation of stretch-induced gene expression in human endothelial cells. Circ. Res. 107 (7), 898–902. http://dx.doi.org/10.1161/CIRCRESAHA.110.227850.

Xu, J.Y., Li, B.X., Cheng, S.Y., 1992. Short-term effects of Angelica sinensis and nifedipine on chronic obstructive pulmonary disease in patients with pulmonary hypertension. Zhongguo Zhong Xi Yi Jie He Za Zhi 12 (12), 716–718. 707. Retrieved from: http://www.ncbi.nlm.nih.gov/pubmed/1304838.

Yakubo, S., Ito, M., Ueda, Y., Okamoto, H., Kimura, Y., Amano, Y., et al., 2014. Pattern classification in kampo medicine. Evid. Based Complement. Alternat. Med. 2014, 535146. http://dx.doi.org/10.1155/2014/535146.

Yamakawa, J., Motoo, Y., Moriya, J., Ogawa, M., Uenishi, H., Akazawa, S., et al., 2013. Role of Kampo medicine in integrative cancer therapy. Evid. Based Complement. Alternat. Med. 2013, 570848. http://dx.doi.org/10.1155/2013/570848.

Yoshihisa, Y., Furuichi, M., Ur Rehman, M., Ueda, C., Makino, T., Shimizu, T., 2010. The traditional Japanese formula keishibukuryogan inhibits the production of inflammatory cytokines by dermal endothelial cells. Mediators Inflamm. 2010, 804298. http://dx.doi.org/10.1155/2010/804298.

Zhang, L., Pu, Z., Wang, J., Zhang, Z., Hu, D., Wang, J., 2014. Baicalin inhibits hypoxia-induced pulmonary artery smooth muscle cell proliferation via the AKT/HIF-1alpha/p27-associated pathway. Int. J. Mol. Sci. 15 (5), 8153–8168. http://dx.doi.org/10.3390/ijms15058153.

Zhao, K.J., Dong, T.T., Tu, P.F., Song, Z.H., Lo, C.K., Tsim, K.W., 2003. Molecular genetic and chemical assessment of radix Angelica (Danggui) in China. J. Agric. Food Chem. 51 (9), 2576–2583. http://dx.doi.org/10.1021/jf026178h.

CHAPTER 8

Japanese Kampo Medicines for Diabetes Mellitus

Hiroshi Suzuki[1,2], Hirohito Sone[2], Kenichi Watanabe[1]
[1]Niigata University of Pharmacy and Applied Life Sciences, Niigata, Japan; [2]Niigata University Graduate School of Medical and Dental Sciences, Niigata, Japan

Introduction

There is a long history of the use of Japanese Kampo medicines for the treatment of diabetes mellitus and these medicines are now gaining favorable attention. Despite better blood glucose level control offered by Western medicine, Japanese Kampo medicines can be adopted for the treatment of diabetes mellitus because of their favorable safety profile over Western medicine. Here we illustrate the disease state of diabetes mellitus and the use of Kampo medicines for the treatment of diabetes mellitus.

The Disease State of Diabetes Mellitus

"Syo-katsu," a term that originated in China and has been used since 50 BCE, refers to symptoms that resemble diabetes mellitus. The symptoms of syo-katsu consist of thirst and polyuria, which are very similar to the symptoms of diabetes mellitus. Diabetes mellitus can be divided into three states of medical conditions: "jou-syou," "chu-syou," and "ka-shou." The disease states of jou-syou are thirst, polyuria, and body weight loss, which are initial symptoms of diabetes mellitus of the nonobese type. Similarly, the disease states of chu-syou are hunger, bulimia, and severe body weight loss, which belong to the obesity type. Finally, the disease states of ka-shou are polyuria, red tongue, and darkish face, which are the advanced symptoms of diabetes mellitus. In general practice, we can use byakkokaninjinto to treat the patients with jou-syou, tyouijoukito to treat the patients with chu-syou, and rokumigan to treat the patients with ka-shou.

Treatment of Diabetes Mellitus Using Japanese Kampo Medicines

We can divide the treatment of diabetes mellitus using Kampo medicines into three patterns: (1) hyperglycemia, (2) subjective symptoms, and (3) complications of diabetes mellitus.

Hyperglycemia

Byakkokaninjinto, made from sekkou, chimo, ninjin, kyoumai, and kanzo, is used to treat patients with the main symptoms, such as thirst and polydipsia, belonging to the jou-syou category. Sekkou and chimo are known for their effect of decreasing blood glucose levels (Suzuki et al., 1984). It is reported that byakkokaninjinto improved the blood glucose levels of diabetes mellitus model mice (Nagayoshi et al., 1966). In addition, it is reported that bofutsusyosan and gosyajinkigan have the effect of improving insulin resistance (Uno et al., 2005).

Subjective Symptoms

Thirst, Polydipsia, and Polyuria

Byakkokaninjinto is used to treat patients having thirst, polydipsia, and polyuria. Goreisan is used to treat patients having thirst, polydipsia, edema, and oliguria. Hachimijiougan is used to treat patients having weakness of the lower limbs, chills, numbness, and nocturnal incontinence. Gosyajinkigan, which is made from goshitsu, syazenshi, and hachimijiougan, is used to treat patients having prominent chills of the lower limbs and edema. Seishinrenshiin is used to treat patients with gastrointestinal weakness, chills, residual urine, frequent urination, oversensitivity, and insomnia (Fukuzawa, 2015).

Fatigue

Juzentaihoto is used to treat patients having fatigue, tendency toward anemia, chillness of the limbs, and drying of the skin and mucosa. Hochuekkito is used to treat patients with fatigue of the limbs, gastrointestinal weakness, appetite loss, and postprandial sleepiness (Fukuzawa, 2015).

Obesity

Daisaikoto is used to treat patients with obesity, shoulder stiffness, and constipation. It is also used to treat patients having hypertension and dyslipidemia. Bofutsusyosan is used to treat patients with obesity, pot belly, rush of blood to the head, and constipation. Bouiougito is used to treat patients having fatigue, flabby skin, edema, excessive sweating, and arthralgia (Shimada et al., 2011).

Yokukansan is reported to significantly decrease the body weight loss of the patients with obesity. It is reported that daisaikoto, bofutsusyosan, and bouiougito decrease body weight by improving lipid metabolism and decreasing fat tissue (Yoshida et al., 1995a,b,c; Li et al., 2009; Akagiri et al., 2008; Ohira et al., 2015). Bofutsusyosan is reported to have the effect of decreasing body weight (Iwasaki et al., 2007; Itoh et al., 2005). In addition, bofutsusyosan also has the effects of decreasing visceral fat, blood glucose levels, and blood cholesterol levels (Hiroki et al., 2004).

Complications of Diabetes Mellitus

Diabetic Neuropathy

The patients with diabetes mellitus also have frequent muscle cramps. Shakuyakukanzoto has been reported to have rapid effects on muscle cramps so that it can be used for the treatment of diabetes-associated muscle cramps (Yoshida et al., 1995a,b,c). Similarly, hachimijiougan has the effect of relieving numbness. There is a report suggesting that gosyajinkigan significantly relieved numbness and was superior to mecobalamin (Sato et al., 2006).

Dysautonomia

Orthostatic Hypotension

Hangebyakujutsutenmato is used to treat patients with gastrointestinal weakness, dizziness, and headache. Similarly, reikeijuchukanto is used to treat patients having dizziness due to bad metabolism, palpitation, rush of blood to the head, headache, and decreased urine volume (Fukuzawa, 2015).

Symptoms of Upper Digestive Tract, Stool Abnormalities

Hangesyakushinto, rikkunshito, and ninjinto are used to treat patients having gastric atony (such as dull feeling in the stomach). Hangesyakushinto, shinbuto, and keishikasyakuyakuto are used to treat patients having diarrhea. Keishikasyakuyakudaioto and mashijingan are used to treat the patients having constipation (Fukuzawa, 2015).

Neogenic Bladder Dysfunction, Impotence

Hachimijiougan, gosyajinkigan, and seishinrennshiin are used to treat patients with neogenic bladder dysfunction. Similarly, hachimijiougan is used to treat patients having impotence and sexual debility (Fukuzawa, 2015).

Diabetic Nephropathy

Saireito, which includes syousaikoto and goreisan, has beneficial effects on the treatment of nephrotic syndrome, and it is reported that saireito treatment has improved the clinical condition of microalbuminuria (Aiso et al., 2011). Saireito is also used to treat patients with thirst, edema, and dizziness. Tokishakuyakusan is used to treat patients with cold hands and feet, edema, and dizziness. Seishinrennshiin is used to treat patients with gastrointestinal weakness, pollakiuria, residual urine, urodynia, and dysuria (Fukuzawa, 2015).

Diabetic Retinopathy

Keishibukuryogan is used to treat patients experiencing chills and rush of blood to the head. Unseiin, which includes shimotsuto and orengedokuto, is used to treat patients with chills, rush of blood to the head, irritation, dry skin and eyes, and cerebral hemorrhage (Fukuzawa, 2015).

Table 8.1: List of Japanese Kampo Medicines for Diabetes Mellitus

Kampo Medicine	Symptoms Treated
Byakkokaninjinto	Thirst, polydipsia, polyuria
Daisaikoto	Obesity, constipation, chest side painfulness
Bofutsushosan	Weight gain, pot belly, rush of blood to the head, constipation
Goreisan	Thirst, edema, polydipsia without polyuria
Hachimijiougan	Pollakiuria, thirst, coldness and numbness of lower half of body, edema
Gosyajinkigan	Pollakiuria, thirst, prominent coldness and edema of lower limbs
Rokumigan	Pollakiuria, thirst, numbness of lower half of body without coldness
Seishinrenshiin	Chills, pollakiuria, gastrointestinal weakness, oversensitivity
Syakuyakukanzoto	Dehydration, leg cramps

Revised edition Fukuzawa, M., Diabetes mellitus and Kampo medicine. J. Jpn. Soc. Med. Func. Foods 2015. 9 (3), 128–130.

Conclusion

The clinical use of Japanese Kampo medicines for the treatment of patients with diabetes mellitus is increasing. There are several reports of the beneficial effects of Kampo medicines in treating patients with diabetes mellitus. We have given a list of a few important Kampo medicines used in the treatment of diabetes mellitus and its symptoms in Table 8.1. The identification of the possible mechanisms of action of these Kampo medicines would further improve their potential usage for the treatment of various disease conditions.

References

Aiso, Y., Ito, K., Sugawara, M., 2011. The examination of clinical usefulness of Saireito to early diabetic Nephropathy. Jpn. J. Med. Pharm. Sci. 65 (6), 751–755.

Akagiri, S., Naito, Y., Ichikawa, H., et al., 2008. Bofutsushosan, an oriental herbal medicine, attenuates the weight gain of white Adipose tissue and the increased size of Adipocytes associated with the increase in their expression of uncoupling protein 1 in high-fat diet-fed male KK/Ta mice. J. Clin. Biochem. Nutr. 42, 158–166.

Fukuzawa, M., 2015. Diabetes mellitus and Kampo medicine. J. Jpn. Soc. Med. Func. Foods 9 (3), 128–130.

Hiroki, C., Yoshimoto, K., Yoshida, T., 2004. Efficacy of Bofu-tsusho-san, an oriental herbal medicine, in obese Japanese women with impaired glucose tolerance. Clin. Exp. Pharmacol. Physiol. 31, 614–619.

Itoh, T., Senda, S., Inoue, H., et al., 2005. The effect of Bofutsusyosan on weight reduction in humans. Kampo Med. 56, 933–939.

Iwasaki, M., Yagi, T., Shichiri, M., 2007. The effect of Bofutsusyosan on the patients have obesity. J. Jpn. Soc. Study Obes. 13, 137–142.

Li, Y., Koikeda, T., Ueda, T., et al., 2009. The effect of general-purpose Daisaikoto on obesity. Jpn. J. Med. Pharm. Sci. 61, 499–509.

Nagayoshi, S., Nishiura, T., Hagiwara, Y., 1966. The effect of Hachimijiogan on alloxan-induced diabetes mellitus. Kampo Med. 17 (1), 236–239.

Ohira, M., Saiki, A., Yamaguchi, T., Imamura, H., Sato, Y., Ban, N., Kawana, H., Nagumo, A., Tatsuno, I., Kosuge, T., Akiba, T., 2015. The efficacy of Yokukansan in obesity patients on overeating due to anger (a retrospective study). Kampo Med. 66 (3), 191–196.

Sato, Y., Uno, T., Oyun, K., Koide, T., Tamagawa, T., Bolin, Q., 2006. Role of herbal medicine (Kampo formulations) on the prevention and treatment of diabetes and diabetic complications. J. Tradit. Med. 23, 185–195.

Shimada, T., Akase, T., Kosugi, M., et al., 2011. Preventive effect of Boiogito on metabolic disorders in the TSOD mouse, a model of spontaneous obese type II diabetes mellitus. Evid. Based Complement. Alternat. Med. 931073.

Suzuki, J., et al., 1984. Folia Pharmacol. Jpn. 83 (1), 1.

Uno, T., Ohsawa, I., Tokudome, M., Sato, Y., 2005. Effects of Gosyajinkigan on insulin resistance in patients with type 2 diabetes. Diabetes Res. Clin. Pract. 69, 129–135.

Yoshida, A., et al., 1995a. Neurolog. Therap. 12, 534–592.

Yoshida, T., et al., 1995b. J. Jpn. Soc. Study Obes. 1 (2), 122–155.

Yoshida, T., et al., 1995c. Int. J. Obes. 19, 717–722.

CHAPTER 9

Japanese Kampo Medicine for Aging-Related Neurological Diseases

Vijayasree V. Giridharan[1], Rajarajan A. Thandavarayan[2], Tetsuya Konishi[3,4,5], J. Quedevo[1,6,7]

[1]The University of Texas Health Science Center at Houston (UTHealth), Houston, TX, United States; [2]Houston Methodist Research Institute, Houston, TX, United States; [3]NUPALS Liaison R/D Promotion Division, Niigata, Japan; [4]Changchun University of Chinese Medicine, Changchun, China; [5]HALD Food Function Research Institute, Niigata, Japan; [6]The University of Texas Graduate School of Biomedical Sciences at Houston, Houston, TX, United States; [7]University of Southern Santa Catarina (UNESC), Criciúma, SC, Brazil

Introduction

Kampo medicine is based on Chinese herbal remedies first introduced into Japan via Korea around the 5th century. It was subsequently modified to suit the environment and cultural practices of the 17th and 18th centuries (the Edo era) and adapted to Japanese culture. During the Edo period (1603–1867), Kampo medicine entered upon a new phase of development after a long period of inner conflict had come to an end. The Edo era was a dynamic period of innovation for Kampo, during which various medical theories and practices evolved. Kampo medicine was the main medical treatment in Japan until the introduction of Western medicine from Europe several hundred years ago (Motoo et al., 2009; Okamoto et al., 2005). Kampo also reads as Kanpo, literally meaning "method from the Han period (206 BCE to AD 220) of ancient China." The Han method refers to the herbal system of China that developed during the Han dynasty. The traditional herbal medicines used in China have more than 2000 years of history. Kampo encompasses acupuncture, moxibustion, and other components of the Chinese medical system, but it relies primarily on prescription of herbal formulas.

Although Kampo medicine has its origins in traditional Chinese medicine (TCM) it differs from TCM in many respects. TCM emphasizes the Yin and Yang theory of five elements, which adopts the traditional concepts of East Asian natural philosophy. Japanese Kampo favors diagnostic methods that directly relate the symptoms to the therapy, bypassing speculative concepts. TCM prescriptions are individualized at the herbal level, whereas Kampo medicine is individualized at the formula level. Kampo medicine has a simplified prescription pattern. Abdominal findings and diagnoses are uniquely developed and used widely in Kampo compared to TCM (Yu et al., 2006). Furthermore, some Japanese physicians have criticized the highly theoretical and speculative nature of Chinese medicine as being inadequate to meet the problems of everyday practice. The strongest critique came from Yoshimasu Todo in the 18th century, who stated that "In clinical medicine, we should only rely on what we actually have observed by examination of the patient." In Kampo therapy, the diagnosis is based on examination of the abdomen, for which a refined palpation technique called fukushin has been developed. Practitioners believe that the results from the abdominal palpation give additional clinical information for selecting the most appropriate herbal prescription for the individual patient. Abdominal palpation as a diagnostic procedure has a strong influence on Kampo therapy even today (Fujikawa, 1979; Otsuka, 1988). Since 1971, traditional Kampo prescriptions have been included in the Japanese national health insurance drugs list. Today, 148 kinds of Kampo formulas are prescribed under the same. According to a survey by the journal *Nikkei Medical*, the application of Kampo has steadily increased, and more than 70% of physicians prescribe Kampo drugs today (Watanabe et al., 2011).

In Western countries, herbal therapies from different origins have received considerable attention. Especially, Chinese herbal medicines, as part of TCM, are receiving increasing interest. Globally, TCM is still far more visible than Kampo. Kampo drugs are available over the counter, meeting Japanese good manufacturing practice criteria. However, as Japanese pharmaceutical companies have started clinical trials in the United States, several drugs have already been registered as investigational new drugs by the Food and Drug Administration. Safety and toxicity data from Japan are generally accepted by the US and European agencies (Watanabe et al., 2011). To increase the visibility and application of Kampo medicine globally, in 2001, the Japanese Ministry of Education, Culture, Sports, Science, and Technology included Kampo medical education as part of the core curriculum of medical schools and today, a total of 80 medical schools provide Kampo medical education (Arai et al., 2012; Nishimura et al., 2009).

Role of Kampo in Age-Related Brain Disorders

Aging is an inevitable complex phenomenon, associated with functional senescence in most organisms (higher organisms). Among the various theories of aging, the free radical theory postulates that lifelong accumulation of oxidative damage and a dwindling antioxidant defense system cause induction of oxidative stress via excessive generation of reactive oxygen species (ROS), which leads to the formation of oxidatively modified macromolecules, including proteins (Uversky and Anthony, 2007). On the other hand, the brain is rich in polyunsaturated fatty acids and catecholamines as oxidizable substrates and relatively deficient in antioxidant defenses, compared with other organs, and therefore is highly susceptible to oxidative damage (Chong et al., 2005). Kampo medicine targets age-related diseases to prevent and ameliorate the "mibyou" condition, also known as the presymptomatic or subhealthy condition. The pathology of mibyou is not well understood; however, oxidative stress is an underlying basic etiology associated with many aging-related diseases, and thus psychologically induced oxidative stress, especially in the brain, is considered one of the pathologies of mibyou (Konishi, 2009). Indeed, ROS are constantly produced through the high consumption of oxygen for energy metabolism and also from the metabolic processes of neurotransmitter molecules. Thus the oxidative stress-induced neuronal damage and cell death play critical roles in the pathogenesis of neurodegenerative disorders such as Alzheimer's disease (AD) (Kidd, 2008; Nunomura et al., 2006) and Parkinson's disease (PD) (Danielson and Andersen, 2008; Ebadi and Sharma, 2006). Because these neurodegenerative diseases are considered serious factors that decrease the quality of life in a long-lived society, the prevention of cerebral oxidative stress is an emergent social task. In this context, Japanese Kampo medicines would be an interesting target of study for their preventive and therapeutic effects on oxidative stress-related brain disorders. In this chapter, we aim to enumerate the various Kampo medicines with evidence for their potential in various age-related neurological disorders such as AD and PD and also in other neuropsychiatric disorders.

Kampo Medicine in Dementia

Dementia refers to a group of symptoms that are of a typically chronic and progressive nature. The dementia syndrome involves disturbances of multiple higher cortical functions, such as memory, thinking, orientation, perception, and behavior, which are severe enough to affect the ability to perform everyday activities. Cognitive decline is often accompanied by deterioration in emotional control, social behavior, or motivation. The most common forms of dementia are AD (60–70% of cases) dementia, vascular dementia (VaD), dementia with Lewy bodies (DLB), PD dementia, and frontotemporal dementia (Burckhardt et al., 2016).

Clinical Studies

In addition to dementia, the descriptive term "behavioral and psychological symptoms of dementia" (BPSD) is used to cover a range of noncognitive disturbances, including anxiety, depression, irritability, aggression, agitation, eating disorders, and inappropriate social or sexual behaviors. BPSD are very frequent, so that 90% of demented patients have at least one. The pathophysiology of BPSD is related to an imbalance between the various neurotransmitters, such as acetylcholine, serotonin, dopamine, and noradrenaline (de Caires and Steenkamp, 2010). Yokukansan (YKS) (TJ-54), also called yi-gan san in Chinese, is composed of seven herbal mixtures (Table 9.1). In 2005, Iwasaki et al., reported the first case-controlled study of YKS on dementia. This study states that 4 weeks of treatment with YKS significantly improved scores on both the Neuropsychiatric Inventory (NPI) for the assessment of BPSD and the Barthel Index (BI) for activities of daily living in 52 patients with mild to severe dementia (Iwasaki et al., 2005a,b). Reports from various studies show the application of YKS in various types of dementia such as AD, PD, VaD, and DLB. In Table 9.3, we have listed various study models that used YKS in patients with different types of dementia. Chotosan (CTS), composed of 11 different crude drugs (Table 9.1), is reported to have beneficial effects on dementia patients. In a clinical study CTS administered at the dose of 7.5 g/kg/day improved both electrophysiological indices related to attention and decision-making and neuropsychological test scores in chronic stroke patients with mild cognitive impairment

Table 9.1: Herbal Constituents of Kampo Medicines

Yokukansan (g) (Okamoto et al., 2014)	Chotosan (Parts) (Okamoto et al., 2014)	Kososan (g) (Ito et al., 2009)	Kamishoyosan (g) (Mizowaki et al., 2001)
Japanese *Angelica* root (3) *Atractylodes lancea* rhizome (4) *Bupleurum* root (2) *Poria* sclerotium (4) *Glycyrrhiza* root (1.5) *Cnidium* rhizome (3) *Uncaria* hook (3)	Uncariae cum uncis ramulus (3) Citri reticulatae pericarpium (3) Pinelliae rhizoma (3) Ophiopogonis radix (3) *Poria* (3) Ginseng radix (2) Saposhnikoviae radix (2) Chrysanthemi flos (2) Glycyrrhizae radix (1) Zingiberis rhizoma (1) Gypsum fibrosum (5)	Cyperi rhizoma (4) Perillae herba (2) Aurantii nobilis pericarpium (3) Glycyrrhizae radix (2) Zingiberis rhizoma (0.5)	*Bupleurum falcatum* (3) *Paeonia lactiflora* (3) *A. lancea* (3) *Angelica acutiloba* (3) *Poria cocos* (3) *Gardenia jasminoides* (2) *Paeonia suffruticosa* (2) *Glycyrrhiza uralensis* (1.5) *Zingiber officinale* (1) *Mentha arvensis* (1)

(Yamaguchi et al., 2004). In another double-blind, randomized, placebo-controlled study, CTS treatment improved the cognitive functions and activities of daily living in AD and VaD patients compared to placebo (Matsumoto et al., 2013).

Preclinical Studies

In Tg2576, AD mouse model, treatment with YKS improved learning and cognitive defects as well as decreased anxiety-like behavior (Tabuchi et al., 2009).

Kampo Medicines in Depression

Depression is a momentary feeling of sadness or despondency, most often related to a perceived loss or sense of helplessness about a particular event, and often involves biological, psychological, and social elements that mainly affect concentration or interest in life. According to the diagnostic criteria for major depression in the *Diagnostic and Statistical Manual of Mental Disorders* (DSM)-IV, the list of symptoms that should be considered for the diagnosis of major depression is as follows: sadness (or irritability in children), loss of interest or pleasure in usual activities, changes in appetite (increased or decreased) or weight, disturbed sleep (insomnia or hypersomnia), psychomotor agitation or retardation, fatigue or loss of energy, feelings of guilt, self-blame, decreased ability to concentrate or make decisions, and thinking about or planning suicide or suicidal behavior (Dobson and David, 2008). Only five symptoms from this list are required for a diagnosis of depression, yet individuals can experience more than this minimum in increasingly severe cases. Diagnostically, at least one of these symptoms must include pervasive sadness or loss of interest, although this requirement could be refined in future versions of the DSM on the basis of recent and future research (Zimmerman et al., 2006). In

Japanese Kampo medicine emotion-related disorders are closely related to the concept of "utsu." Nowadays, utsu is defined as depression, a growing public concern throughout the world. Utsu has a long history as a disease and pathology of emotion-related disorders in Japan. In the Edo period, this term meant "constraint" and was used to describe many of the emotional and psychological sufferings of those times (Daidoji, 2013).

Preclinical Studies

Kososan, a Kampo medicine called xiang-su-san in Chinese, is composed of five herbs as given in Table 9.1 and is clinically used for the treatment of depression-like symptoms. Earlier findings suggest that kososan can alleviate depression induced by interferon (IFN)-α therapy for hepatitis C. In a stress and IFN-α–induced animal model of depression oral administration of kososan showed an antidepressant-like effect by normalizing the dysfunction of the hypothalamic–pituitary–adrenal axis, which is strongly associated with the pathogenesis of depression (Ito et al., 2006, 2016). Furthermore, studies also demonstrated that regulation of the orexinergic system and hippocampal cell proliferation by long-term kososan treatment plays an important role in its antidepressant-like effect in the stress-induced mouse model (Ito et al., 2009). A study by Ito et al. (2012) also demonstrated the antidepressant activity of kososan administered orally at 1.0 g/kg once daily for 28 days. This study highlights the essential role of neuropeptide Y after long-term treatment with kososan in the depressant-like mouse model (Ito et al., 2012).

Kampo Medicine in Anxiety

Anxiety is a feeling of apprehension or fear of future threat. According to Barlow's concepts, anxiety is a future-oriented mood state associated with preparation for possible upcoming negative events. That is, anxiety corresponds to an animal's state during a potential predatory attack (Barlow, 2002). Collapsing mood and anxiety disorders belong to an overarching class of "internalizing" disorders, as follows: bipolar disorders (bipolar I, bipolar II, and cyclothymia), distress or anxious–misery disorders (major depression, dysthymia, generalized anxiety disorder, and post-traumatic stress disorder), and fear disorders (panic disorder, agoraphobia, social phobia, and specific phobia) (Krueger, 1999).

Clinical Studies

YKS at the dose of 7.5 g/day for 12 weeks improved neuropsychiatric symptoms associated with panic disorder, including hallucinations, anxiety, and apathy, without severe adverse events and worsening of the panic disorder (Hatano et al., 2014). In an open-label pilot study of borderline personality disorder (BPD), YKS treatment significantly reduced the number of BPD symptoms, including low mood, impulsivity, and anxiety (Miyaoka et al., 2008). Another study showed that four patients who fulfilled the DSM criteria for panic disorder with

Table 9.2: Herbal Constituents of Kampo Medicines

Hangekobokuto (g) (Kuribara et al., 2000)	Shigyakusan (g) (Ninomiya, 2008)	Ninjinyoeito (g) (Suzuki et al., 2015)	Kamikihito (g) (Egashiral et al., 2007)
Pinelliae rhizoma (6) Hoelen (5) Magnoliae cortex (3) Perillae herba (2) Zingiberis rhizoma (1) Bupleuri radix (1)	Bupleuri radix (5) Paeoniae radix (4) Aurantii fructus immaturus (2) Glycyrrhizae radix (1.5)	Japanese *Angelica* root (4) *Atractylodes* rhizome (4) Uchida-Wakan-yaku (4) *Rehmannia* root (4) *Poria* sclerotium (4) Ginseng (3) Cinnamon bark (2.5) *Citrus unshiu* peel (2) *Polygala* root (2) Peony root (2) *Astragalus* root (1.5) *Schisandra* fruit (1) *Glycyrrhiza* (1)	Astragali radix (3) Bupleuri radix (3) Zizyphi spinosi semen (3) Atractylodis lanceae rhizoma (3) Ginseng radix (3) Hoelen (3) Longan arillus (3), Polygalae radix (2) Gardeniae fructus (2) Zizyphi fructus (2) Angelicae radix (2) Glycyrrhizae radix (1) Zingiberis rhizoma (1)

agoraphobia were relieved of anticipatory anxiety and had no agoraphobic avoidance after therapy with kamishoyosan (TJ-24; composed of 10 herbal constituents given in Table 9.1) at 7.5 g/day for 8 weeks or hangekobokuto (TJ-16; composed of six herbal constituents given in Table 9.2) at 7.5 g/day for 2 weeks (Mantani et al., 2002).

Preclinical Studies

Several studies have shown the anxiolytic effects of YKS. YKS administered singly or repeatedly had an effect on basal or stress-induced levels of serum corticosterone; repeated administration of YKS decreased anxiety-like behavior in an open-field test and an elevated-plus maze test (Shoji and Mizoguchi, 2013). Three months of YKS administration improved aspects of age-related anxiety in F344/N aged rats in a study whose results suggest that this improvement may result from the enhancement of serotonergic and dopaminergic transmission (Mizoguchi et al., 2010). Rats subjected to electrical foot shock as aversive stress were given YKS at a dose of 1.0 g/kg once a day for 14 or 16 days. The effects evaluated using contextual fear conditioning and the elevated-plus maze test showed the anxiolytic property of YKS (Yamaguchi et al., 2012). Another Kampo medicine, shigyakusan (SKS; composed of four herbal constituents given in Table 9.2), is used to treat inflammatory conditions such as cholecystitis and gastritis as well as psychiatric disorders. SKS administered at dose levels of 0.15, 0.3, and 0.45 g/kg was shown to have anxiolytic activity in a mouse model with low side effects (Tanaka et al., 2013).

Kampo Medicine in Working and Spatial Memory

Memory is the term given to the structures and processes involved in the storage and subsequent retrieval of information. Using memory, past experiences can be retrieved to use this information in the present (Sternberg, 1999). Working memory is the process of actively maintaining a representation of information for a brief period of time so that it is available for use (Ungerleider et al., 1998).

Preclinical Studies

The Kampo medicine kamikihito (KKT; composed of 14 herbal constituents given in Table 9.2) has been widely used for treating insomnia, anemia, amnesia, palpitations, and neurosis. It has been reported to increase both the muscarinic receptor density and choline acetyltransferase activity, which is essential for memory retention. A study by Egashira et al. (2007) showed that KKT treatment (1 and 3 mg/kg, po) significantly improved scopolamine (a nonselective muscarinic receptor antagonist)-induced impairment of spatial memory. Further, this study also reported that KKT (30 mg/kg, po) significantly improved the Δ^9-tetrahydrocannabinol psychoactive component–induced impairment of spatial memory. This study reveals that KKT may ameliorate the impairment of spatial memory by enhancing the activity of cholinergic neurons (Egashira et al., 2007). Another study by Mizoguchi et al. (2011) showed that YKS administered to 21-month-old rats for 3 months ameliorated age-related impairments of working memory and reversal learning, which might be mediated by a dopaminergic mechanism in the prefrontal cortex structure (Mizoguchi et al., 2011).

Kampo Medicine in Alzheimer's Disease

AD is an age-related progressive neurodegenerative disorder characterized by a gradual decline in cognition, a decreased ability to perform activities of daily living, and neuropsychiatric and behavioral problems. AD is one of the most common pathological causes of senile dementia (Citron, 2010).

Clinical Studies

A study by Kudoh et al. included 23 outpatients, of whom 11 received treatment with donepezil alone and 12 received a combined treatment with ninjinyoeito (NYT; composed of 13 herbal constituents given in Table 9.2) for 2 years after having received donepezil alone. The results suggest that a combination treatment of NYT and donepezil could be a more reasonable approach for AD patients with a mild depressive mood, compared with donepezil-only treatment (Kudoh et al., 2016). In an open-label study, patients with AD were administered YKS (7.5 g/day) for 4 weeks to investigate changes in neuropsychological test results and care burden from the start to the completion of the study treatment. At the end of the study a clinically significant decrease was seen in terms of hallucinations, agitation, anxiety, irritability, or abnormal behavior in AD patients. The results of this study suggest that YKS might be an effective and well-tolerated drug in the treatment of BPSD in AD patients (Hayashi et al., 2010). A detailed note on YKS in clinical practice for dementia is given in Table 9.3.

Table 9.3: Application of Yokukansan in Various Types of Dementia in Clinical Models

Study Design	Diagnosis	Study Size/Sex/ Dose	Outcome	References
Prospective, randomized, observer blind, multicenter, and open label	Mild to severe dementia	$n = 52$ (YKS = 27; control = 25)/24 men and 28 women/7.5 g/day, 4 weeks	NPI and BI scores showed significant improvement; MMSE results unchanged in both groups	Iwasaki et al. (2005a,b)
Prospective, single arm, and open label	Mild to severe Lewis body dementia	$n = 14$/9 men and 5 women/7.5 g/day, 4 weeks	NPI and BI scores showed significant improvement; MMSE results unchanged in both groups	Iwasaki et al. (2005a,b)
Prospective, single arm, and open label	Mild to severe dementia	$n = 5$/1 man and 4 women/7.5 g/day, 4 weeks	Significant improvement in NPH/NI scores; MMSE results unchanged in both groups	Shinno et al. (2008)
Prospective, randomized, crossover, multi-center, and open label	AD dementia, Lewis body dementia	$n = 106$/7.5 g/day, 4 weeks	NPI scores significantly increased; no change in MMSE, BI, and IADL	Mizukami et al. (2009)
Prospective, randomized, open label	AD dementia	$n = 15$ (YKS = 10; control = 5)/2 men and 13 women/7.5 g/day, 12 weeks	Significant improvement in NPI scores; no change in MMSE	Monji et al. (2009)
Prospective, single arm, multicenter, and open label	AD dementia	$n = 26$/15 men and 11 women/7.5 g/day, 4 weeks	Significant improvement in NPI; no change in MMSE and DAD	Hayashi et al. (2010)
Prospective, nonblinded, randomized, multicenter, and open label	AD dementia	$n = 61$ (YKS = 29; control = 32)/25 men and 36 women/7.5 g/day, 4 weeks	Significant improvement in NPI; no change in MMSE, DAD, and ZBI	Okahara et al. (2010)
Prospective, single arm, and open label	PD dementia	$n = 14$ (PD = 7; PD dementia = 7)/8 men and 6 women/7.5 g/day, 4 weeks	Significant improvement in NPI	Kawanabe et al. (2010)
Prospective, single arm, and open label	Frontotemporal dementia	$n = 20$/7 men and 13 women/7.5 g/day, 4 weeks	Significant improvement in NPI	Kimura et al. (2010)

Continued

Table 9.3: Application of Yokukansan in Various Types of Dementia in Clinical Models—cont'd

Study Design	Diagnosis	Study Size/Sex/ Dose	Outcome	References
Prospective, single arm, multicenter, and open label	Lewis body dementia	$n = 63/30$ men and 33 women/7.5 g/ day, 4 weeks	Significant improvement in NPI and ZBI scores; no change in MMSE	Iwasaki et al. (2012)
Prospective, single arm, multicenter, and open label	Vascular dementia	$n = 13/9$ men and 4 women/7.5 g/day, 4 weeks	Significant improvement in NPI; no change in MMSE, BI, and DAD	Nagata et al. (2012)
Prospective, single arm, and open label	AD dementia, vascular dementia	$n = 11$ (AD = 8; vascular demen- tia = 3)/7.5 g/day, 4 weeks	Significant improvement in NPI; no change in BI	Sumiyoshi et al. (2013)
Prospective, randomized, rater blinded, and triple-group	Mild to severe dementia	$n = 76$ (YKS = 26)/25 men and 51 women/2.5–7.5 g/day	Significant improvement in NPI; no change in MMSE	Teranishi et al. (2013)
Prospective, randomized, multicenter, double blinded, placebo controlled	AD dementia	$n = 147$ (YKS = 75; placebo = 70)/ 61 men and 84 women/7.5 g/day, 4 weeks	No significant difference in NPI total score and MMSE total score	Furukawa et al. (2015)
Prospective, rater blinded, random- ized, flexible dose, triple group	AD dementia, vascular dementia, Lewis body dementia	$n = 82$ (YKS = 27; risperidone = 27; fluvox- amine = 28)/2.5– 7.5 g/day	Significant improvement in NPI; no change in MMSE	Takeyoshi et al. (2016)

AD, Alzheimer-type dementia; *BI*, barthel index; *DAD*, disability assessment for dementia; *IADL*, instrumental activities of daily living; *MMSE*, mini-mental state examination; *NPH/NI*, nursing home version of NPI; *NPI*, neuropsychiatric inventory; *PD*, Parkinson's disease; *YKS*, Yokukansan; *ZBI*, Zarit Burden interview.

Preclinical Studies

A number of studies have reported the efficacy of YKS in dementia models of AD transgenic animals (Fujiwara et al., 2011; Tabuchi et al., 2009). A 2013 study revealed that YKS has an ameliorative effect on spatial memory impairment in an early phase AD rat model, and that its therapeutic mechanism is mediated by an increase in acetylcholine release and the modulation of DMN1 expression, leading to improved synaptic function (Uchida et al., 2013).

Kampo Medicine in Other Neuropsychiatric Diseases

Most brain disorders may cause psychiatric symptoms. The cerebral disorders that cause psychiatric symptoms are called neuropsychiatric disorders. Neuropsychiatric disorders commonly occur in elderly patients and occasionally mimic endogenous psychoses (Lyketsos, 2006).

Antipsychotic drug-induced extrapyramidal disorders have some variations, involving PD dystonia, akathisias, and tardive dyskinesia (TD). A study by Ishikawa et al. (2000) reports that treatment with kamishoyosan (KSS; Table 9.1) effectively reduced the tremor associated with PD. Eight patients with tremor from antipsychotic drug-induced parkinsonism were given KSS 7.5 g/day three times a day orally. Tremor was evaluated on a five-point scale following KSS administration for a given number of days ranging from 1 week to 1 month. Treatment with KSS significantly reduced the tremor associated with PD (Ishikawa et al., 2000).

TD is a serious motor condition predominantly caused by long-term use of antipsychotics associated with the treatment of schizophrenia. This disease is generally characterized by abnormal involuntary movements of the tongue, lips, face, trunk, and extremities. TD is an irreversible condition and as of this writing few effective treatment options exist. In a study including 69 schizophrenia patients (49 presenting with TD, whereas the remaining 20 patients showed no TD), the TD group was treated for 16 weeks with KSS and assessed using the Abnormal Involuntary Movement scale. There was a reduction in total Abnormal Involuntary Movement scale scores in the TD group treated with KSS at 4, 8, and 16 weeks of treatment (Lee et al., 2007).

Studies have shown that dementia patients experience a decrease in the amount of slow-wave sleep and rapid-eye-movement sleep, resulting in sleep disturbances. Treatment with YKS (7.5 g/day, three times daily for 3 days) significantly extended the total sleep time of 20 adult male patients compared with the control group (Aizawa et al., 2002). In another study, treatment with YKS (2.5 g, before meals, three times a day for 4 weeks) for both BPSD and sleep structure in dementia patients showed significant improvements in NPI scores and reduced delusions, hallucinations, agitation/aggression, anxiety, and irritability, as well as increases in total sleep time (Shinno et al., 2008).

YKS is reported to be valuable in the treatment of various emotional symptoms in BPD. A 12-week open-label study investigated the effect of YKS (6.4 ± 1.9 g daily) on 25 female BPD patients. The results from the study showed significant improvements in various symptoms of BPD, including depression, aggression, impulsivity, and anxiety, without significant side effects (Miyaoka et al., 2008).

Conclusion

Since 2005, there has been a global surge in the use of complementary and alternative medicine in both developed and developing countries. As a complementary and alternative medicine, Kampo is a holistic and individualized treatment with a long tradition and history. The aforementioned studies explain the role of Kampo medicine in neurological disorders. Such ancient herbal prescriptions can be effectively used to prevent intractable nervous diseases such as dementia, depression, and anxiety, as they show excellent preventive effects against neuron damage, enforcing action on natural healing forces, and even regulatory action against adverse expression of genes. It is time to protect and promote Japanese Kampo medicine, the unchanging form of knowledge inherited from the past, to future descendants. The development of new potential therapies against neurodegenerative diseases represents a crucial prerequisite for improving and extending the quality of life among older people. These challenges require novel approaches, because current treatments are often symptomatic and do not stop or slow underlying neurodegenerative processes. Kampo medicine rather can be considered as a future medicine, the "third medicine," which is situated in a higher dimension than that of contemporary Oriental and Western medicines. Kampo medicines consumed alone or in combination with Western medicines are shown to have beneficial effects in neurological disorders, in both clinical and preclinical systems. However, to increase the evidence-based knowledge, it is necessary to perform research on the mechanisms of action of Kampo (Japanese herbal) medicine in various neurological disorders.

References

Aizawa, R., Kanbayashi, T., Saito, Y., Ogawa, Y., Sugiyama, T., Kitajima, T., et al., 2002. Effects of Yoku-kan-san-ka-chimpi-hange on the sleep of normal healthy adult subjects. Psychiatry Clin. Neurosci. 56 (3), 303–304. http://dx.doi.org/10.1046/j.1440-1819.2002.01006.x.

Arai, M., Katai, S., Muramatsu, S., Namiki, T., Hanawa, T., Izumi, S., 2012. Current status of Kampo medicine curricula in all Japanese medical schools. BMC Complement. Altern. Med. 12, 207. http://dx.doi.org/10.1186/1472-6882-12-207.

Barlow, D., 2002. The Nature and Treatment of Anxiety and Panic. Anxiety and its Disorders, second ed. Guilford Press, New York.

Burckhardt, M., Herke, M., Wustmann, T., Watzke, S., Langer, G., Fink, A., 2016. Omega-3 fatty acids for the treatment of dementia. Cochrane Database Syst. Rev. 4, CD009002. http://dx.doi.org/10.1002/14651858.CD009002.pub3.

Chong, Z.Z., Li, F., Maiese, K., 2005. Oxidative stress in the brain: novel cellular targets that govern survival during neurodegenerative disease. Prog. Neurobiol. 75 (3), 207–246. http://dx.doi.org/10.1016/j.pneurobio.2005.02.004.

Citron, M., 2010. Alzheimer's disease: strategies for disease modification. Nat. Rev. Drug Discov. 9 (5), 387–398. http://dx.doi.org/10.1038/nrd2896.

Daidoji, K., 2013. Treating emotion-related disorders in Japanese traditional medicine: language, patients and doctors. Cult. Med. Psychiatry 37 (1), 59–80. http://dx.doi.org/10.1007/s11013-012-9297-4.

Danielson, S.R., Andersen, J.K., 2008. Oxidative and nitrative protein modifications in Parkinson's disease. Free Radic. Biol. Med. 44 (10), 1787–1794. http://dx.doi.org/10.1016/j.freeradbiomed.2008.03.005.

de Caires, S., Steenkamp, V., 2010. Use of Yokukansan (TJ-54) in the treatment of neurological disorders: a review. Phytother. Res. 24 (9), 1265–1270. http://dx.doi.org/10.1002/ptr.3146.

Dobson, K.S., David, J., 2008. Introduction: assessing risk and resilience factors in models of depression. Risk Factor. Depression 1–16. http://dx.doi.org/10.1016/B978-0-08-045078-0.00001-0.

Ebadi, M., Sharma, S., 2006. Metallothioneins 1 and 2 attenuate peroxynitrite-induced oxidative stress in Parkinson disease. Exp. Biol. Med. (Maywood) 231 (9), 1576–1583.

Egashira, N., Manome, N., Kurauchi, K., Matsumoto, Y., Iwasaki, K., Mishima, K., et al., 2007. Kamikihi-to, a Kampo medicine, ameliorates impairment of spatial memory in rats. Phytother. Res. 21 (2), 126–129. http://dx.doi.org/10.1002/ptr.2034.

Fujikawa, Y., 1979. Nippon igaku-shi History of Japanese Medicine. Nagayama Shoten.

Fujiwara, H., Takayama, S., Iwasaki, K., Tabuchi, M., Yamaguchi, T., Sekiguchi, K., et al., 2011. Yokukansan, a traditional Japanese medicine, ameliorates memory disturbance and abnormal social interaction with anti-aggregation effect of cerebral amyloid beta proteins in amyloid precursor protein transgenic mice. Neuroscience 180, 305–313. http://dx.doi.org/10.1016/j.neuroscience.2011.01.064.

Furukawa, K., Tomita, N., Uematsu, D., Okahara, K., Shimada, H., Ikeda, M., et al., 2015. Randomized double-blind placebo-controlled multicenter trial of Yokukansan for neuropsychiatric symptoms in Alzheimer's disease. Geriatr. Gerontol. Int. http://dx.doi.org/10.1111/ggi.12696.

Hatano, T., Hattori, N., Kawanabe, T., Terayama, Y., Suzuki, N., Iwasaki, Y., et al., 2014. An exploratory study of the efficacy and safety of yokukansan for neuropsychiatric symptoms in patients with Parkinson's disease. J. Neural Transm. (Vienna) 121 (3), 275–281. http://dx.doi.org/10.1007/s00702-013-1105-y.

Hayashi, Y., Ishida, Y., Inoue, T., Udagawa, M., Takeuchi, K., Yoshimuta, H., et al., 2010. Treatment of behavioral and psychological symptoms of Alzheimer-type dementia with Yokukansan in clinical practice. Prog. Neuropsychopharmacol. Biol. Psychiatry 34 (3), 541–545. http://dx.doi.org/10.1016/j.pnpbp.2010.02.016.

Ishikawa, T., Funahashi, T., Kudo, J., 2000. Effectiveness of the Kampo *kami-shoyo-san* (TJ-24) for tremor of antipsychotic-induced parkinsonism. Psychiatry Clin. Neurosci. 54 (5), 579–582. http://dx.doi.org/10.1046/j.1440-1819.2000.00756.x.

Ito, N., Nagai, T., Yabe, T., Nunome, S., Hanawa, T., Yamada, H., 2006. Antidepressant-like activity of a Kampo (Japanese herbal) medicine, Koso-san (Xiang-Su-San), and its mode of action via the hypothalamic-pituitary-adrenal axis. Phytomedicine 13 (9–10), 658–667. http://dx.doi.org/10.1016/j.phymed.2006.01.002.

Ito, N., Yabe, T., Nagai, T., Oikawa, T., Yamada, H., Hanawa, T., 2009. A possible mechanism underlying an antidepressive-like effect of Kososan, a Kampo medicine, via the hypothalamic orexinergic system in the stress-induced depression-like model mice. Biol. Pharm. Bull. 32 (10), 1716–1722.

Ito, N., Hori, A., Yabe, T., Nagai, T., Oikawa, T., Yamada, H., Hanawa, T., 2012. Involvement of neuropeptide Y signaling in the antidepressant-like effect and hippocampal cell proliferation induced by kososan, a Kampo medicine, in the stress-induced depression-like model mice. Biol. Pharm. Bull. 35 (10), 1775–1783.

Ito, N., Nagai, T., Hirose, E., Kiyohara, H., Oikawa, T., Yamada, H., Hanawa, T., 2016. Antidepressive-like effect of volatile components of kososan in a mouse model of stress-induced depression. Tradit. Kampo Med.

Iwasaki, K., Maruyama, M., Tomita, N., Furukawa, K., Nemoto, M., Fujiwara, H., et al., 2005a. Effects of the traditional Chinese herbal medicine Yi-Gan San for cholinesterase inhibitor-resistant visual hallucinations and neuropsychiatric symptoms in patients with dementia with Lewy bodies. J. Clin. Psychiatry 66 (12), 1612–1613.

Iwasaki, K., Satoh-Nakagawa, T., Maruyama, M., Monma, Y., Nemoto, M., Tomita, N., et al., 2005b. A randomized, observer-blind, controlled trial of the traditional Chinese medicine Yi-Gan San for improvement of behavioral and psychological symptoms and activities of daily living in dementia patients. J. Clin. Psychiatry 66 (2), 248–252.

Iwasaki, K., Kosaka, K., Mori, H., Okitsu, R., Furukawa, K., Manabe, Y., et al., 2012. Improvement in delusions and hallucinations in patients with dementia with Lewy bodies upon administration of yokukansan, a traditional Japanese medicine. Psychogeriatrics 12 (4), 235–241. http://dx.doi.org/10.1111/j.1479-8301.2012.00413.x.

Kawanabe, T., Yoritaka, A., Shimura, H., Oizumi, H., Tanaka, S., Hattori, N., 2010. Successful treatment with Yokukansan for behavioral and psychological symptoms of Parkinsonian dementia. Prog. Neuropsychopharmacol. Biol. Psychiatry 34 (2), 284–287. http://dx.doi.org/10.1016/j.pnpbp.2009.11.019.

Kidd, P.M., 2008. Alzheimer's disease, amnestic mild cognitive impairment, and age-associated memory impairment: current understanding and progress toward integrative prevention. Altern. Med. Rev. 13 (2), 85–115.

Kimura, T., Hayashida, H., Furukawa, H., Takamatsu, J., 2010. Pilot study of pharmacological treatment for frontotemporal dementia: effect of Yokukansan on behavioral symptoms. Psychiatry Clin. Neurosci. 64 (2), 207–210. http://dx.doi.org/10.1111/j.1440-1819.2010.02072.x.

Konishi, T., 2009. Brain oxidative stress as basic target of antioxidant traditional oriental medicines. Neurochem. Res. 34 (4), 711–716. http://dx.doi.org/10.1007/s11064-008-9872-9.

Krueger, R.F., 1999. The structure of common mental disorders. Arch. Gen. Psychiatry 56 (10), 921–926.

Kudoh, C., Arita, R., Honda, M., Kishi, T., Komatsu, Y., Asou, H., Mimura, M., 2016. Effect of ninjin'yoeito, a Kampo (traditional Japanese) medicine, on cognitive impairment and depression in patients with Alzheimer's disease: 2 years of observation. Psychogeriatrics 16 (2), 85–92. http://dx.doi.org/10.1111/psyg.12125.

Kuribara, H., Kishi, E., Hattori, N., Okada, M., Maruyama, Y., 2000. The anxiolytic effect of two oriental herbal drugs in Japan attributed to honokiol from magnolia bark. J. Pharm. Pharmacol. 52 (11), 1425–1429.

Lee, J.G., Shin, B.S., Lee, Y.C., Park, S.W., Kim, Y.H., 2007. Clinical effectiveness of the Kampo medicine kamishoyosan for adjunctive treatment of tardive dyskinesia in patients with schizophrenia: a 16-week open trial. Psychiatry Clin. Neurosci. 61 (5), 509–514. http://dx.doi.org/10.1111/j.1440-1819.2007.01700.x.

Lyketsos, C.G., 2006. Lessons from neuropsychiatry. J. Neuropsychiatry Clin. Neurosci. 18 (4), 445–449. http://dx.doi.org/10.1176/jnp.2006.18.4.445.

Mantani, N., Hisanaga, A., Kogure, T., Kita, T., Shimada, Y., Terasawa, K., 2002. Four cases of panic disorder successfully treated with Kampo (Japanese herbal) medicines: kami-shoyo-san and Hange-koboku-to. Psychiatry Clin. Neurosci. 56 (6), 617–620. http://dx.doi.org/10.1046/j.1440-1819.2002.01064.x.

Matsumoto, K., Zhao, Q., Niu, Y., Fujiwara, H., Tanaka, K., Sasaki-Hamada, S., et al., 2013. Kampo formulations, chotosan, and yokukansan, for dementia therapy: existing clinical and preclinical evidence. J. Pharmacol. Sci. 122 (4), 257–269.

Miyaoka, T., Furuya, M., Yasuda, H., Hayashia, M., Inagaki, T., Horiguchi, J., 2008. Yi-gan san for the treatment of borderline personality disorder: an open-label study. Prog. Neuropsychopharmacol. Biol. Psychiatry 32 (1), 150–154. http://dx.doi.org/10.1016/j.pnpbp.2007.07.026.

Mizoguchi, K., Tanaka, Y., Tabira, T., 2010. Anxiolytic effect of a herbal medicine, yokukansan, in aged rats: involvement of serotonergic and dopaminergic transmissions in the prefrontal cortex. J. Ethnopharmacol. 127 (1), 70–76. http://dx.doi.org/10.1016/j.jep.2009.09.048.

Mizoguchi, K., Shoji, H., Tanaka, Y., Tabira, T., 2011. Ameliorative effect of traditional Japanese medicine yokukansan on age-related impairments of working memory and reversal learning in rats. Neuroscience 177, 127–137. http://dx.doi.org/10.1016/j.neuroscience.2010.12.045.

Mizowaki, M., Toriizuka, K., Hanawa, T., 2001. Anxiolytic effect of Kami-Shoyo-San (TJ-24) in mice: possible mediation of neurosteroid synthesis. Life Sci. 69 (18), 2167–2177.

Mizukami, K., Asada, T., Kinoshita, T., Tanaka, K., Sonohara, K., Nakai, R., et al., 2009. A randomized cross-over study of a traditional Japanese medicine (kampo), yokukansan, in the treatment of the behavioural and psychological symptoms of dementia. Int. J. Neuropsychopharmacol. 12 (2), 191–199. http://dx.doi.org/10.1017/S146114570800970X.

Monji, A., Takita, M., Samejima, T., Takaishi, T., Hashimoto, K., Matsunaga, H., et al., 2009. Effect of yokukan-san on the behavioral and psychological symptoms of dementia in elderly patients with Alzheimer's disease. Prog. Neuropsychopharmacol. Biol. Psychiatry 33 (2), 308–311. http://dx.doi.org/10.1016/j.pnpbp.2008.12.008.

Motoo, Y., Arai, I., Hyodo, I., Tsutani, K., 2009. Current status of Kampo (Japanese herbal) medicines in Japanese clinical practice guidelines. Complement. Ther. Med. 17 (3), 147–154. http://dx.doi.org/10.1016/j.ctim.2008.09.003.

Nagata, K., Yokoyama, E., Yamazaki, T., Takano, D., Maeda, T., Takahashi, S., Terayama, Y., 2012. Effects of yokukansan on behavioral and psychological symptoms of vascular dementia: an open-label trial. Phytomedicine 19 (6), 524–528. http://dx.doi.org/10.1016/j.phymed.2012.02.008.

Ninomiya, F., 2008. Clinical evaluation of perspiration reducing effects of a kampo formula, Shigyaku-san, on Palmoplantar Hidrosis. Evid. Based Complement. Alternat. Med. 5 (2), 199–203. http://dx.doi.org/10.1093/ecam/nem008.

Nishimura, K., Plotnikoff, G., Watanabe, K., 2009. Kampo medicine as an integrative medicine in Japan. JMAJ 52 (3), 147–149.

Nunomura, A., Castellani, R.J., Zhu, X., Moreira, P.I., Perry, G., Smith, M.A., 2006. Involvement of oxidative stress in Alzheimer disease. J. Neuropathol. Exp. Neurol. 65 (7), 631–641. http://dx.doi.org/10.1097/01.jnen.0000228136.58062.bf.

Okahara, K., Ishida, Y., Hayashi, Y., Inoue, T., Tsuruta, K., Takeuchi, K., et al., 2010. Effects of Yokukansan on behavioral and psychological symptoms of dementia in regular treatment for Alzheimer's disease. Prog. Neuropsychopharmacol. Biol. Psychiatry 34 (3), 532–536. http://dx.doi.org/10.1016/j.pnpbp.2010.02.013.

Okamoto, H., Okami, T., Ikeda, M., Takeuchi, T., 2005. Effects of Yoku-kan-san on undifferentiated somatoform disorder with tinnitus. Eur. Psychiatry 20 (1), 74–75. http://dx.doi.org/10.1016/j.eurpsy.2004.09.034.

Okamoto, H., Iyo, M., Ueda, K., Han, C., Hirasaki, Y., Namiki, T., 2014. Yokukan-san: a review of the evidence for use of this Kampo herbal formula in dementia and psychiatric conditions. Neuropsychiatr. Dis. Treat. 10, 1727–1742. http://dx.doi.org/10.2147/NDT.S65257.

Otsuka, Y., 1988. Pharmacotherapy in Oriental Medicine. Excerpta Medica.

Shinno, H., Inami, Y., Inagaki, T., Nakamura, Y., Horiguchi, J., 2008. Effect of Yi-Gan San on psychiatric symptoms and sleep structure at patients with behavioral and psychological symptoms of dementia. Prog. Neuropsychopharmacol. Biol. Psychiatry 32 (3), 881–885. http://dx.doi.org/10.1016/j.pnpbp.2007.12.027.

Shoji, H., Mizoguchi, K., 2013. Brain region-specific reduction in c-Fos expression associated with an anxiolytic effect of yokukansan in rats. J. Ethnopharmacol. 149 (1), 93–102. http://dx.doi.org/10.1016/j.jep.2013.06.005.

Sternberg, R., 1999. Cognitive psychology. Cogn. Psychol.

Sumiyoshi, H., Mantani, A., Nishiyama, S., Fujiwaki, S., Ohta, S., Masuda, Y., et al., 2013. Yokukansan treatment of chronic renal failure patients receiving hemodialysis, with behavioral and psychological symptoms of dementia: an open-label study. Am. J. Geriatr. Psychiatry 21 (11), 1082–1085. http://dx.doi.org/10.1016/j.jagp.2011.06.001.

Suzuki, T., Yamamoto, A., Ohsawa, M., Motoo, Y., Mizukami, H., Makino, T., 2015. Ninjin'yoeito and ginseng extract prevent oxaliplatin-induced neurodegeneration in PC12 cells. J. Nat. Med. 69 (4), 531–537. http://dx.doi.org/10.1007/s11418-015-0921-9.

Tabuchi, M., Yamaguchi, T., Iizuka, S., Imamura, S., Ikarashi, Y., Kase, Y., 2009. Ameliorative effects of *yokukansan*, a traditional Japanese medicine, on learning and non-cognitive disturbances in the Tg2576 mouse model of Alzheimer's disease. J. Ethnopharmacol. 122 (1), 157–162. http://dx.doi.org/10.1016/j.jep.2008.12.010.

Takeyoshi, K., Kurita, M., Nishino, S., Teranishi, M., Numata, Y., Sato, T., Okubo, Y., 2016. Yokukansan improves behavioral and psychological symptoms of dementia by suppressing dopaminergic function. Neuropsychiatr. Dis. Treat. 12, 641–649. http://dx.doi.org/10.2147/NDT.S99032.

Tanaka, M., Satou, T., Koike, K., 2013. Anxiolytic-like effect of Shigyakusan extract with low side effects in mice. J. Nat. Med. 67 (4), 862–866. http://dx.doi.org/10.1007/s11418-013-0746-3.

Teranishi, M., Kurita, M., Nishino, S., Takeyoshi, K., Numata, Y., Sato, T., et al., 2013. Efficacy and tolerability of risperidone, yokukansan, and fluvoxamine for the treatment of behavioral and psychological symptoms of dementia: a blinded, randomized trial. J. Clin. Psychopharmacol. 33 (5), 600–607. http://dx.doi.org/10.1097/JCP.0b013e31829798d5.

Uchida, N., Takasaki, K., Sakata, Y., Nogami, A., Oishi, H., Watanabe, T., et al., 2013. Cholinergic involvement and synaptic dynamin 1 expression in Yokukansan-mediated improvement of spatial memory in a rat model of early Alzheimer's disease. Phytother. Res. 27 (7), 966–972. http://dx.doi.org/10.1002/ptr.4818.

Ungerleider, L.G., Courtney, S.M., Haxby, J.V., 1998. A neural system for human visual working memory. Proc. Natl. Acad. Sci. U. S. A. 95 (3), 883–890.

Uversky, V., Anthony, F., 2007. α-Synuclein aggregation and Parkinson's disease. Aggregation 61–110.

Watanabe, K., Matsuura, K., Gao, P., Hottenbacher, L., Tokunaga, H., Nishimura, K., et al., 2011. Traditional Japanese kampo medicine: clinical research between modernity and traditional medicine—the state of research and methodological suggestions for the future. Evid. Based Complement. Alternat. Med. 2011, 513842. http://dx.doi.org/10.1093/ecam/neq067.

Yamaguchi, S., Matsubara, M., Kobayashi, S., 2004. Event-related brain potential changes after Choto-san administration in stroke patients with mild cognitive impairments. Psychopharmacology (Berl) 171 (3), 241–249. http://dx.doi.org/10.1007/s00213-003-1593-9.

Yamaguchi, T., Tsujimatsu, A., Kumamoto, H., Izumi, T., Ohmura, Y., Yoshida, T., Yoshioka, M., 2012. Anxiolytic effects of yokukansan, a traditional Japanese medicine, via serotonin 5-HT$_{1A}$ receptors on anxiety-related behaviors in rats experienced aversive stress. J. Ethnopharmacol. 143 (2), 533–539. http://dx.doi.org/10.1016/j.jep.2012.07.007.

Yu, F., Takahashi, T., Moriya, J., Kawaura, K., Yamakawa, J., Kusaka, K., et al., 2006. Traditional Chinese medicine and Kampo: a review from the distant past for the future. J. Int. Med. Res. 34 (3), 231–239.

Zimmerman, M., McGlinchey, J.B., Young, D., Chelminski, I., 2006. Diagnosing major depressive disorder IV: relationship between number of symptoms and the diagnosis of disorder. J. Nerv. Ment. Dis. 194 (6), 450–453. http://dx.doi.org/10.1097/01.nmd.0000221425.04436.46.

CHAPTER 10

Antiinflammatory Effects of Kampo Medicines in Atopic Dermatitis

Vengadeshprabhu Karuppagounder, Mayumi Nomoto, Kenichi Watanabe
Niigata University of Pharmacy and Applied Life Sciences, Niigata, Japan

Introduction

Atopic dermatitis (AD) is a chronic, relapsing, and inflammatory skin disease in humans, caused by a complex interrelationship among genetic, psychological, pharmacological, environmental, skin barrier dysfunctional, and immunological factors (Udompataikul and Limpa-o-vart, 2012). Disease onset typically occurs by 6 months of age in 45%, 1 year of age in 60%, and 5 years of age in 85% of affected infants and children. Up to 70% of children have a spontaneous remission before adolescence. The skin is an important interface between the body and its environment. Moreover, a leaky skin epithelial barrier combined with abnormal immune responsiveness probably contributes to the pathophysiology of AD (Kuo et al., 2013). The pathogenesis of AD is a complex mechanism. Environmental allergens such as the house dust mite, *Dermatophagoides farinae*, cause AD in humans (Matsuoka et al., 2003). AD is mainly associated with the T helper cell (Th) 2 phenotype, in which interleukin (IL)-4, IL-6, and IL-13 secretion and Th2-type cytokine-mediated immunoglobulin (Ig) E production are dominant (Leung et al., 2003). In addition, the accumulation of large numbers of eosinophils, mast cells, and dendritic cells has been observed in both dermis and epidermis of patients with AD (Leung and Bieber, 2003).

Topical or systemic corticosteroids are the first-line treatment option for AD. However, long-term use of corticosteroids causes severe adverse effects (Furue et al., 2003). Recently, medicinal herbs have emerged as a therapeutic alternative for the treatment of AD and have been proven safe (Yang et al., 2013). Moreover, traditional Kampo medicines have attracted considerable attention. Because they usually contain many different herbal medicines, interactions among their constituents are likely to play an important role in their effects. It can be difficult to identify the active constituents and to elucidate the mechanism of their action (Makino, 2005). Many patients currently visit physicians seeking Kampo medicine treatment for AD (Shimizu, 2013).

Possible Mechanisms Underlying the Pathogenesis of Atopic Dermatitis

Genetics

The pathogenesis of AD involves many genes, particularly those encoding epidermal structural proteins and those encoding key elements of the immune system. A 2006 genetic discovery documented the strong association between AD and mutations in the filaggrin gene (Palmer et al., 2006), which give rise to functional impairments thereby interrupting the skin barrier. Mutations of filaggrin occur mainly in early onset AD and indicate a propensity toward asthma. There is, however, no association between mutant filaggrin and allergic airway diseases without AD (Bieber, 2008). Several candidate genes have been identified in AD, notably on chromosome 5q31–q33. All of them encode cytokines in the regulation of IgE synthesis: IL-4, IL-5, IL-12, and IL-13. These and other cytokines are produced from two main types of T lymphocytes, Th1 and Th2 cells. The activation of Th2 cells produces IL-4 as well as IL-5 and IL-13 cytokines and upregulates the production of IgE (Hoffjan and Epplen, 2005). Th1 cells produce mainly interferon (IFN)-γ and IL-12, which suppress the production of IgE and enhance the production of IgG. Polymorphisms of the gene encoding the cytokine IL-18, which contribute to the shift of Th1 and Th2 cross-regulation toward Th1-mediated response or the innate immune system, may contribute to the imbalance between Th1 and Th2 immune response in AD (Novak et al., 2005).

Skin Barrier Dysfunction

An intact epidermal compartment is a prerequisite for the skin to function as a physical and chemical barrier. The barrier itself is the stratum corneum, the brick and mortar–like structure of the upper epidermal layer. An alteration in the barrier that causes increased transepidermal water loss is a hallmark of AD (Proksch et al., 2003). The theory of skin barrier effects is more recent, and has its origin in the observation that individuals with mutations in the filaggrin gene are at increased risk of developing AD (Palmer et al., 2006). The filaggrin gene encodes structural proteins in the stratum corneum and the stratum granulosum that help bind the keratinocytes together. This holds the intact skin barrier and hydrated stratum corneum. Mutation of filaggrin leads to transepidermal water loss and skin barrier dysfunction, which causes eczema. There is evidence to suggest that the impaired skin barrier, which results in dry skin, leads to increased penetration of allergens into the skin, resulting in AD, asthma, and hay fever (De Benedetto et al., 2012).

Kampo Medicines

Herbal medicines are used as adjunctive therapy for AD and inflammatory skin diseases. Kampo medicines are composed of herbal, animal, and mineral crude drugs and are prepared according to formulas mentioned in the Japanese and Chinese classical literature

(Yamashita et al., 2013). Kampo medicines were originally introduced to Japan from China more than 100 decades ago. Because of its unique development in Japan, Kampo is quite different from traditional Chinese medicine and Kampo prescriptions have been used to treat various diseases for centuries in Japan. The Japanese government has approved 148 Kampo prescription products for use in clinical practice (Shimizu, 2013). Moreover, Kampo medicines have also become popular in Western countries.

Kampo medicines are useful for treating inflammatory skin diseases such as AD. Extensive clinical and preclinical data suggest that the Kampo formulas byakkokaninjinto, yokukansan, rokumigan, hochuekkito, and jumihaidokuto can be used effectively against AD and inflammatory skin diseases.

Byakkokaninjinto

Byakkokaninjinto (bai-hu-jia-ren-sheng-tang) is composed of five crude drugs (Gypsum fibrosum, Anemarrhenae rhizoma, Glycyrrhizae radix, Ginseng radix, and Oryzae semen). It is commonly used to improve symptoms of dry mouth, hot flashes, perspiration, and pruritus. A previous report suggests that byakkokaninjinto treatment increases or restores aquaporin 5 expression, which is known to regulate salivary secretion from the submandibular gland (Yanagi et al., 2008). One to two weeks of treatment with byakkokaninjinto effectively suppressed severe facial erythema in AD patients (Shimizu, 2013). In addition, byakkokaninjinto significantly attenuated tumor necrosis factor-α, IFN-γ, and histamine production in contact dermatitis. Moreover, oral administration of byakkokaninjinto suppressed IgE-mediated triphasic skin reaction (Tatsumi et al., 2001). Three main crude constituents, Gypsum fibrosum, Glycyrrhizae radix, and Oryzae semen, were primarily responsible for the efficacy of byakkokaninjinto, for which the interaction between Gypsum fibrosum and other crude drugs might be essential. These findings seem to reflect the beneficial effect of the oral use of byakkokaninjinto on AD of dry and warm skin.

Yokukansan

Yokukansan is a traditional Japanese Kampo medicine composed of seven crude medical herbs (*Atractylodes lancea* rhizoma, *Poria* sclerotium, *Cnidium* rhizoma, Japanese *Angelica* radix, *Bupleurum* radix, *Glycyrrhiza* radix, and *Uncaria* thorn) (Wakabayashi et al., 2014). Yokukansan has been approved by the Ministry of Health, Labor, and Welfare of Japan as a remedy for insomnia, neurosis, and irritability in children. Yokukansan treatment alleviates the behavioral and psychological symptoms of dementia, such as hallucinations and aggressiveness, in patients with Alzheimer's disease. It regulates glutamate signaling in the central nervous system, and it is a novel glutamate receptor antagonist (Kawakami et al., 2011). Moreover, yokukansan reportedly exerts antiallergy effects on IgE-mediated triphasic cutaneous inflammation in socially associated mice. Furthermore, yokukansan treatment effectively attenuated scratching behavior and ameliorated AD-like lesions in NC/Nga mice. In addition, yokukansan inhibited the activity of glutamate receptors and decreased transepidermal water loss in the skin of NC/Nga mice (Funakushi et al., 2011). Wakabayashi et al. (2014) reported that yokukansan affects peripheral glutamate signaling in keratinocytes. Glutamine is essential as a transmitter, and AD lesions may produce excess glutamate. The investigation indicated that the source of the glutamate was the keratinocytes and yokukansan controls extracellular glutamate concentrations, suppresses its receptors, and activates glutamate transport in keratinocytes (Wakabayashi et al., 2014). These results suggest that yokukansan affects both the epidermis and the central nervous system. Yokukansan might be an alternative or a complementary therapeutic option for the treatment of AD and inflammatory skin disease.

Rokumigan

Rokumigan is composed of six different crude herbs, *Rehmannia* radix, *Dioscorea* rhizoma, Corni fructus, hoelen, Moutan cortex, and *Alisma* rhizoma (Liao et al., 2014). It is one of the most common herbal formulas used for kidney complaints, edema, and body enrichment. Moreover, this Kampo formula has been reported to possess antiinflammatory, antioxidant, and free radical scavenging activities (Kang et al., 2006). In addition, rokumigan acts by preventing bacterial adhesion rather than by inhibiting growth, which may represent an advantage because bacteria are unlikely to develop resistance. Rokumigan effectively attenuated lipopolysaccharide-induced IL-6 secretion in gingival fibroblasts and epithelial cells and also promoted wound-healing properties (Liao et al., 2014). These attributes suggest that rokumigan may be seen as a powerful adjunctive therapy for inflammatory diseases.

Hochuekkito

Hochuekkito is composed of 10 medicinal plants (Astragali radix, Atractylodis lanceae rhizoma, Ginseng radix, Angelicae radix, Bupleuri radix, Zizyphi fructus, Aurantii nobilis pericarpium, Glycyrrhizae radix, Cimicifugae rhizoma, and Zingiberis rhizoma) (Shimizu, 2013). In experiments using animal models, orally administered hochuekkito exhibited various immunopharmacological effects, particularly antiallergy properties. Moreover, hochuekkito treatment dramatically suppressed serum IgE level and eosinophil infiltration and alleviated AD by controlling Th1/Th2 balance, possibly by the induction of IFN-γ production from intraepithelial lymphocytes (Kobayashi et al., 2003). In addition, it also helps to mitigate leukocytopenia of mice treated with anticancer agents and augments resistance against bacterial infections (Kaneko et al., 1999). A 2010 double-blind, placebo-controlled study showed considerably effective benefits in managing the clinical signs of AD patients with hochuekkito (Kobayashi et al., 2010). In addition, hochuekkito effectively suppressed the dose of topical steroids and/or tacrolimus in AD patients without aggravating AD. Another study demonstrated that hochuekkito treatment alleviated skin damage by reducing oxidative stress in UVB-induced skin damage (Yanagihara et al., 2013). Based on these clinical and preclinical data we can suggest that hochuekkito promotes the recovery of skin impairment and alleviates inflammatory skin diseases and AD.

Jumihaidokuto

Jumihaidokuto, a pharmaceutical-grade traditional Japanese Kampo medicine, is composed of 10 crude components: Platycodi radix, Bupleuri radix, Cnidii rhizoma, *Poria* sclerotium, *Quercus* cortex, Araliae cordatae rhizoma, Schizonepetae radix, Glycyrrhizae radix, Schizonepetae, and Zingiberis rhizoma (Matsumoto et al., 2015). It has been used for the treatment of skin symptoms such as swelling, burning sensation, and reddening in the clinical setting of both acute and chronic skin diseases (Higaki et al., 2002). Jumihaidokuto treatment effectively suppressed inflammation in hapten-induced allergic dermatitis in mouse models and also improved inflammatory acne in patients. In addition, jumihaidokuto attenuated ear thickness in two models of acute dermatitis developed using phorbol myristate acetate or *Propionibacterium acnes*, a gram-positive anaerobic microbe (Nose et al., 1999). Moreover, recently, we have reported that jumihaidokuto treatment effectively suppressed oxidative stress, apoptosis, and inflammatory markers such as IL-4, IL-1β, and IL-2Rα in an acute colitis model (Sreedhar et al., 2015). Furthermore, Pruni cortex (Rosaceae), which is one of the components of jumihaidokuto (Kracie Pharma Ltd., Japan) and is also called the bark of "sakura," has been used in Japan and other Asian countries as a traditional medicine to treat several diseases. We reported that Pruni cortex ameliorates skin inflammation, possibly through the high-mobility group box-1–nuclear factor κB pathway in house dust mite–induced AD in the NC/Nga mouse model (Watanabe et al., 2015). All these findings strongly suggest the use of jumihaidokuto as a therapeutic option for AD and inflammatory skin diseases.

Concluding Remarks

The experimental data discussed in this review show that various Kampo formulas may successfully alleviate or prevent various biochemical and structural alterations in inflammatory skin diseases, including AD. Although the results of human trials are somewhat variable, some studies have provided promising results, especially those using a combination of herbal crude drugs. Nevertheless, more controlled, randomized human clinical trials are required to confirm the efficacy and optimal dosage of Kampo medicines, to further confirm their promise for the treatment of AD and other inflammatory skin diseases.

References

Bieber, T., 2008. Atopic dermatitis. N. Engl. J. Med. 358 (14), 1483–1494.

De Benedetto, A., Kubo, A., Beck, L.A., 2012. Skin barrier disruption: a requirement for allergen sensitization? J. Investig. Dermatol. 132 (3 Pt 2), 949–963.

Funakushi, N., Yamaguchi, T., Jiang, J., Imamura, S., Kuhara, T., Suto, H., Ueki, R., Kase, Y., Kobayashi, H., Ogawa, H., Ikeda, S., 2011. Ameliorating effect of Yokukansan on the development of atopic dermatitis-like lesions and scratching behavior in socially isolated NC/Nga mice. Arch. Dermatol. Res. 303 (9), 659–667.

Furue, M., Terao, H., Rikihisa, W., Urabe, K., Kinukawa, N., Nose, Y., Koga, T., 2003. Clinical dose and adverse effects of topical steroids in daily management of atopic dermatitis. Br. J. Dermatol. 148 (1), 128–133.

Higaki, S., Toyomoto, T., Morohashi, M., 2002. Seijo-bofu-to, Jumi-haidoku-to and Toki-shakuyaku-san suppress rashes and incidental symptoms in acne patients. Drugs Exp. Clin. Res. 28 (5), 193–196.

Hoffjan, S., Epplen, J.T., 2005. The genetics of atopic dermatitis: recent findings and future options. J. Mol. Med. 83 (9), 682–692.

Kaneko, M., Kawakita, T., Kumazawa, Y., Takimoto, H., Nomoto, K., Yoshikawa, T., 1999. Accelerated recovery from cyclophosphamide-induced leukopenia in mice administered a Japanese ethical herbal drug, *Hochu-ekki-to*. Immunopharmacology 44 (3), 223–231.

Kang, D.G., Sohn, E.J., Moon, M.K., Mun, Y.J., Woo, W.H., Kim, M.K., Lee, H.S., 2006. Yukmijihwang-tang ameliorates ischemia/reperfusion-induced renal injury in rats. J. Ethnopharmacol. 104 (1–2), 47–53.

Kawakami, Z., Ikarashi, Y., Kase, Y., 2011. Isoliquiritigenin is a novel NMDA receptor antagonist in kampo medicine yokukansan. Cell. Mol. Neurobiol. 31 (8), 1203–1212.

Kobayashi, H., Ishii, M., Takeuchi, S., Tanaka, Y., Shintani, T., Yamatodani, A., Kusunoki, T., Furue, M., 2010. Efficacy and safety of a traditional herbal medicine, *Hochu-ekki-to* in the long-term management of *Kikyo* (delicate constitution) patients with atopic dermatitis: a 6-month, multicenter, double-blind, randomized, placebo-controlled study. Evid. Based Complement. Alternat. Med. 7 (3), 367–373.

Kobayashi, H., Mizuno, N., Kutsuna, H., Teramae, H., Ueoku, S., Onoyama, J., Yamanaka, K., Fujita, N., Ishii, M., 2003. *Hochu-ekki-to* suppresses development of dermatitis and elevation of serum IgE level in NC/Nga mice. Drugs Exp. Clin. Res. 29 (2), 81–84.

Kuo, I.H., Yoshida, T., De Benedetto, A., Beck, L.A., 2013. The cutaneous innate immune response in patients with atopic dermatitis. J. Allergy Clin. Immunol. 131 (2), 266–278.

Leung, D.Y., Bieber, T., 2003. Atopic dermatitis. Lancet 361 (9352), 151–160.

Leung, D.Y., Jain, N., Leo, H.L., 2003. New concepts in the pathogenesis of atopic dermatitis. Curr. Opin. Immunol. 15 (6), 634–638.

Liao, J., Azelmat, J., Zhao, L., Yoshioka, M., Hinode, D., Grenier, D., 2014. The Kampo medicine Rokumigan possesses antibiofilm, anti-inflammatory, and wound healing properties. BioMed Res. Int. 2014, 436206.

Makino, T., 2005. Pharmacological properties of Gyokuheifusan, a traditional Kampo medicinal formula. Yakugaku Zasshi 125 (4), 349–354.

Matsumoto, T., Matsubara, Y., Mizuhara, Y., Sekiguchi, K., Koseki, J., Tsuchiya, K., Nishimura, H., Watanabe, J., Kaneko, A., Maemura, K., Hattori, T., Kase, Y., 2015. Plasma pharmacokinetics of polyphenols in a traditional Japanese medicine, jumihaidokuto, which suppresses propionibacterium acnes-induced dermatitis in rats. Molecules 20 (10), 18031–18046.

Matsuoka, H., Maki, N., Yoshida, S., Arai, M., Wang, J., Oikawa, Y., Ikeda, T., Hirota, N., Nakagawa, H., Ishii, A., 2003. A mouse model of the atopic eczema/dermatitis syndrome by repeated application of a crude extract of house-dust mite Dermatophagoides farinae. Allergy 58 (2), 139–145.

Nose, M., Sakushima, J., Harada, D., Ogihara, Y., 1999. Comparison of immunopharmacological actions of 8 kinds of kampo-hozais clinically used in atopic dermatitis on delayed-type hypersensitivity in mice. Biol. Pharm. Bull. 22 (1), 48–54.

Novak, N., Kruse, S., Potreck, J., Maintz, L., Jenneck, C., Weidinger, S., Fimmers, R., Bieber, T., 2005. Single nucleotide polymorphisms of the IL18 gene are associated with atopic eczema. J. Allergy Clin. Immunol. 115 (4), 828–833.

Palmer, C.N., Irvine, A.D., Terron-Kwiatkowski, A., Zhao, Y., Liao, H., Lee, S.P., Goudie, D.R., Sandilands, A., Campbell, L.E., Smith, F.J., O'Regan, G.M., Watson, R.M., Cecil, J.E., Bale, S.J., Compton, J.G., DiGiovanna, J.J., Fleckman, P., Lewis-Jones, S., Arseculeratne, G., Sergeant, A., Munro, C.S., El Houate, B., McElreavey, K., Halkjaer, L.B., Bisgaard, H., Mukhopadhyay, S., McLean, W.H., 2006. Common loss-of-function variants of the epidermal barrier protein filaggrin are a major predisposing factor for atopic dermatitis. Nat. Genet. 38 (4), 441–446.

Proksch, E., Jensen, J.M., Elias, P.M., 2003. Skin lipids and epidermal differentiation in atopic dermatitis. Clin. Dermatol. 21 (2), 134–144.

Shimizu, T., 2013. Efficacy of kampo medicine in treating atopic dermatitis: an overview. Evid. Based Complement. Altern. Med. 2013, 260235.

Sreedhar, R., Arumugam, S., Karuppagounder, V., Thandavarayan, R.A., Giridharan, V.V., Pitchaimani, V., Afrin, M.R., Harima, M., Nakamura, T., Nakamura, M., Suzuki, K., Watanabe, K., 2015. Jumihaidokuto effectively inhibits colon inflammation and apoptosis in mice with acute colitis. Int. Immunopharmacol. 29 (2), 957–963.

Tatsumi, T., Yamada, T., Nagai, H., Terasawa, K., Tani, T., Nunome, S., Saiki, I., 2001. A Kampo formulation: byakko-ka-ninjin-to (Bai-Hu-Jia-Ren-Sheng-Tang) inhibits IgE-mediated triphasic skin reaction in mice: the role of its constituents in expression of the efficacy. Biol. Pharm. Bull. 24 (3), 284–290.

Udompataikul, M., Limpa-o-vart, D., 2012. Comparative trial of 5% dexpanthenol in water-in-oil formulation with 1% hydrocortisone ointment in the treatment of childhood atopic dermatitis: a pilot study. J. Drugs Dermatol. 11 (3), 366–374.

Wakabayashi, M., Hasegawa, T., Yamaguchi, T., Funakushi, N., Suto, H., Ueki, R., Kobayashi, H., Ogawa, H., Ikeda, S., 2014. Yokukansan, a traditional Japanese medicine, adjusts glutamate signaling in cultured keratinocytes. BioMed Res. Int. 2014, 364092.

Watanabe, K., Karuppagounder, V., Arumugam, S., Thandavarayan, R.A., Pitchaimani, V., Sreedhar, R., Afrin, R., Harima, M., Suzuki, H., Suzuki, K., Nakamura, T., Nomoto, M., Miyashita, S., Fukumoto, K., Ueno, K., 2015. Pruni cortex ameliorates skin inflammation possibly through HMGB1-NFkappaB pathway in house dust mite induced atopic dermatitis NC/Nga transgenic mice. J. Clin. Biochem. Nutr. 56 (3), 186–194.

Yamashita, H., Tanaka, H., Inagaki, N., 2013. Treatment of the chronic itch of atopic dermatitis using standard drugs and kampo medicines. Biol. Pharm. Bull. 36 (8), 1253–1257.

Yanagi, Y., Yasuda, M., Hashida, K., Kadokura, Y., Yamamoto, T., Suzaki, H., 2008. Mechanism of salivary secretion enhancement by Byakkokaninjinto. Biol. Pharm. Bull. 31 (3), 431–435.

Yanagihara, S., Kobayashi, H., Tamiya, H., Tsuruta, D., Okano, Y., Takahashi, K., Masaki, H., Yamada, T., Hasegawa, S., Akamatsu, H., Ishii, M., 2013. Protective effect of hochuekkito, a Kampo prescription, against ultraviolet B irradiation-induced skin damage in hairless mice. J. Dermatol. 40 (3), 201–206.

Yang, G., Choi, C.H., Lee, K., Lee, M., Ham, I., Choi, H.Y., 2013. Effects of Catalpa ovata stem bark on atopic dermatitis-like skin lesions in NC/Nga mice. J. Ethnopharmacol. 145 (2), 416–423.

CHAPTER 11

Japanese Kampo Medicine for Hepatic Inflammation

Remya Sreedhar[1], Geetha Kandasamy[2], Shanish Antony[3], Somasundaram Arumugam[1]

[1]Niigata University of Pharmacy and Applied Life Sciences, Niigata, Japan; [2]KMCH College of Pharmacy, Coimbatore, Tamilnadu, India; [3]Government Medical College, Kottayam, India

Introduction

Hepatic inflammatory conditions are mostly multifactorial diseases having close correlations with metabolic disorders. This makes their treatment difficult using a single pharmacological drug. The use of plant extracts/decoctions or polyherbal formulations to treat various liver diseases is very common in various traditional systems of medicine (Ayurveda, traditional Chinese, and Japanese Kampo medicine). Medicinal herbs are known for their multifaceted implications and thus can make up an effective treatment schedule against hepatic inflammation (Jadeja et al., 2014). In this chapter, we discuss the available reports classified based on Kampo medicine along with their identified uses for various liver inflammation–related disorders.

Daikenchuto

Daikenchuto is a Japanese Kampo medicine prepared by Tsumura & Co., containing processed ginger, ginseng, and *Zanthoxylum* fruit. Daikenchuto treatment suppresses the inflammatory reaction, stimulates bowel movement, and improves oral intake after hepatic resection, which may decrease serious morbidity after hepatic resection (Nishi et al., 2012). Sinusoidal obstruction syndrome is drug-induced liver injury that occurs in patients who receive hematopoietic cell transplantation and chemotherapy with oxaliplatin. Daikenchuto attenuates monocrotaline-induced liver injury by preventing neutrophil-mediated liver damage through blockage of the upregulation of cytokine-induced neutrophil chemoattractant and intracellular adhesion molecule-1 mRNA levels (Narita et al., 2009). Daikenchuto prevents bacterial translocation in rats exposed to the stress of fasting, activation of hepatic stellate cells, and subsequent hepatic fibrosis. It may prevent the progression of hepatic fibrosis in children with biliary atresia and improve their prognosis (Yada et al., 2016).

Despite these favorable results with daikenchuto treatment, caution should be practiced while prescribing to patients with hepatic dysfunction, as it may aggravate the condition. The patient's progress should be carefully monitored, and if no improvement in symptoms/ findings is observed, continuous treatment should be avoided ("TSUMURA Daikenchuto Extract Granules for Ethical Use," 2014).

Shosaikoto

Shosaikoto, one of the most frequently prescribed Kampo medicines, is used to treat chronic hepatitis and has shown confirmed clinical efficacy. It is a mixture of seven herbal preparations; *Bupleurum* root, *Pinellia* tuber, *Scutellaria* root, ginseng, jujube, licorice, and ginger. It is widely administered in Japan to patients with chronic hepatitis and cirrhosis. In a prospective study, this herbal medicine was found to play a chemopreventive role in the development of hepatocellular carcinoma in cirrhotic patients. It functions as a potent antifibrosuppressant via the inhibition of oxidative stress in hepatocytes and hepatic stellate cells, and its active components are baicalin and baicalein (Shimizu, 2000). Shosaikoto treatment to rats prevented endotoxin-induced hypoferremia and inhibited the activity of hepatic δ-aminolevulinate synthetase and cytochrome P-450 level 18 h after endotoxin injection. Similarly, shosaikoto significantly depressed the endotoxin-induced increase in heme oxygenase activity in liver microsomes. Shosaikoto may therefore protect rats against lethality caused by endotoxin through its ability to regulate the heme metabolism in septic shock (Sakaguchi et al., 2005).

However, caution must be exercised in conditions such as existing lung impairment, concurrent interferon usage, additional glycyrrhizin intake, and serious preexisting liver damage. Its intake is contraindicated during pregnancy and lactation, migraine, very high blood pressure (systolic over 180 mm Hg), and epistaxis (nose bleeds) (Wen, 2006).

Keishibukuryogan

Keishibukuryogan is one of the Kampo medicines and has been widely administered to patients with blood stagnation for improving blood circulation. It is now one of the most frequently used medicines in Japan. It is composed of five medicinal plants, *Cinnamomum cassia* Blume (Cinnamomi cortex), *Paeonia lactiflora* Pallas (Paeoniae radix), *Paeonia suffruticosa* Andrews (Moutan cortex), *Prunus persica* Batsch (Persicae semen), and *Poria cocos* Wolf (hoelen). Paeoniae radix and Moutan cortex have many known active components in common, including paeoniflorin, paeonol, oxypaeoniflorin, benzoylpaeoniflorin, and palbinone (Yoshihisa et al., 2010). This formula is frequently used in traditional Japanese and Chinese medicine to treat several symptoms and manifests antiinflammatory and scavenging effects. Treatment with keishibukuryogan led to a significant reduction in liver injury tests and blood cholesterol but had no effects on body weight in all nonalcoholic fatty liver disease cases tested. Further, liver tests and lipid profiles returned to baseline values when keishibukuryogan treatment was stopped (Fujimoto et al., 2010).

Despite these beneficial effects, keishibukuryogan treatment may cause hepatic dysfunction, with increased aspartate transaminase (AST/GOT), alanine aminotransferase (ALT/GPT), plasma alkaline phosphatase (Al-P), and gamma glutamyl-transpeptidase (γ-GTP) levels, and/or jaundice may occur. The patient should be carefully monitored for abnormal findings. Administration should be discontinued and appropriate therapeutic measures should be taken, if abnormalities are observed. Hypersensitivity reactions such as rashes, redness, and pruritis and gastrointestinal abnormalities such as anorexia, epigastric distress, nausea, and diarrhea may occur as adverse effects. Caution must be exercised in elderly patients and during pregnancy (peach kernel and Moutan bark may cause premature birth or abortion) ("TSUMURA Keishibukuryogan Extract Granules for Ethical Use," 2007).

Juzentaihoto

Juzentaihoto is a Kampo medicine and is a nourishing agent, a so-called "hozai" (in Japanese), that is used for improving disturbances and imbalances in the homeostatic condition of the body. It contains *Astragalus* root, cinnamon bark, *Rehmannia* root, peony root, *Cnidium* rhizome, *Atractylodes lancea* rhizome, Japanese *Angelica* root, ginseng, *Poria* sclerotium, and *Glycyrrhiza* ("TSUMURA Juzentaihoto Extract Granules for Ethical Use," 2014). This drug is administered to patients with various debilitating conditions, including postsurgery patients and patients with chronic illnesses, for whom it can alleviate general symptoms such as extreme fatigue, pale complexion, loss of appetite, dry or scaly skin, night sweating, and dryness of the mouth (Saiki, 2000). Juzentaihoto inhibits the progression of liver tumors in a dose-dependent manner and contributes to long-term survival (Okumi and Koyama, 2014).

Care must be taken when treating patients with a weak gastrointestinal tract and with anorexia, nausea, and vomiting. Eczema and dermatitis may be aggravated by its use ("TSUMURA Juzentaihoto Extract Granules for Ethical Use," 2014).

Ninjinyoeito

Most physicians who practice Kampo medicine in Japan have observed that Kampo medicine therapy can be as effective as interferon therapy in the treatment of chronic hepatitis C. Ninjinyoeito (TJ-108) was very effective on chronic hepatitis C virus (HCV) infection, and its therapeutic effect is due to the inhibitory effect on HCV infection and also the protective effect on immunological hepatopathy of *Schisandra* fruit and its lignan component, gomisin A. Gomishi is the dried fruit of *Schisandra chinensis* Baillon (Fructus Schisandrae chinensis, FSC) and has been used as a Japanese Kampo medicine to treat inflammatory and liver diseases. It is included as one of the components of seishoekkito, ninjinyoeito, and seihaito. The antiinflammatory activity of FSC and its constituents was analyzed, and it was demonstrated that gomisin N and γ-schizandrin are involved in the hepatoprotective effect of the FSC extract, which has therapeutic potential for liver disease (Takimoto et al., 2013).

Caution must be exercised in patients with a weak gastrointestinal tract and with anorexia, nausea, and vomiting. Eczema and dermatitis may be aggravated by its use ("TSUMURA Ninjin'yoeito Extract Granules for Ethical Use," 2013).

Inchinkoto

Inchinkoto (TJ-135) is an herbal medicine consisting of three kinds of crude drugs, and in Japan it is administered mainly to patients with cholestasis. Administration of inchinkoto may be useful in patients with severe acute hepatitis accompanying cholestasis or in those with autoimmune hepatitis, by inhibiting the production of inflammatory cytokines and enhancing the production of antiinflammatory cytokines (Yamashiki et al., 2000). This traditional Japanese Kampo medicine is used in eastern Asia as a choleretic and hepatoprotective agent. Inchinkoto ameliorates murine concanavalin A–induced hepatitis via suppression of interferon-γ and interleukin-12 production. Its major components, inchinko and sanshishi, both may contribute to the protective effects of inchinkoto against concanavalin A hepatitis. Capillarisin was found to be potently hepatoprotective, and genipin may also contribute, especially via modulation of cytokine production (Mase et al., 2010). Adverse effects and contraindications are similar to those of keishibukuryogan ("TSUMURA Inchinkoto Extract Granules for Ethical Use," 2014).

Others

Ampelopsis brevipedunculata (Maxim.) Trautv. (Vitaceae) has been used in Japanese herbal folk medicine to treat liver disease. A feeding regimen with *A. brevipedunculata* extract inhibited the progression of hepatic injury induced by carbon tetrachloride in mice (Yabe and Matsui, 2000).

Herbal compound 861, which is made of 10 herbs, with *Salvia miltiorrhiza* as its chief component, has been shown experimentally to be effective in suppressing fibrogenesis, enhancing collagen degradation, and inhibiting tissue inhibitor of metallopeptidase expression. Clinically, an open trial of 2000 patients showed improvement of symptoms in 83% and normalization of serum ALT in 82%. In a controlled study of 107 patients with hepatitis B virus-related disease, double liver biopsies showed that the fibrosis reversal rate after 6 months of treatment with compound 861 was 78% in S2, 82% in S3 (precirrhotic stage), and 75% in S4 (early cirrhosis), as assessed by Scheuer and Chevallier's criterion (Wang, 2000). In addition, compound 861 prevents hepatocarcinogenesis in diethylnitrosamine and 2-acetylaminofluorene–induced liver preneoplastic lesions in rats (Cui et al., 2003).

Caution

The combined use of Kampo medicines with Western medicines may cause unexpected adverse events including undesirable drug–drug interactions. This may be because they were originally developed for their individual use and not in combination with any Western medicine. Although adverse effects of Kampo medicines are rare compared with those of Western medicines, severe events such as liver dysfunction and interstitial pneumonia have been reported in increasing trends. Medical staff, including pharmacists, therefore, should be aware of the onset of adverse events before the patient's symptoms become severe. These issues should also be addressed in educational materials for students of clinical pharmacy and pharmacy practice (Homma, 2016).

References

Cui, R., Wang, B., Zhang, F., Chen, G., Yin, S., 2003. Suppressive effect of herbal compound 861 on chemical hepatocarcinogenesis in rats. Chin. Med. J. (Engl.) 116 (3), 378–382. Retrieved from: http://www.ncbi.nlm.nih.gov/pubmed/12781041.

Fujimoto, M., Tsuneyama, K., Kinoshita, H., Goto, H., Takano, Y., Selmi, C., et al., 2010. The traditional Japanese formula keishibukuryogan reduces liver injury and inflammation in patients with nonalcoholic fatty liver disease. Ann. N. Y Acad. Sci. 1190, 151–158. http://dx.doi.org/10.1111/j.1749-6632.2009.05265.x.

Homma, M., 2016. Education Program of kampo-medicine for Undergraduates in preparation for clinical Setting. Yakugaku Zasshi 136 (3), 417–422. http://dx.doi.org/10.1248/yakushi.15-00232-4.

Jadeja, R., Devkar, R.V., Nammi, S., 2014. Herbal medicines for the treatment of nonalcoholic steatohepatitis: current scenario and future prospects. Evid. Based Complement. Alternat. Med. 2014, 648308. http://dx.doi.org/10.1155/2014/648308.

Mase, A., Makino, B., Tsuchiya, N., Yamamoto, M., Kase, Y., Takeda, S., Hasegawa, T., 2010. Active ingredients of traditional Japanese (kampo) medicine, inchinkoto, in murine concanavalin A-induced hepatitis. J. Ethnopharmacol. 127 (3), 742–749. http://dx.doi.org/10.1016/j.jep.2009.11.029.

Narita, M., Hatano, E., Tamaki, N., Yamanaka, K., Yanagida, A., Nagata, H., et al., 2009. Dai-kenchu-to attenuates rat sinusoidal obstruction syndrome by inhibiting the accumulation of neutrophils in the liver. J. Gastroenterol. Hepatol. 24 (6), 1051–1057. http://dx.doi.org/10.1111/j.1440-1746.2009.05795.x.

Nishi, M., Shimada, M., Uchiyama, H., Ikegami, T., Arakawa, Y., Hanaoka, J., et al., 2012. The beneficial effects of kampo medicine Dai-ken-chu-to after hepatic resection: a prospective randomized control study. Hepatogastroenterology 59 (119), 2290–2294. http://dx.doi.org/10.5754/hge10115.

Okumi, H., Koyama, A., 2014. Kampo medicine for palliative care in Japan. Biopsychosoc. Med. 8 (1), 6. http://dx.doi.org/10.1186/1751-0759-8-6.

Saiki, I., 2000. A kampo medicine "Juzen-taiho-to"—prevention of malignant progression and metastasis of tumor cells and the mechanism of action. Biol. Pharm. Bull. 23 (6), 677–688. Retrieved from: http://www.ncbi.nlm.nih.gov/pubmed/10864015.

Sakaguchi, S., Furusawa, S., Iizuka, Y., 2005. Preventive effects of a traditional Chinese medicine (Sho-saiko-to) on septic shock symptoms; approached from heme metabolic disorders in endotoxemia. Biol. Pharm. Bull. 28 (1), 165–168. Retrieved from: http://www.ncbi.nlm.nih.gov/pubmed/15635185.

Shimizu, I., 2000. Sho-saiko-to: Japanese herbal medicine for protection against hepatic fibrosis and carcinoma. J. Gastroenterol. Hepatol. 15 (Suppl.), D84–D90. Retrieved from: http://www.ncbi.nlm.nih.gov/pubmed/10759225.

Takimoto, Y., Qian, H.Y., Yoshigai, E., Okumura, T., Ikeya, Y., Nishizawa, M., 2013. Gomisin N in the herbal drug gomishi (*Schisandra chinensis*) suppresses inducible nitric oxide synthase gene via C/EBPbeta and NF-kappaB in rat hepatocytes. Nitric Oxide 28, 47–56. http://dx.doi.org/10.1016/j.niox.2012.10.003.

Tsumura & Co. (Ed.), 2014. TSUMURA Daikenchuto Extract Granules for Ethical Use, tenth ed.

Tsumura & Co. (Ed.), 2014. TSUMURA Inchinkoto Extract Granules for Ethical Use, seventh ed.

Tsumura & Co. (Ed.), 2014. TSUMURA Juzentaihoto Extract Granules for Ethical Use, seventh ed.

Tsumura & Co. (Ed.), 2007. TSUMURA Keishibukuryogan Extract Granules for Ethical Use, sixth ed.

Tsumura & Co. (Ed.), 2013. TSUMURA Ninjin'yoeito Extract Granules for Ethical Use, sixth ed.

Wang, B.E., 2000. Treatment of chronic liver diseases with traditional Chinese medicine. J. Gastroenterol. Hepatol. 15 (Suppl.), E67–E70. Retrieved from: http://www.ncbi.nlm.nih.gov/pubmed/10921385.

Wen, D., 2006. Announcing SST (Sho-saiko-to): The All Natural Prescription-strength Liver Remedy from Japan. Retrieved from: http://www.shosaikoto.com/cautions.php.

Yabe, N., Matsui, H., 2000. Ampelopsis brevipedunculata (Vitaceae) extract inhibits a progression of carbon tetrachloride-induced hepatic injury in the mice. Phytomedicine 7 (6), 493–498. http://dx.doi.org/10.1016/S0944-7113(00)80035-5.

Yada, K., Ishibashi, H., Mori, H., Morine, Y., Zhu, C., Feng, R., et al., 2016. The Kampo medicine "Daikenchuto (TU-100)" prevents bacterial translocation and hepatic fibrosis in a rat model of biliary atresia. Surgery 159 (6), 1600–1611. http://dx.doi.org/10.1016/j.surg.2016.02.002.

Yamashiki, M., Mase, A., Arai, I., Huang, X.X., Nobori, T., Nishimura, A., et al., 2000. Effects of the Japanese herbal medicine "Inchinko-to" (TJ-135) on concanavalin A-induced hepatitis in mice. Clin. Sci. (Lond.) 99 (5), 421–431. Retrieved from: http://www.ncbi.nlm.nih.gov/pubmed/11052923.

Yoshihisa, Y., Furuichi, M., Ur Rehman, M., Ueda, C., Makino, T., Shimizu, T., 2010. The traditional Japanese formula keishibukuryogan inhibits the production of inflammatory cytokines by dermal endothelial cells. Mediators Inflamm. 2010, 804298. http://dx.doi.org/10.1155/2010/804298.

CHAPTER 12

Kampo Medicines for Autoimmune Disorders: Rheumatoid Arthritis and Autoimmune Diabetes Mellitus

Kenichi Watanabe, Vengadeshprabhu Karuppagounder, Remya Sreedhar, Meilei Harima, Somasundaram Arumugam
Niigata University of Pharmacy and Applied Life Sciences, Niigata, Japan

Introduction

Autoimmune diseases (AIDs) are characterized by irregular functioning of the immune system that causes an individual immune system to generate antibodies that attack their own body tissues. Approximately 75% or more of those affected by AIDs are women (Smith and Germolec, 1999). The initiation of attack against the body's self-molecules in most instances is unknown, but a number of studies suggest that they are powerfully linked with factors such as genetics, infections, and the environment. It is now deemed probable that many chronic inflammatory and destructive diseases are autoimmune, including rheumatoid arthritis (RA), Graves' disease, Sjogren's syndrome, and Hashimoto's thyroiditis, all affecting about 1% of the world population. In addition, AIDs comprise less common diseases such as type 1 diabetes, Crohn's disease, vitiligo, systemic lupus erythematosus, multiple sclerosis, autoimmune myocarditis, pernicious anemia, and primary biliary cirrhosis. More than 80 types of AIDs have been identified worldwide (Cho and Feldman, 2015). These diseases are known by their primary target organ, such as skin, central nervous system, intestine, and pancreas. For type 1 diabetes mellitus and autoimmune thyroid disease, extensive tissue destruction antedates disease presentation; hence the primary therapy remains hormone replacement, as opposed to antiinflammatory agents, in both of these diseases.

In some instances, the antibodies may not be aimed at a specific tissue or organ; for instance, antiphospholipid antibodies can react with substances such as phospholipids that are the normal components of platelets, and the outermost layer of cellular telephones, which can contribute to the establishment of blood clots within the blood vessels as in thrombosis. Autoimmunity is most commonly exhibited in late childhood to early maturity; additional phenotypic variability probably arises from factors that emerge during evolution, such as autoantibody formation and epigenetic programming, as well as from environmental agents. However, the differentiating features of AIDs provide a conceptual framework within which to accelerate the development and application of novel therapeutic agents (Cho and Feldman, 2015). The background of AIDs is multifactorial and remains unclear. Nevertheless, the existence of a strong genetic component determining susceptibility to these diseases is well recognized. Recently, medicinal herbs have come forth as a therapeutic option for the treatment of AIDs with minimal side effects, compared with modern drugs. Moreover, Japanese traditional Kampo medicines have attracted considerable attention (Venkatesha et al., 2011). Thus, here we discuss the evidence that supports the use of Kampo medicines as an antiinflammatory agent. We also discuss the possible molecular targets of Kampo formulas in AIDs.

Possible Mechanisms Underlying the Pathogenesis of Autoimmune Diseases

Immune System

Various parts of the immune system may be involved in AID pathology. Antigens are taken up by antigen-presenting cells (APCs) such as dendritic cells (DCs) and processed into peptides, which are loaded onto the major histocompatibility complex (MHC) molecules for presentation to T cells via their receptors. Cytotoxic T cells can directly damage a target, whereas T helper cells (Th; activated by MHC class II) release cytokines that can cause direct effects or activate macrophages, monocytes, and B cells. Surface antigens bind to B-cell receptors; upon receiving signals from Th cells, the B cell secretes antibodies specific for antigens. An antibody may bind to its specific target alone or may bind to and activate macrophages simultaneously via the Fc receptor (Ercolini and Miller, 2009).

A nonprofessional APC does not constitutively express the MHC class II proteins required for binding to native T cells; these are expressed only once the nonprofessional APCs are stimulated by cytokines such as interferon (IFN)-γ. Other key players in AIDs are messenger molecules called cytokines and chemokines (Ercolini and Miller, 2009). Cytokines are proteins that can trigger immune cells and affect nonimmune processes and thereby cause inflammation and harm. Chemokines are small particles that attract other immune cells and can lead to the invasion and inflammation of the target organ. For instance, overproduction of cytokines and chemokines leads to autoimmune myocarditis and RA.

Toll-Like Receptors in Autoimmunity

Toll-like receptors (TLRs), the best-characterized pattern recognition receptors, were first reported in humans in 1998. TLRs can be classified based on their localization in the cell, so that TLR1, 2, 4, 5, and 6 are expressed on the cell membrane, whereas TLR3, 7, 8, and 9 are localized mainly in the endosomal compartment (Kawai and Akira, 2007). Moreover, ligands binding to TLRs lead to the expression of some immune response genes, including inflammatory cytokines, stimulatory immune cytokines, chemokines, and costimulatory molecules

(Li et al., 2009). Considering the role of TLRs as a vital connection between the natural and the adaptive immune responses, the idea has occurred that continuous activation or dysregulation of TLR signaling may lead to the pathogenesis of autoimmunity (Abdollahi-Roodsaz et al., 2007; Fischer and Ehlers, 2008).

Systemic AIDs are frequently connected with the production of autoantibodies that react with nuclear or cytosolic cellular components, which are mainly involved in the immunopathogenesis of various AIDs (Green and Marshak-Rothstein, 2011). Numerous previous studies demonstrated that Th17 and Th1 cells or the interleukin (IL)-17$^+$IFN-γ^+ cluster of differentiation (CD)-4$^+$ T cells may have pathogenic roles in chronic inflammation and AIDs. Before the discovery of Th17 cells, it was believed that Th1 cells were the primary pathogenic cell population in T-cell-mediated AIDs. Moreover, mice deficient in IFN-γ or IL-12 were found to have enhanced susceptibility to collagen-induced arthritis and experimental autoimmune encephalomyelitis (Cua et al., 2003; Mohammad Hosseini et al., 2015).

Role of High-Mobility Group Protein-1 in Autoimmunity

The nuclear protein high-mobility group protein-1 (HMGB1) is a proinflammatory cytokine associated with the development of several AIDs. It is mainly secreted from immune cells, such as DCs, monocytes, and macrophages, and damaged cells. Extracellular HMGB1 can interact with the receptor for advanced glycation endproducts, TLR2, and TLR4; there is also a possibility that different regions in HMGB1 interact with different receptors (Karuppagounder et al., 2016). In acute inflammatory events like sepsis, HMGB1 plays a significant part in the course of systemic immune reaction. In vitro and in a mouse model, administration of endotoxin led to the release of HMGB1 from macrophages with measurably augmented extracellular levels (Pilzweger and Holdenrieder, 2015). The same effect occurs after addition of tumor necrosis factor (TNF) or IL-1 in vitro. Likewise, in RA, a positive proinflammatory feedback loop was found, in which HMGB1 induces release of TNFα from activated macrophages, which in turn induces translocation to the cytosol in macrophages. HMGB1 was also shown to promote angiogenesis in RA via enhanced expression of vascular endothelial growth factor and hypoxia-inducible factor-1α activation (Park et al., 2015).

Kampo Medicines for Autoimmune Diseases

Herbal medicines have been used in Japan for more than 1500 years, and traditional Japanese Kampo medicines are now fully integrated into the modern health care system. In addition, more than 100 Kampo medicines are officially approved as prescription drugs and covered by the national health insurance system in Japan. Moreover, Kampo medicines are dispensed at all the university, national, and foundation hospitals in Japan as prescription drugs, frequently in combination with Western drugs. Rooted in Chinese medicine, the knowledge of Kampo medicine has been transmitted from generation to generation for

1500 years (Motoo et al., 2011). Nevertheless, because of the problem of cultivating and procuring identical species of some of the herbs in the Chinese formulas, together with the limited maritime commerce at the time, Kampo followed a decidedly unique path of development in the Japanese archipelago. Consequently, there is a stark difference between Chinese and Japanese herbal formulas (Kono et al., 2015). A study showed that, of 900 physicians surveyed, 92.4% reported having prescribed Kampo medicines, 73.5% of which were for cancer patients. Only 9.7% of the physicians reported that they considered Kampo medicines to be harmful (Ito et al., 2012).

Furthermore, Kampo medicines are useful for treating AIDs such as RA and type 1 diabetes. Extensive clinical and preclinical data suggest that Kampo formulas have been used effectively against AIDs and immune disorders. In the following, we discuss the antiinflammatory and immune-regulating activities of Kampo medicines in preventing and alleviating the complications of AIDs, with a focus on RA and diabetes.

Kampo Medicines for Rheumatoid Arthritis

RA is a common AID characterized by continual inflammatory synovitis usually involving peripheral joints in a symmetric distribution, the cause of which lies in immune regulatory factors such as the loss of tolerance (Verbrugge et al., 2015). The synovial inflammation, if uncontrolled, may contribute to cartilage damage, bone erosion, and ankylosis of the affected joints (Gorman and Cope, 2008). In this case mostly women are affected compared with men. The usual age of onset is between the late 1920s and the early 1950s, although no age is immune to the disease (Venkatesha et al., 2011). Moreover, a previous study reported that RA is a genetic immune disorder and about 70% of patients have an HLA-DR4 or DR1 allele or both (Gorman and Cope, 2008). Nevertheless, the precise mechanisms or target autoantigens have not been distinguished for RA. HMGB1, type II collagen, aggrecan, immunoglobulin-binding protein, and heat shock protein 65 are among the antigens that have been implicated in the pathogenesis of RA. The nonsteroidal antiinflammatory drugs are the mainstay of therapy for a large proportion of patients with RA. However, because of the severe adverse reactions, high cost, and limited efficacy of these drugs in many patients, the use of complementary and alternative medicines by RA patients is becoming increasingly popular in developed and developing countries (Cibere et al., 2003). Since ancient times, many kinds of Kampo medicines have been used traditionally and are found to be clinically effective for RA treatment. These formulas usually contain ingredients from various medicinal plants that are supposed to exert antiinflammatory and immune-regulator effects and are efficient for treating RA.

Keishinieppiittokaryojutsubu

Keishinieppiittokaryojutsubu (KER) is composed of 12 crude medicinal herbs: Atractylodis lanceae rhizoma, hoelen, Gypsum fibrosum, Zizyphi fructus, Cinnamomi cortex, Ephedrae herba, Paeoniae radix, Glycyrrhizae radix, Zingiberis rhizoma, Aconiti tuber, Sinomeni caulis et rhizoma, and Astragali radix (Kogure et al., 2010). It is one of the representative Kampo formulas for the treatment of RA. Moreover, this Kampo formula is reported to possess antiinflammatory properties. In addition, KER treatment effectively suppresses serum IL-6, TNFα, and IL-17 in patients with RA (Kogure et al., 2009).

Keishibukuryogan

Keishibukuryogan (KBG) is a Kampo formula composed of five crude medicinal herbs: Cinnamomi cortex, Paeoniae radix, Moutan cortex, Persicae semen, and hoelen. It is usually applied to treat thrombotic disease and coronary artery disease. Moreover, KBG improves microcirculation in patients with multiple old lacunar infarction (Hikiami et al., 2003), and also prevents the progression of atherosclerosis and preserves endothelium-dependent vasorelaxation in a cholesterol-fed rabbit model (Sekiya et al., 1999). Another study performed with 16 RA patients who received KBG (12 g/day) for 12 weeks showed that KBG treatment effectively decreased disease activity, tender joint count, soluble CD106, and lipid peroxide (Nozaki et al., 2006). A similar study reported that KBG treatment effectively ameliorated RA (Ogawa et al., 2007). Furthermore, the plasma and endothelial nitric oxide synthase (NOS) and CD106 levels were significantly attenuated by KBG treatment in adjuvant-induced arthritis rats (Nozaki et al., 2007).

Kanzobushito

Kanzobushito (KBT) is also one of the Japanese traditional Kampo medicines for AIDs such as RA. It is composed of the following crude herbs: Cinnamomi cortex, Glycyrrhizae radix, Atractylodis lanceae rhizoma, and Aconiti tuber. Treatment with KBT effectively decreased tartrate-resistant acid phosphatase-positive cells at the synovium–bone interface and at the sites of focal bone erosion, coincident with the findings that the receptor activator of nuclear factor-κB ligand (RANKL)/osteoprotegerin (OPG) mRNA ratio was significantly reduced by KBT treatment. It also decreased mRNA levels of macrophage colony-stimulating factor (M-CSF) and inducible NOS in peritoneal macrophages and joints of collagen-induced arthritic mice (Ono et al., 2004). These findings suggest that KBT is a potential new therapeutic agent for the treatment of RA.

Daibofuto

Daibofuto (DBT) is a Kampo medicine composed of 15 crude herbs: Glycyrrhizae radix, Atractylodis lanceae rhizoma, Zingiberis rhizoma, Paeoniae radix, Zizyphi fructus, Aconiti tuber, Glehniae radix cum rhizoma, Angelicae radix, Rehmanniae radix, Cnidii rhizome, Ginseng radix, Achyranthis radix, Eucommiae cortex, Notopterygii rhizoma, and Astragali radix. It is given to patients who have been afflicted with RA for a long time and as a result have reduced physical strength. DBT treatment effectively reduced the ratio of RANKL/OPG and suppressed M-CSF mRNA levels (Inoue et al., 2004). These outcomes indicate that antiosteoclastogenic and immuno-modulatory effects of DBT effectively suppressed collagen-induced arthritis in mice.

Kampo Medicines for Autoimmune Diabetes

Insulin-dependent diabetes mellitus (IDDM) is the classical life-threatening kind of diabetes. Most patients with IDDM present when young, and the peak age of onset is 11–13 years (Neil et al., 1987). It is characterized by the progressive and selective destruction of β cells in the islets of Langerhans and is believed to involve a crucial role of the autoimmune reaction (Cooke and Mandell, 1994; Tisch et al., 1993). The islets of Langerhans of diabetic patients and animals are heavily infiltrated with mononuclear cells, most of which are T cells and macrophages. Infiltrating T cells include both CD4+ and CD8+ cells and mainly produce cytokines and proinflammatory factors (O'Reilly et al., 1991). Activated cytokines lead to the development of diabetes, which may be due to either a direct toxic effect on β cells or their use in determining the differentiation and function of T cells (Ploix et al., 1998).

Ninjinto

Ninjinto (NJT) is a Kampo medicine composed of four crude herbs: Zingiberis siccatum rhizoma, Glycyrrhizae radix, Atractylodis lanceae rhizoma, and Ginseng radix. Long-term administration of NJT prevents the progression of insulitis and the development of diabetes in the spontaneous model of nonobese diabetes (NOD) mice. Moreover, NJT treatment effectively suppresses blood glucose and IFN-γ levels, followed by increased IL-4 levels, in the NOD mouse model (Kobayashi et al., 2000). All these findings suggest that the Kampo medicine NJT has the ability to modulate cytokine production in the autoimmune diabetic condition.

Concluding Remarks

The preclinical and clinical data discussed in this chapter show that some Kampo formulas might successfully mitigate or prevent various biochemical and structural alterations in AIDs, including RA and autoimmune diabetes. Although the effects in human trials are somewhat variable, some studies have provided promising results, particularly those using a compounding of different herbal crude drugs.

References

Abdollahi-Roodsaz, S., Joosten, L.A., Roelofs, M.F., Radstake, T.R., Matera, G., Popa, C., et al., 2007. Inhibition of Toll-like receptor 4 breaks the inflammatory loop in autoimmune destructive arthritis. Arthritis Rheum. 56 (9), 2957–2967. http://dx.doi.org/10.1002/art.22848.

Cho, J.H., Feldman, M., 2015. Heterogeneity of autoimmune diseases: pathophysiologic insights from genetics and implications for new therapies. Nat. Med. 21 (7), 730–738. http://dx.doi.org/10.1038/nm.3897.

Cibere, J., Deng, Z., Lin, Y., Ou, R., He, Y., Wang, Z., et al., 2003. A randomized double blind, placebo controlled trial of topical *Tripterygium wilfordii* in rheumatoid arthritis: reanalysis using logistic regression analysis. J. Rheumatol. 30 (3), 465–467. Retrieved from: http://www.ncbi.nlm.nih.gov/pubmed/12610802.

Cooke, A., Mandell, T., 1994. Spontaneous loss of T-cell tolerance to glutamic acid decarboxylase in murine insulin-dependent diabetes. J. Endocrinol. Invest. 17 (7), 585–593. Retrieved from: http://www.ncbi.nlm.nih.gov/pubmed/7829834.

Cua, D.J., Sherlock, J., Chen, Y., Murphy, C.A., Joyce, B., Seymour, B., et al., 2003. Interleukin-23 rather than interleukin-12 is the critical cytokine for autoimmune inflammation of the brain. Nature 421 (6924), 744–748. http://dx.doi.org/10.1038/nature01355.

Ercolini, A.M., Miller, S.D., 2009. The role of infections in autoimmune disease. Clin. Exp. Immunol. 155 (1), 1–15. http://dx.doi.org/10.1111/j.1365-2249.2008.03834.x.

Fischer, M., Ehlers, M., 2008. Toll-like receptors in autoimmunity. Ann. N. Y. Acad. Sci. 1143, 21–34. http://dx.doi.org/10.1196/annals.1443.012.

Gorman, C.L., Cope, A.P., 2008. Immune-mediated pathways in chronic inflammatory arthritis. Best Pract. Res. Clin. Rheumatol. 22 (2), 221–238. http://dx.doi.org/10.1016/j.berh.2008.01.003.

Green, N.M., Marshak-Rothstein, A., 2011. Toll-like receptor driven B cell activation in the induction of systemic autoimmunity. Semin. Immunol. 23 (2), 106–112. http://dx.doi.org/10.1016/j.smim.2011.01.016.

Hikiami, H., Goto, H., Sekiya, N., Hattori, N., Sakakibara, I., Shimada, Y., Terasawa, K., 2003. Comparative efficacy of Keishi-bukuryo-gan and pentoxifylline on RBC deformability in patients with "oketsu" syndrome. Phytomedicine 10 (6–7), 459–466. http://dx.doi.org/10.1078/094471103322331395.

Inoue, M., Ono, Y., Mizukami, H., 2004. Suppressive effect of Dai-bofu-to on collagen-induced arthritis. Biol. Pharm. Bull. 27 (6), 857–862. Retrieved from: http://www.ncbi.nlm.nih.gov/pubmed/15187433.

Ito, A., Munakata, K., Imazu, Y., Watanabe, K., 2012. First nationwide attitude survey of Japanese physicians on the use of traditional Japanese medicine (kampo) in cancer treatment. Evid. Based Complement. Altern. Med. 2012, 957082. http://dx.doi.org/10.1155/2012/957082.

Karuppagounder, V., Arumugam, S., Thandavarayan, R.A., Sreedhar, R., Giridharan, V.V., Watanabe, K., 2016. Molecular targets of quercetin with anti-inflammatory properties in atopic dermatitis. Drug Discov. Today 21 (4), 632–639. http://dx.doi.org/10.1016/j.drudis.2016.02.011.

Kawai, T., Akira, S., 2007. TLR signaling. Semin. Immunol. 19 (1), 24–32. http://dx.doi.org/10.1016/j.smim.2006.12.004.

Kobayashi, T., Song, Q.H., Hong, T., Kitamura, H., Cyong, J.C., 2000. Preventive effect of Ninjin-to (Ren-Shen-Tang), a Kampo (Japanese traditional) formulation, on spontaneous autoimmune diabetes in non-obese diabetic (NOD) mice. Microbiol. Immunol. 44 (4), 299–305. Retrieved from: http://www.ncbi.nlm.nih.gov/pubmed/10832976.

Kogure, T., Sato, H., Kishi, D., Ito, T., Tatsumi, T., 2009. Serum levels of anti-cyclic citrullinated peptide antibodies are associated with a beneficial response to traditional herbal medicine (kampo) in rheumatoid arthritis. Rheumatol. Int. 29 (12), 1441–1447. http://dx.doi.org/10.1007/s00296-009-0877-8.

Kogure, T., Tatsumi, T., Sato, H., Oku, Y., Kishi, D., Ito, T., 2010. Traditional herbal medicines (kampo) for patients with rheumatoid arthritis receiving concomitant methotrexate: a preliminary study. Altern. Ther. Health Med. 16 (1), 46–51. Retrieved from: http://www.ncbi.nlm.nih.gov/pubmed/20085177.

Kono, T., Shimada, M., Yamamoto, M., Kaneko, A., Oomiya, Y., Kubota, K., et al., 2015. Complementary and synergistic therapeutic effects of compounds found in Kampo medicine: analysis of daikenchuto. Front Pharmacol. 6, 159. http://dx.doi.org/10.3389/fphar.2015.00159.

Li, M., Zhou, Y., Feng, G., Su, S.B., 2009. The critical role of Toll-like receptor signaling pathways in the induction and progression of autoimmune diseases. Curr. Mol. Med. 9 (3), 365–374. Retrieved from: http://www.ncbi.nlm.nih.gov/pubmed/19355917.

Mohammad Hosseini, A., Majidi, J., Baradaran, B., Yousefi, M., 2015. Toll-like receptors in the pathogenesis of autoimmune diseases. Adv. Pharm. Bull. 5 (Suppl. 1), 605–614. http://dx.doi.org/10.15171/apb.2015.082.

Motoo, Y., Seki, T., Tsutani, K., 2011. Traditional Japanese medicine, Kampo: its history and current status. Chin. J. Integr. Med. 17 (2), 85–87. http://dx.doi.org/10.1007/s11655-011-0653-y.

Neil, H.A., Gatling, W., Mather, H.M., Thompson, A.V., Thorogood, M., Fowler, G.H., et al., 1987. The Oxford Community diabetes study: evidence for an increase in the prevalence of known diabetes in Great Britain. Diabet. Med. 4 (6), 539–543. Retrieved from http://www.ncbi.nlm.nih.gov/pubmed/2962810.

Nozaki, K., Goto, H., Nakagawa, T., Hikiami, H., Koizumi, K., Shibahara, N., Shimada, Y., 2007. Effects of keishibukuryogan on vascular function in adjuvant-induced arthritis rats. Biol. Pharm. Bull. 30 (6), 1042–1047. Retrieved from: http://www.ncbi.nlm.nih.gov/pubmed/17541151.

Nozaki, K., Hikiami, H., Goto, H., Nakagawa, T., Shibahara, N., Shimada, Y., 2006. Keishibukuryogan (gui-zhi-fu-ling-wan), a Kampo formula, decreases disease activity and soluble vascular adhesion molecule-1 in patients with rheumatoid arthritis. Evid. Based Complement. Altern. Med. 3 (3), 359–364. http://dx.doi.org/10.1093/ecam/nel025.

O'Reilly, L.A., Hutchings, P.R., Crocker, P.R., Simpson, E., Lund, T., Kioussis, D., et al., 1991. Characterization of pancreatic islet cell infiltrates in NOD mice: effect of cell transfer and transgene expression. Eur. J. Immunol. 21 (5), 1171–1180. http://dx.doi.org/10.1002/eji.1830210512.

Ogawa, K., Kojima, T., Matsumoto, C., Kamegai, S., Oyama, T., Shibagaki, Y., et al., 2007. Identification of a predictive biomarker for the beneficial effect of a Kampo (Japanese traditional) medicine keishibukuryogan in rheumatoid arthritis patients. Clin. Biochem. 40 (15), 1113–1121. http://dx.doi.org/10.1016/j.clinbiochem.2007.06.005.

Ono, Y., Inoue, M., Mizukami, H., Ogihara, Y., 2004. Suppressive effect of Kanzo-bushi-to, a Kampo medicine, on collagen-induced arthritis. Biol. Pharm. Bull. 27 (9), 1406–1413. Retrieved from: http://www.ncbi.nlm.nih.gov/pubmed/15340228.

Park, S.Y., Lee, S.W., Kim, H.Y., Lee, W.S., Hong, K.W., Kim, C.D., 2015. HMGB1 induces angiogenesis in rheumatoid arthritis via HIF-1alpha activation. Eur. J. Immunol. 45 (4), 1216–1227. http://dx.doi.org/10.1002/eji.201444908.

Pilzweger, C., Holdenrieder, S., 2015. Circulating HMGB1 and RAGE as clinical biomarkers in malignant and autoimmune diseases. Diagnostics 5 (2), 219–253. http://dx.doi.org/10.3390/diagnostics5020219.

Ploix, C., Bergerot, I., Fabien, N., Perche, S., Moulin, V., Thivolet, C., 1998. Protection against autoimmune diabetes with oral insulin is associated with the presence of IL-4 type 2 T-cells in the pancreas and pancreatic lymph nodes. Diabetes 47 (1), 39–44. Retrieved from: http://www.ncbi.nlm.nih.gov/pubmed/9421372.

Sekiya, N., Tanaka, N., Itoh, T., Shimada, Y., Goto, H., Terasawa, K., 1999. Keishi-bukuryo-gan prevents the progression of atherosclerosis in cholesterol-fed rabbit. Phytother. Res. 13 (3), 192–196. http://dx.doi.org/10.1002/(SICI)1099-1573(199905)13:3<192::AID-PTR412>3.0.CO;2-2.

Smith, D.A., Germolec, D.R., 1999. Introduction to immunology and autoimmunity. Environ. Health Perspect. 107 (Suppl. 5), 661–665. Retrieved from: http://www.ncbi.nlm.nih.gov/pubmed/10502528.

Tisch, R., Yang, X.D., Singer, S.M., Liblau, R.S., Fugger, L., McDevitt, H.O., 1993. Immune response to glutamic acid decarboxylase correlates with insulitis in non-obese diabetic mice. Nature 366 (6450), 72–75. http://dx.doi.org/10.1038/366072a0.

Venkatesha, S.H., Rajaiah, R., Berman, B.M., Moudgil, K.D., 2011. Immunomodulation of autoimmune arthritis by herbal CAM. Evid. Based Complement. Altern. Med. 2011, 986797. http://dx.doi.org/10.1155/2011/986797.

Verbrugge, S.E., Scheper, R.J., Lems, W.F., de Gruijl, T.D., Jansen, G., 2015. Proteasome inhibitors as experimental therapeutics of autoimmune diseases. Arthritis Res. Ther. 17, 17. http://dx.doi.org/10.1186/s13075-015-0529-1.

CHAPTER 13

Kampo Medicine for Renal Inflammatory Conditions

V. Ravichandiran[1], Murugan Veerapandian[1], K.T. Manisenthil Kumar[2]
[1]*National Institute of Pharmaceutical Education and Research, Kolkata, India;* [2]*KMCH College of Pharmacy, Coimbatore, Tamilnadu, India*

Introduction

Kampo, the Japanese traditional multiherbal medicine, has been effectively practiced in Asia and other parts of the world for a long time. The Japanese Ministry of Health, Labor, and Welfare standardizes the quality and quantity of its active components. According to 2014 statistics, around 90% of medical practitioners in Japan prescribe Kampo medicine in daily practice (Mogami and Hattori, 2014). In general Kampo formulations are composed of mixtures of crude extracts prepared from the various parts of herbs, viz., roots, bark, leaves, and rhizomes, which are formulated by several pharmaceutical industries in Japan and are under strict Japanese governmental regulations (Watanabe et al., 2011; Yakubo et al., 2014). Owing to their well-known therapeutic functions, Kampo medicines are often supplied in combination with Western drugs. Therefore the evaluation of interactions between Western drugs and Kampo herbal components is now widely advised. Peer-reviewed articles published in the subject area of Kampo medicine have also dramatically increased, which is evidenced by a PubMed survey (Fig. 13.1). For this review, a survey based on the keywords "Kampo medicine" was performed considering only English-language journals. From the available literature it is indeed clear that research on the pharmacological functions of various Kampo formulations is progressively increasing.

Literature describing the role of Kampo therapy integrated with Western drugs for treatment of various clinical conditions such as gastrointestinal disorders, depressive disorder, gastric cancer, esophageal cancer, and pancreatic cancer with ascites is available (Mogami and Hattori, 2014). Zhong et al. (2015) have reviewed the recent advances in the clinical practice of traditional Chinese herbal medicine for kidney disease. Chronic kidney disease (CKD) is known to be a worldwide public health issue. Owing to the lack of effective medicines, many patients with CKD across the globe hunt for alternative treatments, such as traditional medicines. The clinical practice of traditional herbs based on single or multiple components depends on the collective experimental knowledge of previous practitioners, documented in the historical textbooks. The therapeutic principle of traditional herbal medicines in CKD is

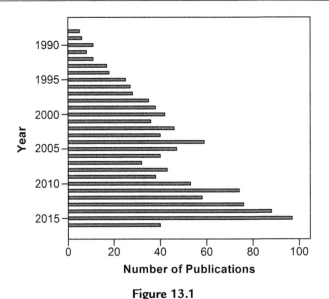

Figure 13.1

The number of articles on Kampo medicine published in English from 1988 through 2016. *This information was derived from PubMed by searching the keywords "Kampo medicine."*

to "drain damp" (promoting urination by regulating the immune system), activate anticoagulation, support the nourishment of the blood, and maintain antianemia. Further, the traditional herbal therapy coordinates the natural stabilization of the body ("Yin and Yang") (Li and Wang, 2005; Zhong et al., 2015). Mechanistic investigations for implementing the usage of traditional Chinese herbal medicines in the treatment of renal-associated diseases that were reported earlier than 2013 are reviewed elsewhere by Zhong et al. (2013). More recent studies have identified the structure–function relationship and the molecular mechanisms of traditional medicines, which are significant advancements in this field. Such studies suggest that the majority of the traditional medicines including Chinese and Japanese herbs are related to antiinflammatory, antifibrotic, immunomodulatory, and antioxidative functions (Table 13.1).

Corticosteroid and immunosuppressive drugs are the general medications prescribed for glomerular disease. But, these medications are known for associated adverse side effects. Further, development of resistance to therapy and relapse of disease after the end of medication are frequent issues. For CKD patients, only partial salutary effects are achieved by modulation of the renin–angiotensin system, which does not essentially avoid the progression to last-stage renal disorder and the requirement of renal replacement (de Zeeuw, 2011). Because of limited therapeutic choices for CKD, several Asian countries are seriously looking for alternative treatments, considering Chinese and Japanese herbal formulations, which have a valuable heritage in the clinical aspect. The therapeutic efficacy of these agents is well supported by a great number of animal investigations, but lacks randomized clinical trials, particularly in patients with CKD. Even though the pharmacologically active herb and its

Table 13.1: Mechanisms of Therapeutic Actions of Commonly Used Herbal Medicines

Herb Name	Active Compounds	Mechanism[a]				Indications	Side Effects
		Antiinflammatory	Antioxidative	Antifibrotic	Immunomodulation		
Astragalus membranaceus	Astragalosides I–VII, flavonoids, etc.	+++	+++	+++	++	Primary glomerular disease (Zhang et al., 2014c), diabetic nephropathy (Li et al., 2011), membranous nephropathy (Ahmed et al., 2007)	No reported side effects
Tripterygium wilfordii Hook F	Triptolide	+++	+	+++	+++	Primary glomerular disease (Zhu et al., 2013; Chen et al., 2013a,b), PKD (Chen et al., 2014), Henoch–Schonlein purpura (Wu et al., 2013)	GI disorders, liver toxicity, infertility, hematopoietic disorders (Liu et al., 2011; Yang et al., 1998)
Radix Bupleuri	Saikosaponin a and d (Ashour et al., 2011)	++	++	++	+	IgA nephropathy (Yoshikawa et al., 1997)	Interstitial pneumonia, liver toxicity, edema, hypertension, cystitis, GI disorders, immunodeficiency (Asano et al., 2006; Lu et al., 2008)
Radix Puerariae	Puerarin		+++			Early diabetic nephropathy (Zhong et al., 2014)	No reported side effects

Continued

Table 13.1: Mechanisms of Therapeutic Actions of Commonly Used Herbal Medicines—cont'd

Herb Name	Active Compounds	Mechanism[a]					Indications	Side Effects
		Antiinflammatory	Antioxidative	Antifibrotic	Immunomodulation			
Abelmoschus manihot	Myricetin, cannabiscitrin, etc. (Lai et al., 2006)	+ +		+ +			Primary glomerular disease (Zhang et al., 2014b), diabetic nephropathy (Chen et al., 2015)	Upper respiratory tract infection, hyperlipidemia, liver toxicity (Zhang et al., 2014b)
Ophiocordyceps sinensis	Cyclic peptides and H1-A (Paterson et al., 2008)	+ +	+ + +				Chronic kidney injury (Zhang et al., 2014a), chronic allograft nephropathy (Li et al., 2009)	Overall only a few side effects reported (dry mouth, nausea, stomach discomfort) (Shao et al., 1985; Xu et al., 1992)
Rheum palmatum L	Emodin or rhein (Li et al., 2014)	+		+ +	+		To improve kidney function in CKD patients (Wang et al., 2012a,b)	GI disorders; long-term use causes electrolyte disorders and liver toxicity (Yang et al., 2012)
Cortex Moutan	Paeonol (Wu et al., 2003)	+ +	+ +				CKD[b]	May affect clotting (Koo et al., 2010)

CKD, chronic kidney disease; GI, gastrointestinal; IgA, immunoglobulin A; PKD, polycystic kidney disease.

[a]+ + +, biological effects were confirmed by multiple in vitro and in vivo studies; + +, effects were shown in only two to four studies (one or two in vitro and one or two in vivo); +, effects were shown in only one study (either in vitro or in vivo).

[b]Used by traditional medicine practitioners without clinical studies.

Adapted with permission from Zhong, Y., Menon, M.C., Deng, Y., Chen, Y., He, J.C. 2015. Recent advances in traditional Chinese medicine for kidney disease. Am. J. Kidney Dis. 66 (3), 513–S22, Copyright 2015, Elsevier Publications.

derived components have not been evaluated in large randomized clinical trials, there is a cumulative practice of herbal components complementing the existing therapies for renal-associated diseases (Zhong et al., 2013). This review is an attempt to study the literature describing the characteristics of Japanese Kampo medicine particularly in renal inflammatory conditions. In addition to the clinical functions in glomerulonephritis and stone diseases, the key principles of traditional Chinese herbal treatment of CKD are also highlighted.

Characteristics of Japanese Kampo Medicine

Kampo medicinal practice in Japan differs from traditional Chinese herbal medicine in some aspects. Traditional Chinese medicines are theoretically derived from various medical texts, viz., *Huangdi Neijing, Shennong Ben Cao Jing,* and *Shan Hang Lung,* which were documented during the Han Dynasty, whereas Japanese medical practitioners decided to follow the theories of *Shan Hang Lung* (Nishimura et al., 2009). Although traditional Chinese medicine and Japanese Kampo have similar original features, in time the two forms of clinical practice diverged significantly according to the individual culture. It has been documented that Chinese medicine and Kampo have three major distinct features. First, traditional Chinese medicines are modified at the herbal level, whereas Kampo prescriptions are adapted at the formula level; second, the prescription style is simplified in Kampo medicine; and third, abdominal examination is important for Kampo practice. Such abdominal diagnosis is not prioritized in Chinese and Korean traditional medicine (Nishimura et al., 2009).

There are more than 210 varieties of Kampo formulas prescribed in Japan; the proportions and precise recipes differ from one another. The crude extract of a single plant is a mixture of complex active constituents, which creates difficulties in most of the pharmacological studies. Such complex mixture is potentiated in Kampo medicine, in which usually 3 to 10 or even more plant extracts are united. Researchers have attempted to evaluate the key principles and mechanisms of the therapeutic actions of Kampo formulas. Indications for Kampo medicine are multiplied by fine-tuning the combination of other plant extracts, and a wide range of pharmacological benefits is observed (Iizuka et al., 1998). Table 13.2 presents a list of common indications for the widely prescribed Kampo formulas. In Japan, roughly US$1 billion is spent on Kampo medicinal products. A "Standard Kampo Formula Nomenclature" (Tsutani et al., 2005) was established in 2005 by three major academic societies in Japan, viz., the Japan Society for Oriental Medicine (JSOM), the Medical and Pharmaceutical Society for WAKAN-YAKU (WAKAN), and the Japanese Society of Pharmacognosy (JSP). The *Japanese Pharmacopeia,* 15th edition (2006), has adopted a nomenclature for Kampo formulations, for instance, shosaikoto, kakkonto, etc. Motoo et al. (2009) have classified three types of Kampo products based on how the medicines are handled. Type A describes the clinical practice guidelines (CPG) for Kampo medicines with both strength of evidence and recommendations. Type B describes the CPG with records of references, but deficient in evidence-based recommendations. Type C denotes CPG with information on the Kampo practice or Kampo-associated terminology, but lacking any relevant references (Motoo et al., 2009).

Table 13.2: Clinical Indications of Seven Commonly Used Kampo Formulas

Compound	Clinical Indications
Juzen-taiho-to	Anemia, general fatigue, loss of appetite, chronic disease, chemotherapy or surgery, colds
Keishi-bushi-to	Rheumatoid arthritis
Keishi-ni-eppi-ichi-to	Colds, rheumatoid arthritis, osteoarthritis, eczema
Keishi-ni-eppi-ichi-to-ka-ryo-jutsubu	Rheumatoid arthritis, Behcet's disease, eczema
Shosaiko-to	Chronic gastroenteritis, chronic hepatitis, chronic tonsillitis, orthostatic hypotension, bronchial asthma, psychological problems
Toki-shakuyaku-san	General fatigue, cold limbs, anemia, headache, menopausal syndrome, sterility, chronic nephritis, edema
Unsei-in	Allergic dermatitis, psoriasis, eczema, gastritis, Behcet's disease, urticaria

Adapted with permission from Borchers, A.T., Sakai, S., Henderson, G.L., Harkey, M.R., Keen, C.L., Stern, J.S., Terasawa, K., Gershwin, M.E. 2000. Shosaiko-to and other Kampo (Japanese herbal) medicines: a review of their immunomodulatory activities. J. Ethnopharmacol. 73, 1–13, Copyright 2000, Elsevier Publications.

Inflammatory Pathways in Renal Diseases

Immune response and inflammatory factors play a vital role in the pathogenesis of renal disease (Imig and Ryan, 2013; Kurts et al., 2013). Macrophages and dendritic cells are the innate immune moieties having significant functions in mediating renal inflammation and injury (Kurts et al., 2013). In an infection, innate immune cells recognize microbial products through pattern recognition receptors, such as TLRs (Toll-like receptors), and are triggered to secrete proinflammatory cytokines and chemokines (Kurts et al., 2013; Anders and Schlondorff, 2007).

Initiation and progression of inflammation due to acute renal injury is mediated by the release of various cytokines by leukocytes and renal tubular cells into the damaged kidney. Some of the proinflammatory cytokines/chemokines are increased in ischemic acute kidney injury, viz., IFN-γ, interleukin-2 (IL-2), IL-10, GM-CSF, transforming growth factor-β (TGF-β), CXCL1, IL-6, MIP-2, and monocyte chemoattractant protein-1 (MCP-1) (Goes et al., 1995; Kielar et al., 2005; Akcay et al., 2009). TLRs are known for responding to pathogen-associated molecular patterns and damage-associated molecular patterns (DAMPs), which are endogenous ligands produced as a result of tissue damage. DAMPs act as an important trigger for activation of innate immune cell and inflammation in the kidney. Renal cells, such as mesangial and tubular epithelial cells, also mediate TLRs and generate proinflammatory cytokines and chemokines, contributing to renal damage (Anders et al., 2007; Schroppel and He, 2006). Likewise, autoimmune disorders are a major cause of renal inflammation and damage. For instance, systemic lupus erythematosus and lupus nephritis engage both innate and adaptive immune cells, including renal cells, T cells, B cells, dendritic cells, and macrophages (Lech and Anders, 2013; Kurts et al., 2013; Sterner et al., 2014; Davidson and Aranow, 2010;

Bagavant and Fu, 2009). Lupus nephritis is featured by the presence of several autoantibodies that build immune complexes and deposit in the glomeruli of the kidney (Sterner et al., 2014). There are several mechanisms associated with the immune complexes and the derived inflammation, such as activation of Fc receptors and recruitment of inflammatory cells (Clynes et al., 1998; Turnberg and Cook, 2005). Immune complexes formed in the renal cells also act as an endogenous trigger of TLRs and activate the proinflammatory cytokines (Anders et al., 2007). Patients with clinical conditions of immunoglobulin A (IgA) nephropathy generate high levels of abnormal glycosylated IgA and anti-glycan autoantibodies, resulting in the formation of IgA-immune complexes and deposits in the kidney glomeruli, which progressively induce kidney damage. Nuclear factor κB (NF-κB) is an essential mediator of signal transduction stimulated by various major inflammatory cytokines, viz., tumor necrosis factor-α (TNFα) and IL-1, thereby participating in the effector phase of inflammation (Kiryluk and Novak, 2014). Angiotensin has a physiological role of regulating vasoconstriction and blood pressure, but it is deregulated in inflammatory conditions and the pathogenesis of hypertension, atherosclerosis, and cardiac and renal injuries (Kiryluk and Novak, 2014). Activation of NF-κB has a significant role in angiotensin II-induced expression of chemokines and its associated renal inflammation. Diabetes-induced renal disease also remains as the most common cause of CKD. The pathological pathways associated with the clinical condition of diabetic nephropathy are activated by oxidative stress that affects various kidney cells. However, kidney fibrosis is the most fundamental and prominent feature in the cause of inflammation, which is derived by TGF-β (Anguiano et al., 2015). Important literature relevant to Kampo medicine and its specific applications in CKD and urinary stone diseases is discussed in the following sections.

Kampo Medicine in Chronic Kidney Disease

Diabetic nephropathy in patients often results in chronic glomerulonephritis and nephrosclerosis, which are the major root cause of renal failure. Renal injury in CKD could be generally prevented using angiotensin-converting enzyme inhibitors and angiotensin II receptor blockers (Li and Wang, 2005). Investigations into Kampo medicine revealed that the efficacy of the herbal formulas is promising in the treatment of CKD. Saireito, a Kampo formula, was shown to have the property of reducing urinary protein and promoting proliferation of cell nuclear antigen. Further, saireito has shown the suppression of ED-1-positive cells (macrophages) together with the deposition of extracellular matrix protein in a rat model of glomerulonephritis induced by anti-rat thymocyte serum (Liu et al., 2004; Ono et al., 2005). Saireito has a significant role in the suppression of upregulated mRNA expression in glomeruli associated with TGF-β and connective tissue growth factor. In another study with HIGA mice (Makino et al., 2003), the effects of Perillae herba (perilla) and rosmarinic acid were found to significantly suppress proteinuria and mesangial cell proliferation. Further, the serum levels of IgA, glomerular IgA, and IgG deposition were also reduced in HIGA mice. An in vitro study suggested that cultured Peyer's patch cells and spleen cells from perilla-treated mice exhibited considerably less IgA than those of the control group. Rosmarinic acid, a polyphenolic constituent of perilla, also showed considerable suppression of serum IgA and glomerular IgA deposition in HIGA mice. These results suggest that perilla has a partial effect in the suppression of IgA nephropathy via immune modulation of the intestinal mucosal system. Shichimosukokato and saibokuto are two other Kampo medicines shown to have significant effects in the reduction of proteinuria in IgA nephropathic conditions with focal mesangial proliferation. The efficacy of saibokuto was similar to that of dilazep hydrochloride on proteinuria, and slightly predominant on hematuria (Ono and Makino, 2009). Similarly, decoctions made from the Chinese herb *Astragalus mongholicus* or *Astragalus membranaceus* derived from the Leguminose plant had an effect in decreasing proteinuria and pathological injury and enhanced the total cholesterol and albumin levels in plasma. These results confirm that *Astragalus* decreases glomerular hyperfusion and improves kidney function. The mechanism associated with these benefits may be attributed to the inactivation of free radicals and inhibition of nitric oxide and TNFα synthesis (Ma et al., 1999; Xu et al., 1997). In another study on adriamycin-induced nephrosis in rats, *Astragalus* exhibited a therapeutic function on diuresis partly through the downregulation of the gene associated with hypothalamic vasopressin, the renal V2 receptor, and aquaporin 2 (Shi et al., 1996). Observed results suggested that *Astragalus* has definite therapeutic effects in the early stages of CKD. Likewise, the medicinal herb rhubarb derived from the root of the plant *Rheum palmatum* L has significant function in the treatment of CKD. The chemical components of rhubarb include over 20 anthraquinones, of which emodin, rhein, and aloe-emodin have been investigated much in China. For instance, in an in vitro study, emodin exhibited a suppression of lipopolysaccharide (LPS)-induced cell proliferation via inhibition of c-myc oncogene expression and blocked IL-6 production. Further, emodin has an inhibitory effect on LPS-stimulated IL-1 secretion in human macrophages and decreased the activity of Na-K-ATP and Ca-ATP in renal tubular epithelial cells. Some of the other Chinese herbs used in the aid of CKD are reviewed elsewhere (Li and Wang, 2005), such as *Cordyceps sinensis*; tetrandrine, an active component of *Stephania tetrandra*; and *Tripterygium wilfordii*.

Keishibukuryogan is the traditional Japanese formulation known for improving blood circulation. This herbal formulation was shown to improve conjunctional microcirculation in cerebrospinal vascular conditions (Itoh et al., 1992), suggesting the benefits of enhanced hemorheological factors such as blood viscosity, red blood cell aggregability, and deformability (Hikiami et al., 2003). A report by Nakagawa et al. (2007) demonstrated the therapeutic functions of keishibukuryogan in the kidney of diabetic rats, which evidenced the suppression of fibronectin deposition associated with TGF-β1. In another study an additional property of keishibukuryogan toward decreasing lipid peroxidation and elevating superoxide dismutase activity in the kidney was reported by Nakagawa et al. (2003). In this report, the research group of Nakagawa et al. (2011) also attempted to reveal the pharmacological effect of keishibukuryogan on the early stage of renal failure in the remnant kidney model. The chemical structure of

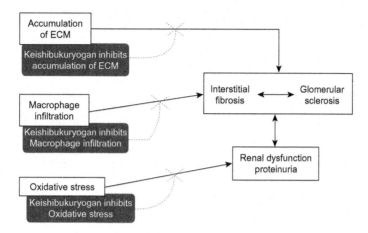

Figure 13.2

Hypothetical representation of the effects of keishibukuryogan on renal failure. *ECM*, extracellular matrix. *Reproduced from Nakagawa, T., Tashiro, I., Fujimoto, M., Jo, M., Sakai, S., Oka, H., Goto, H., Shimada, Y., Shibahara, N., 2011. Keishibukuryogan reduces renal injury in the early stage of renal failure in the remnant kidney model. Evid. Based Complement. Altern. Med. 914249, 1–8, an open access article, Copyright, 2011, Hindawi Publications.*

the methanolic extract of keishibukuryogan was investigated using the HPLC technique, which revealed important constituents, viz., oxypaeoniflorin, albiflorin, paeoniflorin, pentagalloyl glucose, benzoic acid, cinnamic acid, benzoyl paeoniflorin, cinnamaldehyde, amygdalin, and paeonol. This study reported that a 3% keishibukuryogan formulation significantly suppressed osteopontin mRNA levels, and MCP-1 and vascular cell adhesion molecule-1 mRNA levels exhibited a tendency to decrease, but without statistical significance. Further, 3% keishibukuryogan attenuated the serum urea nitrogen and proteinuria excretion levels. Observed results supported the usefulness of keishibukuryogan in slowing the development of chronic renal failure. Fig. 13.2 summarizes the hypothetical illustration proposed by Nakagawa et al. (2011) for the effects of keishibukuryogan on renal failure.

Kampo Medicine in Urinary Stone Disease

Urolithiasis is the formation of urinary calculi in the bladder or urinary tract resulting from various factors such as diet, water intake, biochemical metabolism, and genetic risk factors. Kidney stone disease affects approximately 10–12% of the general population and often results in renal inflammation, which results in a significant medical expenditure for individuals (Miyaoka and Monga, 2009). In general, kidney stones are made of calcium salts such as calcium oxalate and calcium phosphate. Other chemical components include struvite (magnesium ammonium phosphate), uric acid, and cystine. Compared to Western therapies, herbal combinations of Kampo medicines are shown to have positive effects in long-term use for the treatment of stone disease with little or no adverse side effects (Gürocak and Küpeli, 2006). An effective herbal therapy for the management of urolithiasis may inhibit the nucleation and formation of crystals or might promote the exclusion of small crystals through an effect on urothelial adherence or by diuresis (Gohel and Wong, 2006).

Choreito, a Kampo medicine, comprises an herbal blend and is assumed to be a valuable remedy for nephritis and nephrolithiasis (Hidaka et al., 1991). Although choreito extract had no inhibitory effect on the growth of amorphous calcium phosphate, it does have an active role in the inhibition of hydroxyapatite in vitro (Hidaka et al., 1991). Another in vitro study using a synthetic urine model was done to evaluate the roles of two choreito components, takusya (Alismatis rhizoma) and kagosou (Prunellae spica), in the inhibition of calcium oxalate growth and aggregation (Koide et al., 1995). These in vitro experiments revealed that kagosou has a weaker effect compared to takusya. In an in vivo model, Wistar rats were treated with $0.5\,\mu g$ of ethylene glycol (5%) daily for a period of 4 weeks, during which takusya at a low dose (relative to human daily dosage per unit body weight) prominently decreased the calcium concentration in the kidney tissues, compared to the control group, and significantly reduced the calcium oxalate deposits distinctly inside the tubular lumen (Koide et al., 1995). Further studies on takusya have shown significant suppression of osteopontin, which is the known stone matrix influencing the nucleation and aggregative formation of stones (McKee et al., 1995). Likewise, wullingsan (WLS), a multicomponent herbal composite containing *Alisma orientale, Polyporus umbellatus, Poria cocos,* and *Cinnamomum cassia,* was shown to have a diuretic effect. The pharmacological study of WLS extract revealed that it is capable of inhibiting calcium oxalate nucleation by prolonging the induction time in a dose-dependent fashion. An in vivo study of WLS on ethylene glycol–induced nephrocalcinosis in a rat model showed lower crystal deposit scores. The observed result was coherent with another rat model of nephrocalcinosis in which the animals were fed a high phosphorus diet. Some of the other active herbal combinations used in the treatment of stone disease are jin qian cao (*Desmodium styracifolium* Merr) and niao shi mixture (NSM). The mechanism of action derived from jin qian cao was found to be lowering of calcium excretion and increased urine citrate and 24-h creatinine excretion in an oxalate stone model (Miyaoka and Monga, 2009). In the case of NSM, it blocks the formation of 4-hydroxy-L-proline-induced stones and decreases serum calcium and uric acid (Miyaoka and Monga, 2009). Although Kampo medicines are observed to have potential effects on stone disease in in vitro and animal studies, earlier literature reviews have identified that clinical trials are still lacking. The claims of effectiveness in humans should be subjected to comprehensive evaluation.

Randomized Clinical Trials of Traditional Medicines in Kidney Disease

Several small-scale clinical investigations of herbal medicines in the treatment of kidney disease are disseminated in Chinese journals. However, large and well-organized randomized controlled clinical trials are still not sufficient. A 2015 review by Zhong et al. (2015)

highlighted the available well-designed randomized clinical trials related to traditional herbal medicines in various kidney diseases, which are reproduced here in Table 13.3. In 2007, the JSOM Committee for Evidence-Based Medicine started to compile evidence reports of Kampo treatment (EKAT project). The main role of EKAT is to compile structured abstracts of randomized controlled trials along with remarks by an external reviewer. As of December 31, 2012, there were 378 controlled randomized clinical trials of Kampo medicines reported in Japan (Motoo et al., 2014). But further studies to determine the good randomized controlled clinical trials conforming to CONSORT (consolidated standards of reporting trials) and PRISMA (preferred reporting items for systematic reviews and meta-analyses) requirements are needed to explain the importance of Kampo diagnosis and treatment (Motoo et al., 2014).

Table 13.3: Trials Investigating the Use of Traditional Medicines in Kidney Disease

References	No.	Disease	Therapeutic Arms	Primary Outcome	Study Period (Months)	Outcome
Wang et al. (2012)	573	Primary glomerulonephritis with CKD stage 3	Traditional medicines[a]/placebo versus benazepril/placebo versus traditional medicines/benazepril	Mean eGFR	6	48.5 ± 15.9 versus 43.0 ± 12.4 versus 48.3 ± 17.5 mL/min ($p < .05$)
Chen et al. (2013)	190	Membranous nephropathy	Shenqi particle versus cyclophosphamide/steroid	CR + PR	11	46/63 (73.0%) versus 54/69 (78.3%); $p = .5$
[b]Wu et al. (2013)	58	Henoch–Schonlein purpura	Triptolide/prednisone versus prednisone	CR + PR	6	40/42 (95%) versus 10/14 (72%); $p = .029$
Zhang et al. (2014c)	417	Primary glomerular disease	AM versus losartan versus AM/losartan combination	Mean change in proteinuria	6	−508 versus −376 mg/day ($p = .003$) versus −545 mg/day ($p < .001$)
[c]Chen et al. (2014)	9	ADPKD with proteinuria >1 g/day	*Tripterygium*	Reduction in proteinuria	12	6/9 patients to <0.5 g/day

ADPKD, autosomal dominant polycystic kidney disease; *AM*, Abohelmus manicot; *CKD*, chronic kidney disease; *CR*, complete remission; *eGFR*, estimated glomerular filtration rate; *PR*, partial remission.
[a]Traditional Chinese medicine mixture that was formulated and titrated according to symptoms.
[b]Pediatric patients (this study reported longer term outcomes).
[c]Prospective single-center observational experience; all patients had experienced treatment failure with losartan.
Adapted with permission from Zhong, Y., Menon, M.C., Deng, Y., Chen, Y., He, J.C. 2015. Recent advances in traditional Chinese medicine for kidney disease. Am. J. Kidney Dis. 66 (3), 513–522, Copyright 2015, Elsevier Publications.

Summary and Outlook

Therapeutic efficiencies of Kampo medicinal compositions are mainly supported by physicians' clinical expertise and clinical evaluation. From the recent research contributions it is indeed promising that Kampo medicines have clinical value and in some cases resulted in better health care in comparison to modern therapies, especially in long-term use for CKDs and their associated conditions. Several potential therapeutic Kampo formulas could be identified in single or hybrid extract forms, which have multiple pharmacological actions, viz., antiinflammatory, antioxidative, antifibrotic, or immunomodulatory. Although promising results have been derived from the literature discussed in this chapter, Kampo medicinal practice still has limitations, which need adequate attention for rationalized therapy. For instance, the active individual components of Kampo medicines and the percentage of dose for follow-up visits vary according to patients' symptoms and signs. Clinical trials with single and multiple combinations are needed. Understanding the interactions of Kampo herbs with Western medicine is an area of wide interest, which needs special attention for improving existing practice. Further, the development of resistance among CKD patients toward herbal treatment should also be taken into account for better care. Some of the existing clinical investigations of traditional Chinese or Japanese herbal medicines for renal inflammatory conditions have issues, including limited size, suboptimal reports, and flawed protocols. Modern informatics in health care and its allied systems could help to achieve effective and structurally well-characterized clinical trials.

Acknowledgments

Dr. M. Veerapandian is supported by the Department of Science and Technology, Government of India, through DST-Inspire Faculty (DST/INSPIRE/04/2015/002081).

References

Ahmed, M.S., Hou, S.H., Battaglia, M.C., Picken, M.M., Leehey, D.J., 2007. Treatment of idiopathic membranous nephropathy with the herb *Astragalus membranaceus*. Am. J. Kidney Dis. 50, 1028–1032.

Akcay, A., Nguyen, Q., Edelstein, C.L., 2009. Mediators of inflammation in acute kidney injury. Mediators Inflamm. 137072, 1–12.

Anders, H.J., Schlondorff, D., 2007. Toll-like receptors: emerging concepts in kidney disease. Curr. Opin. Nephrol. Hypertens. 16 (3), 177–183.

Anguiano, L., Riera, M., Pascual, J., José Soler, M., 2015. Endothelin blockade in diabetic kidney disease. J. Clin. Med. 4, 1171–1192.

Asano, T., Fujii, Y., Numao, N., Kageyama, Y., Kihara, K., 2006. The efficiency of Sairei-to for retroperitoneal fibrosis: two case reports. Hinyokika Kiyo 52, 543–547.

Ashour, M.L., Wink, M., 2011. Genus *Bupleurum*: a review of its phytochemistry, pharmacology and modes of action. J. Pharm. Pharmacol. 63, 305–321.

Bagavant, H., Fu, S.M., 2009. Pathogenesis of kidney disease in systemic lupus erythematosus. Curr. Opin. Rheumatol. 21 (5), 489–494.

Borchers, A.T., Sakai, S., Henderson, G.L., Harkey, M.R., Keen, C.L., Stern, J.S., Terasawa, K., Gershwin, M.E., 2000. Shosaiko-to and other Kampo (Japanese herbal) medicines: a review of their immunomodulatory activities. J. Ethnopharmacol. 73, 1–13.

Chen, Y., Deng, Y., Ni, Z., et al., 2013a. Efficacy and safety of traditional Chinese medicine (Shenqi particle) for patients with idiopathic membranous nephropathy: a multicenter randomized controlled clinical trial. Am. J. Kidney Dis. 62, 1068–1076.

Chen, Y., Gong, Z., Chen, X., et al., 2013b. *Tripterygium wilfordii* Hook F (a traditional Chinese medicine) for primary nephritic syndrome. Cochrane Database Syst. Rev. 8, CD008568.

Chen, D., Ma, Y., Wang, X., et al., 2014. Triptolide-containing formulation in patients with autosomal dominant polycystic kidney disease and proteinuria: an uncontrolled trial. Am. J. Kidney Dis. 63, 1070–1072.

Chen, Y.Z., Gong, Z.X., Cai, G.Y., et al., 2015. Efficacy and safety of *Flos Abelmoschus manihot* (Malvaceae) on type 2 diabetic nephropathy: a systematic review. Chin. J. Integr. Med. 6, 464–472.

Clynes, R., Dumitru, C., Ravetch, J.V., 1998. Uncoupling of immune complex formation and kidney damage in autoimmune glomerulonephritis. Science 279 (5353), 1052–1054.

Davidson, A., Aranow, C., 2010. Lupus nephritis: lessons from murine models. Nat. Rev. Rheumatol. 6 (1), 13–20.

de Zeeuw, D., 2011. Unmet need in renal protection-do we need a more comprehensive approach? Contrib. Nephrol. 171, 157–160.

Goes, N., Urmson, J., Ramassar, V., Halloran, P.F., 1995. Ischemic acute tubular necrosis induces an extensive local cytokine response: evidence for induction of interferon-γ, transforming growth factor-β 1, granulocyte-macrophage colony-stimulating factor, interleukin-2, and interleukin-10. Transplantation 59, 565–572.

Gohel, M.D., Wong, S.P., 2006. Chinese herbal medicines and their efficacy in treating renal stones. Urol. Res. 34, 365–372.

Gürocak, S., Küpeli, B., 2006. Consumption of historical and current phytotherapeutic agents for urolithiasis: a critical review. J. Urol. 176, 450–455.

Hidaka, S., Abe, K., Liu, S.Y., 1991. A new method for the study of the formation and transformation of calcium phosphte precipitates: effects of several chemical agents and Chinese folk medicines. Arch. Oral Biol. 36, 49–54.

Hikiami, H., Goto, H., Sekiya, N., Hattori, N., Sakakibara, I., Shimada, Y., et al., 2003. Comparative efficacy of Keishi-bukuryogan and pentoxifylline on RBC deformability in patients with ''oketsu'' syndrome. Phytomedicine 10, 459–466.

Iizuka, S., Ishige, A., Komatsu, Y., Matsumiya, T., Inazu, M., Takeda, H., 1998. Effects of Toki-shakuyaku-san on electric footshock stress in overiectomized mice. Methodol. Find. Exp. Clin. Pharmacol. 20, 39–46.

Imig, J.D., Ryan, M.J., 2013. Immune and inflammatory role in renal disease. Compr. Physiol. 3 (2), 957–976.

Itoh, T., Terasawa, K., Kohta, K., Shibahara, N., Tosa, H., Hiyama, Y., 1992. Effects of Keishi-bukuryo-gan and Trapidil on the microcirculation in patients with cerebro-spinal vascular disease. J. Med. Pharm. Soc. WAKAN-YAKU 9, 40–46.

Kielar, M.L., John, R., Bennett, M., et al., 2005. Maladaptive role of IL-6 in ischemic acute renal failure. J. Am. Soc. Nephrol. 16, 3315–3325.

Kiryluk, K., Novak, J., 2014. The genetics and immunobiology of IgA nephropathy. J. Clin. Investig. 124 (6), 2325–2332.

Koide, T., Yamaguchi, S., Utsunomiya, M., Yoshioka, T., Sugiyama, K., 1995. The inhibitory effect of kampou extracts on in vitro calcium oxalate crystallization and in vivo stone formation in an animal model. Int. J. Urol. 2, 81–86.

Koo, Y.K., Kim, J.M., Koo, J.Y., et al., 2010. Platelet anti-aggregatory and blood anti-coagulant effects of compounds isolated from *Paeonia lactiflora* and *Paeonia suffruticosa*. Pharmazie 65, 624–628.

Kurts, C., Panzer, U., Anders, H.J., Rees, A.J., 2013. The immune system and kidney disease: basic concepts and clinical implications. Nat. Rev. Immunol. 13 (10), 738–753.

Lai, X.Y., Zhao, Y.Y., Liang, H., 2006. Studies on chemical constituents in flower of *Abelmoschus manihot*. Zhongguo Zhong Yao ZaZhi 31, 1597–1600.

Lech, M., Anders, H.J., 2013. The pathogenesis of lupus nephritis. J. Am. Soc. Nephrol. 24 (9), 1357–1366.

Li, X., Wang, H., 2005. Chinese herbal medicine in the treatment of chronic kidney disease. Adv. Chronic Kidney Dis. 12 (3), 276–281.

Li, Y., Xue, W.J., Tian, P.X., et al., 2009. Clinical application of *Cordyceps sinensis* on immunosuppressive therapy in renal transplantation. Transplant. Proc. 41, 1565–1569.

Li, M., Wang, W., Xue, J., Gu, Y., Lin, S., 2011. Meta-analysis of the clinical value of *Astragalus membranaceus* in diabetic nephropathy. J. Ethnopharmacol. 133, 412–419.

Li, Z., Zhang, L., He, W., Zhu, C., Yang, J., Sheng, M., 2014. *Astragalus membranaceus* inhibits peritoneal fibrosis *via* monocyte chemoattractant protein (MCP)-1 and the transforming growth factor-beta1 (TGF-beta1) pathway in rats submitted to peritoneal dialysis. Int. J. Mol. Sci. 15, 12959–12971.

Liu, N., Makino, T., Honda, G., Muso, E., Kita, T., Ono, T., 2004. Suppressive effects of sairei-to on nesangial proliferation in a rat model of glomerulonephritis. Clin. Exp. Nephrol. 8, 216–222.

Liu, J., Jiang, Z., Liu, L., et al., 2011. Triptolide induces adverse effect on reproductive parameters of female Sprague–Dawley rats. Drug Chem. Toxicol. 34, 1–7.

Lu, PaW., Chiu, H., 2008. Discussion on Xiao Chai Hu Tang clinical application and its side effects. Chin. Prim. Health Care 22, 80–82.

Ma, J., Fan, S., Chen, J., et al., 1999. Messenger RNA expressions of vasopressin system and aquaporin-2 in adriamycin-induced nephrotic rats and effects of *Astragalus membranaceus*. Chin. Med. J. 112, 1068–1072.

Makino, T., Ono, T., Matsuyama, K., Nogaki, F., Miyawaki, S., Honda, G., Muso, E., 2003. Suppressive effects of *Perilla frutescens* on IgA nephropathy in HIGA mice. Nephrol. Dial. Transplant. 18, 484–490.

McKee, M.D., Nanci, A., Khan, S.R., 1995. Ultrastructural immunodetection of osteopontin and osteocalcin as major matrix components of renal calculi. J. Bone Miner. Res. 10, 1913–1929.

Miyaoka, R., Monga, M., 2009. Use of traditional Chinese medicine in the management of urinary stone disease. Int. Braz. J. Urol. 35 (4), 396–405.

Mogami, S., Hattori, T., 2014. Beneficial effects of Rikkunshito, a Japanese kampo medicine, on gastrointestinal Dysfunction and Anorexia in combination with Western drug: a systematic review. Evid. Based Complement. Altern. Med. 519035, 1–7.

Motoo, Y., Arai, I., Hyodo, I., Tsutani, K., 2009. Current status of Kampo (Japanese herbal) medicines in Japanese clinical practice guidelines. Complement. Ther. Med. 17, 147–154.

Motoo, Y., Arai, I., Tsutani, K., 2014. Use of Kampo diagnosis in randomized controlled trials of Kampo products in Japan: a systematic review. PLoS One 9, e104422.

Nakagawa, T., Yokozawa, T., Oowada, S., Goto, H., Shibahara, N., Shimada, Y., et al., 2003. Amelioration of kidney damage in spontaneously diabetic WBN/Kob rats after treatment with Keishi-bukuryo-gan. J. Tradit. Med. 20, 156–164.

Nakagawa, T., Goto, H., Hikiami, H., Yokozawa, T., Shibahara, N., Shimada, Y., 2007. Protective effects of keishibukuryogan on the kidney of spontaneously diabetic WBN/Kob rats. J. Ethnopharmacol. 110, 311–317.

Nakagawa, T., Tashiro, I., Fujimoto, M., Jo, M., Sakai, S., Oka, H., Goto, H., Shimada, Y., Shibahara, N., 2011. Keishibukuryogan reduces renal injury in the early stage of renal failure in the remnant kidney model. Evid. Based Complement. Altern. Med. 914249, 1–8.

Nishimura, K., Plotnikoff, G.A., Watanabe, K., 2009. Kampo medicine as an integrative medicine in Japan. Japan Med. Assoc. J. 52 (3), 147–149.

Ono, T., Makino, T., 2009. Basic study and clinical practice of Kampo medicines in chronic kidney disease (CKD): chronic glomerulonephritis and nephrosclerosis. J. Tradit. Med. 26, 230–234.

Ono, T., Liu, N., Makino, T., Nogaki, F., Muso, E., Honda, G., Kita, T., 2005. Suppressive mechanisms of sairei-to on mesangial matrix expansion in rat mesangio proliferative glomerulonephritis. Nephron Exp. Nephrol. 100, e132–e142.

Paterson, R.R., 2008. Cordyceps: a traditional Chinese medicine and another fungal therapeutic biofactory? Phytochemistry 69, 1469–1495.

Schroppel, B., He, J.C., 2006. Expression of Toll-like receptors in the kidney: their potential role beyond infection. Kidney Int. 69 (5), 785–787.

Shao, G., 1985. Treatment of hyperlipidemia with cultivated Cordyceps—a double-blind, randomized placebo control trial. Zhong Xi Yi Jie He ZaZhi 5, 652–654.

Shi, H., Qian, T., Jiang, J., et al., 1996. Experiment study of BHD and AM treatment on adriamycin nephropathy in rats [in Chinese]. J. Nan Tong Med. Coll. 16, 503–505.

Sterner, R.M., Hartono, S.P., Grande, J.P., 2014. The pathogenesis of lupus nephritis. J. Clin. Cell. Immunol. 5 (2), 205.

Tsutani, K., Satake, M., Toriizuka, K., Hikiami, H., Yamada, K., 2005. Standard Kampo formula nomenclature. Nihon Toyo Igaku Zasshi (Kampo Med.) 56 (4), 611–622. [in Japanese] http://www.jsom.or.jp/pdf/standard kampo.pdf.

Turnberg, D., Cook, H.T., 2005. Complement and glomerulonephritis: new insights. Curr. Opin. Nephrol. Hypertens. 14 (3), 223–228.

Wang, H., Song, H., Yue, J., Li, J., Hou, Y.B., Deng, J.L., 2012a. Rheum officinale (a traditional Chinese medicine) for chronic kidney disease. Cochrane Database Syst. Rev. 7, CD008000.

Wang, Y.J., He, L.Q., Sun, W., et al., 2012b. Optimized project of traditional Chinese medicine in treating chronic kidney disease stage 3: a multicenter double-blinded randomized controlled trial. J. Ethnopharmacol. 139, 757–764.

Watanabe, K., Matsuura, K., Gao, P., Hottenbacher, L., Tokunaga, H., Nishimura, K., et al., 2011. Traditional Japanese kampo medicine: clinical research between modernity and traditional medicine—The state of research and methodological suggestions for the future. Evid. Based Complement. Altern. Med. 513842, 1–19.

Wu, X., Chen, H., Chen, X., Hu, Z., 2003. Determination of paeonol in rat plasma by high-performance liquid chromatography and its application to pharmacokinetic studies following oral administration of Moutan cortex decoction. Biomed. Chromatogr. 17, 504–508.

Wu, L., Mao, J., Jin, X., et al., 2013. Efficacy of triptolide for children with moderately severe Henoch–Schönlein purpura nephritis presenting with nephrotic range proteinuria: a prospective and controlled study in China. BioMed Res. Int. 292865, 1–5.

Xu, R.H., Peng, X.E., Chen, G.Z., Chen, G.L., 1992. Effects of Cordyceps sinensis on natural killer activity and colony formation of B16 melanoma. Chin. Med. J. 105, 97–101.

Xu, Y., Zhang, Q., Wu, Q., 1997. Effect of *Astragalus membranaceus* on experimental diabetic renal hypertrophy and microalbminuria. Acta Univ. Med. Sec. Shanghai 17, 357–359.

Yakubo, S., Ito, M., Ueda, Y., Okamoto, H., Kimura, Y., Amano, Y., et al., 2014. Pattern classification in Kampo medicine. Evid. Based Complement. Altern. Med. 535146, 1–5.

Yang, Y., Liu, Z., Tolosa, E., Yang, J., Li, L., 1998. Triptolide induces apoptotic death of T lymphocyte. Immunopharmacology 40, 139–149.

Yang, J., 2012. Clinical use and side effects of Rheum palmatum L. China Clin. Pract. Med. 7 230–231.

Yoshikawa, N., Ito, H., Sakai, T., et al., 1997. A prospective controlled study of sairei-to in childhood IgA nephropathy with focal/minimal mesangial proliferation. Japanese Pediatric IgA Nephropathy Treatment Study Group. Nihon Jinzo Gakkai Shi 39, 503–506.

Zhang, H.W., Lin, Z.X., Tung, Y.S., et al., 2014a. *Cordyceps sinensis* (a traditional Chinese medicine) for treating chronic kidney disease. Cochrane Database Syst. Rev. 12, CD008353.

Zhang, H.W., Lin, Z.X., Xu, C., Leung, C., Chan, L.S., 2014b. *Astragalus* (a traditional Chinese medicine) for treating chronic kidney disease. Cochrane Database Syst. Rev. 10, CD008369.

Zhang, L., Li, P., Xing, C.Y., et al., 2014c. Efficacy and safety of *Abelmoschus manihot* for primary glomerular disease: a prospective, multicenter randomized controlled clinical trial. Am. J. Kidney Dis. 64, 57–65.

Zhong, Y., Deng, Y., Chen, Y., Chuang, P.Y., He, J.C., 2013. Therapeutic use of traditional Chinese herbal medications for chronic kidney diseases. Kidney Int. 84, 1108–1118.

Zhong, Y., Zhang, X., Cai, X., Wang, K., Chen, Y., Deng, Y., 2014. Puerarin attenuated early diabetic kidney injury through down regulation of matrix metalloproteinase 9 in streptozotocin induced diabetic rats. PLoS One 9, e85690.

Zhong, Y., Menon, M.C., Deng, Y., Chen, Y., He, J.C., 2015. Recent advances in traditional Chinese medicine for kidney disease. Am. J. Kidney Dis. 66 (3), 513–522.

Zhu, B., Wang, Y., Jardine, M., et al., 2013. *Tripterygium* preparations for the treatment of CKD: a systematic review and metaanalysis. Am. J. Kidney Dis. 62, 515–530.

CHAPTER 14

Kampo Medicines for Infectious Diseases

Akihiko Komuro
Niigata University of Pharmacy and Applied Life Sciences, Niigata, Japan

Introduction

Numerous Kampo medicines and Oriental herbs have been used for the treatment of infectious diseases for several reasons, such as genetic background, economical reasons, fewer adverse effects, and so on. This chapter describes Kampo medicines and related Oriental herbs that are effective or promising in the treatment of infectious diseases at the clinical level and/or in animal models. In addition, effective Kampo medicines tested in vitro in cultured-cell studies are also included in this chapter. Each section is categorized by infectious disease and according to the popularity of the Kampo medicine.

Influenza Virus Infection

Influenza virus infection causes annual epidemics and recurring pandemics that have a serious impact on public health and the global economy. Antiinfluenza agents such as oseltamivir and zanamivir have been very effective, but neuraminidase-resistant viruses due to cumulative mutation of neuraminidase have been found (Moscona, 2009; Weinstock and Zuccotti, 2009), and these drugs can be expensive for low-income countries. Several Kampo medicines have been proposed to be effective complementary and alternative medicines against viral infections by stimulating host immune systems or directly acting on virus growth.

Shoseiryuto

Shoseiryuto is used for symptoms such as runny nose, cough, allergic rhinitis, bronchitis, and so on (Ikeda et al., 1994). It has been reported that shoseiryuto possesses antiinfluenza activity in vivo. It was first described that replication of the virus in the nasal cavity and spread of the virus to the lung are efficiently inhibited in intranasal infection with a mouse-adapted influenza strain, A/PR/8/34, in BALB/c mice when shoseiryuto is orally administered (Nagai and Yamada, 1994). Shoseiryuto increases the antiviral IgA antibody in nasal and bronchoalveolar washes of infected mice. It did not stimulate type I interferon (IFN) induction in this study (Nagai and Yamada, 1994); however, other in vitro studies with human cell lines have suggested that shoseiryuto shows type I IFN–mediated inhibition of other viruses such as ganciclovir-resistant human cytomegalovirus (Murayama et al., 2006) and human respiratory syncytial virus (Chang et al., 2013). Regarding influenza virus infection, there have been no reports on inhibitory effects on viral growth by shoseiryuto in a cultured-cell system. Antiinfluenza activity of shoseiryuto is most likely through immunostimulative adjuvant-like activity but not direct action on the virus in any case. Therefore, it is proposed that shoseiryuto is useful for the treatment of influenza virus infection with a history of influenza virus infection and/or as an influenza vaccine adjuvant (Nagai and Yamada, 1998; Yamada and Nagai, 1998). In fact, the same group explored the active ingredient in shoseiryuto and tested for influenza adjuvant activity. Oral administration of one of the ingredients, pinellic acid, to mice with influenza hemagglutinin (HA) vaccine enhanced antiviral IgA antibody in nasal and bronchoalveolar washes, suggesting that pinellic acid may provide a safe and potent oral adjuvant for nasal influenza HA vaccine (Nagai et al., 2002).

Juzentaihoto

The involvement of adjuvant activity of another Kampo medicine has also been investigated for human subjects who are in a high-risk group for influenza infection. Juzentaihoto is a Kampo medicine traditionally used for patients with anemia, anorexia, or fatigue and also has an ability to accelerate recovery from hematopoietic injury induced by radiation and the anticancer drug mitomycin C (Hisha et al., 1997). The influenza adjuvant activity of juzentaihoto was tested using 91 subjects with a minimum age of 65 years by measuring the antibody titer after influenza vaccination (Saiki et al., 2013). The investigation indicated a significant increase in hemagglutination inhibition titer against A/Victoria/210/2009 (H3N2) among the tested vaccine strains, A/California/7/2009 (H1N1), H3N2, and B/Brisbane/60/2008. However, the mechanisms underlying the specificity of juzentaihoto for the H3N2 strain remain to be discovered, although a study has reported that juzentaihoto stimulates the IFN-α response by affecting the responsible transcription factors, IRF-3/7 (Munakata et al., 2012).

Hochuekkito

An antiinfluenza Kampo medicine that affects cytokine and antimicrobial peptide production has been reported. Hochuekkito is a Kampo medicine that is used for treating functional conditions such as general fatigue, compromised state, and gastrointestinal motility disorder (Yanagihara et al., 2013). Hochuekkito administered orally before, on the day of, or after influenza virus infection is found to increase survival rate, suppress viral growth in bronchoalveolar lavage fluid, and inhibit the lung index in mice. Administration of hochuekkito in mice elevates the concentration of IFN-α in bronchoalveolar lavage fluid and decreases inflammatory cytokines such as interleukin (IL)-1α, IL-6, and granulocyte–macrophage colony stimulation factor, but not tumor necrosis factor α (TNFα) and IFN-γ (Mori et al., 1999). Furthermore, it has been reported that hochuekkito enhances the expression of antimicrobial peptides, defensins, in mice compared to control subjects (Dan et al., 2013). Synergistic antiinfluenza effects of hochuekkito with oseltamivir phosphate also have been reported in mice (Ohgitani et al., 2014). Furthermore, a clinical study has indicated that preoperative administration of hochuekkito may ameliorate an excessive postoperative inflammatory response and prolonged immunosuppressed state, resulting in fewer postoperative infectious complications (Iwagaki and Saito, 2013).

Shahakusan

Another antiinfluenza Kampo medicine, shahakusan, has been reported to affect cytokine mRNA expression levels in mandibular lymph node or lung in an influenza-infected mouse model. This Kampo medicine is prescribed in the late phase of infection that causes inflammation in the lung. Shahakusan administered orally from 7 days before to 4 days after infection with the influenza A/PR/8/34 strain in the upper respiratory tract significantly decreases the virus titer in nasal lavage fluid and lowers IL-4, IL-1β, and IL-10 mRNA. In contrast, IL-12 mRNA is increased in infected mice under the same conditions. In addition, shahakusan decreases infiltration of inflammatory cells in the bronchiole and stimulates natural killer (NK) cell activity. However, shahakusan has no direct effect on influenza growth or life cycle (Hokari et al., 2012).

Maoto

Several studies of Kampo medicines that directly act on the influenza life cycle have been reported. The herbal extract of *Ephedra* has an inhibitory effect on the growth of influenza virus (Mantani et al., 1999). For entry of influenza virus into host cells, acidification of lysosomes and endosomes is a well-known factor (Yoshimura et al., 1982). The extract of Ephedrae herba inhibits acidification of endosomes and lysosomes in Madin–Darby canine kidney (MDCK) cells, leading to growth inhibition of the influenza virus A/PR/8/34 when treated immediately or 5–10 min after infection. Chemical inhibition experiments suggest that tannin is one of the active components of inhibition in the extract.

Maoto, which contains *Ephedra*, is used for the early phase of influenza infection, and its efficacy against influenza virus infection has been demonstrated. Oral administration of maoto 4–52 h postinfection significantly reduces virus titers in both nasal and bronchoalveolar lavage fluids of A/J mice (Nagai et al., 2014). The treatment increases antiinfluenza virus IgM, IgA, and IgG1 antibody titers in nasal fluid, bronchoalveolar lavage fluid, and serum, respectively, showing effects similar to those of shoseiryuto. Clinical and randomized studies have also claimed that maoto may be effective in cases of influenza with low sensitivity to oseltamivir and younger patients under 5 years of age (Kubo and Nishimura, 2007; Toriumi et al., 2012).

Cinnamomi Cortex

Trans-cinnamaldehyde (CA), one of the principal components of essential oil derived from Cinnamomi cortex, has antiinfluenza activity in vitro and in vivo (Hayashi et al., 2007). Micromolar levels (20–200 μM) of CA significantly inhibit viral growth in MDCK cells infected with influenza A/PR/8/34 virus. Inhalation in mouse cages (50 mg/cage per day) and intranasal administration of CA (250 μg/mouse per day) significantly increase the survival rate of influenza virus-infected mice. Virus yield in bronchoalveolar lavage fluids is 10 times lower in inhalation treatments of CA compared to control treatments. These findings suggest that Cinnamomi cortex—containing Kampo medicines are effective for acute respiratory infectious diseases.

Hepatitis C Virus Infection

Hepatitis C virus (HCV) infection is a significant worldwide problem in public health. The standard care for HCV is a combination therapy with PEGylated IFN-α and ribavirin, but ribavirin/IFN treatment is not effective enough for some HCV genotypes and shows serious side effects, such as influenza-like symptoms, mental health problems, and hematological abnormalities. Although the IFN-free ledipasvir–sofosbuvir medication had an enormous impact and is very effective for the treatment of chronic HCV genotype 1 (Smith et al., 2015), this therapy could still be expensive for low-income countries with a high prevalence of HCV. Several Kampo medicines and/or natural products have been reported as anti-HCV-agent complementary and alternative medicines.

Ninjinyoeito/Gomisin A

Ninjinyoeito is a Kampo medicine that is used for the treatment of athrepsia due to surgery, anorexia, cold constitution, and anemia. An active component, gomisin A, in Schisandra fruit, among the herbs included in ninjinyoeito, has been reported to have inhibitory effects on HCV and protective effects on immunological hepatopathy against HCV infection (Cyong et al., 2000). Ninjinyoeito is reported to have antiinflammatory properties by suppressing phagocytosis of alveolar macrophages (Aoki et al., 1994) and to increase NK activity in healthy individuals (Kamei et al., 1998). It also has antioxidant and hepatoprotective activities in a cell culture system (Kamei et al., 1998) and an in vivo model (Egashira et al., 2003). Based on these findings, Cyong et al. (2000) have identified an active anti-HCV component in ninjinyoeito as gomisin A in a cultured-cell system and an animal model of immunologically induced acute hepatic failure. The study also demonstrated clinical effects of using ninjin-yoeito to treat chronic HCV; however, the results were not conclusive and further studies are needed to assess the promise of ninjinyoeito for the treatment of chronic HCV (Azzam et al., 2007), as it may reduce viral load or contribute to delaying HCV progress.

Shosaikoto

Shosaikoto has been used for patients with liver diseases in Japan because of its suppressive effect against cancer development in the liver and its macrobiotic effects. To assess its mechanistic aspects, an in vitro study has tested the effects of shosaikoto on the production of IL-12 in circulating mononuclear cells from liver cirrhosis patients (Yamashiki et al., 1999). The group determined IL-12 levels in the monocyte/macrophage fraction and the lymphocyte fraction of peripheral blood obtained from 11 HCV-positive liver cirrhosis patients and 12 healthy subjects and found that IL-12 produced by the patients was significantly lower than that produced by healthy subjects. Shosaikoto stimulation of the monocyte/macrophage fraction or the lymphocyte fraction increased the levels of IL-12 about threefold, which was almost the same level as that of healthy subjects. The study concluded that one of the possible mechanisms of the macrobiotic effects of shosaikoto in liver cirrhosis patients may be the improvement in IL-12 production.

A phase II trial of shosaikoto was conducted in HCV patients who were not candidates for IFN-based therapy to determine the effectiveness for further study (Deng et al., 2011). In the trial, 24 chronic HCV patients were orally administered 2.5 g shosaikoto three times daily for 12 months. Improvement of aspartate aminotransferase and alanine aminotransferase was observed in 16 (67%) and 18 (75%) patients in the study, respectively. Viral load was reduced in 7 patients, increased in 10 patients, and not affected in 7 patients. The study concluded that shosaikoto may improve liver pathology in selected HCV patients who are not candidates for IFN-based treatment, but larger and controlled studies are necessary.

Oxymatrine

Oxymatrine is one of the major alkaloid components of *Sophora flavescens*. It was first described to have anti-HCV and anti-hepatitis B virus (HBV) effects in a cell culture model (Chen et al., 2001b) and an animal model (Chen et al., 2001a). A mouse study indicated that oxymatrine has hepatoprotective activity against acute liver injury induced by allyl alcohol (Liu et al., 1994). Antifibrotic activity of oxymatrine in D-galactosamine-induced rat liver fibrosis has been predicted to be partly through inhibition of lipid peroxidation. Immune-stimulative activity that changes the immune response of HBV-transgenic mice from a Th2 (IL-4 and IL-10) to a Th1 (IFN-γ and IL-2) response has been also reported (Dong et al., 2002; Yang et al., 2002). Because these animal studies and cell-based experiments showed promising effects against HCV infection, several clinical studies have been conducted (Li et al., 1998; Mao et al., 2004). A review paper has evaluated the efficacy of several natural products reported in the treatment of chronic HCV subjects. The paper concluded that the results are promising and indicate the need for further evaluation in HCV cases (Azzam et al., 2007).

Maoto and Daiseiryuto

Maoto and daiseiryuto have been used for the common cold in Japan. Clinical studies have been conducted to assess whether maoto and daiseiryuto reduce the adverse effect of IFN-β in the treatment of chronic HCV patients. In these studies, patients were treated with a combination of IFN-β and either maoto or daiseiryuto and the combinations with Kampo were compared to treatment with IFN-β alone (Kainuma et al., 2002a,b). Adverse effects of IFN-β were evaluated based on the severity of symptoms self-classified into four categories using a questionnaire consisting of 29 items. Scores of symptoms such as discomfort were significantly lower with the combination therapy of IFN-β and Kampo compared to IFN-β alone and none of the patients needed to interrupt therapy because of side effects of IFN-β. Biochemical parameters such as serum alanine aminotransferase and serum hyaluronic acid levels were better compared to IFN-β alone. The authors proposed that administration of these Kampo medicines together with IFN-β treatment could increase the sustained biochemical response rate and reduce liver fibrosis.

Other Herbal Mixtures

There are two studies of the effects of herbal mixtures on HCV infection. EH202 is a mixture of four herbal extracts that have IFN-inducing effects, although information about the ingredients of EH202 is not clearly indicated. A group has conducted an uncontrolled clinical study on E202 in 35 patients with chronic HCV (Kaji et al., 2004). The study claimed that after 3 months of daily EH202 administration, HCV RNA levels in patients were decreased, and improvements in malaise, bloating sensation in the abdomen, and nausea and vomiting were observed in a significant number of patients without showing any serious adverse effects. The authors concluded that EH202 may be safe and useful for the treatment of chronic HCV, although further investigations need to be performed to obtain a definitive conclusion. Another study has reported anti-HCV activity of extracts of *Citrus unshiu* peel (Aurantii nobilis pericarpium) through inhibition of viral absorption in the human acute lymphoblastic leukemia cell line MOLT-4 (Suzuki et al., 2005).

Human Immunodeficiency Virus Infection

Shosaikoto has been widely used for patients with chronic hepatitis and cirrhosis in Japan (Shimizu, 2000). A study has examined the inhibitory effect of shosaikoto on human immunodeficiency virus type 1 (HIV-1) replication in peripheral blood mononuclear cells

(Piras et al., 1997). In the study, the anti-HIV activity of shosaikoto was tested when combined with known anti-HIV drugs such as zidovudine (AZT), lamivudine (3TC), or a combination of AZT/3TC. In vitro experiments indicated that shosaikoto enhanced anti-HIV activity of 3TC among the tested combinations. The authors suggested that a combination therapy of shosaikoto and 3TC has potential as a chemotherapeutic modality for HIV-1 infection. Because it has been reported that shosaikoto inhibits the reverse transcriptase of murine leukemia virus and HIV in vitro (Ono et al., 1990), this activity may be the underlying mechanism of its anti-HIV activity. Another in vitro study has reported that *Polyporus* sclerotium, gardenia fruit, *Atractylodes lancea* rhizoma, *Cnidium* rhizoma, and Japanese *Angelica* root have some anti-HIV activity (Kato et al., 2012). However, no clinical trials of shosaikoto or other Kampo medicines against HIV infection have been reported so far.

Hepatitis B Virus Infection

Shosaikoto was initially tested in 1992 for anti-HBV infection in vitro and in clinical studies. The in vitro study tested peripheral blood mononuclear cells (PBMCs) from patients with chronic active hepatitis and indicated that shosaikoto increased IFN-γ and anti-HBV antibodies produced in PBMCs in a dose-dependent manner (Kakumu et al., 1991). The clinical study investigated the efficacy of shosaikoto in children with chronic HBV infection and with sustained liver disease (Tajiri et al., 1991). Seven of 14 patients (50%) became negative for hepatitis B antigen within a year in the study. The hepatitis B antigen clearance rate in the shosaikoto-treated group was higher than the control annual hepatitis B antigen clearance rate (22.7%) in 22 untreated patients. Other groups also have confirmed similar effects of shosaikoto on HBV infection (Akbar et al., 1999; Chen et al., 2001a; Dong et al., 2002). In addition, a 2007 study demonstrated that shosaikoto directly inhibits viral growth in a HepG2 cell model (Chang et al., 2007). Therefore, the group has proposed shosaikoto as a supplementary to nucleotide analogs to minimize the recurrence of viremia after its discontinuation.

Herpes Simplex *Virus Type 1 Infection*

The effects of kakkonto against cutaneous herpes simplex type 1 (HSV-1) infection in mice have been described (Nagasaka et al., 1995). Kakkonto, at a dose corresponding to that in humans, reduces the mortality of HSV-1-infected mice and reduces localized skin lesions. Kakkonto does not inhibit viral growth in vitro and does not affect cytokine production, NK cell activity, natural cytotoxic killer cell activity, or the population of T-cell subsets in spleen cells of infected mice. Because the delayed-type hypersensitivity (DTH) response to HSV-1 antigen is stronger in kakkonto-treated mice than in untreated mice, the authors attributed the reduction in the mortality of kakkonto-treated mice to an induction of a strong DTH to HSV-1.

Another study has investigated the protective effects of hochuekkito on mitomycin C–immunosuppressed mice. An HSV-1 lethal infection caused by mitomycin C treatment in mice was prevented by oral hochuekkito administration. The authors concluded that hochuekkito may be beneficial for the treatment of infectious diseases in immunocompromised patients receiving chemotherapeutic drugs (Kido et al., 2000). No clinical trials of hochuekkito against HSV-1 infection have been reported.

Severe Acute Respiratory Syndrome Coronavirus Infection

Two in vitro studies of the inhibitory effects of herbal extracts against severe acute respiratory syndrome coronavirus (SARS-CoV) infection have been reported. Extract from a vegetable, the tender leaf of *Toona sinensis* Roem, inhibits growth of SARS-CoV in vitro (Chen et al., 2008). Another study also demonstrated that six herbal extracts from Gentianae radix (long dan; the dried rhizome of *Gentiana scabra*), *Dioscoreae* rhizoma (shan yao; the tuber of *Dioscorea batatas*), Cassiae semen (jue ming zi; the dried seed of *Cassia tora*), and Loranthi ramus (sang ji sheng; the dried stem with leaf of *Taxillus chinensis*) and two from Cibotii rhizoma (gou ji; the dried rhizome of *Cibotium barometz*) inhibit replication of SARS-CoV at 25 to 200 µg/mL concentrations in Vero E6 cells (Wen et al., 2011). Interestingly, extracts from Dioscoreae Rhizome and Rhizome Cibotii were found to inhibit SARS-CoV 3CL protease activity among the extracts tested.

BK Virus–Associated Hemorrhagic Cystitis

BK virus–associated hemorrhagic cystitis (BKV-HC) is a common problem arising occasionally after hematopoietic stem cell transplantation. A group examined the efficacy of choreito for treating BKV-HC in children who underwent allogeneic hematopoietic stem cell transplantation (Kawashima et al., 2015). The duration until complete resolution of hematuria was significantly shorter in the choreito-treated group (median 9 days, range 4–17 days) compared to the nonchoreito group (median 17 days, range 15–66 days; $p = .037$). The BKV load in urine was decreased a month after choreito treatment and no adverse effect was observed. Therefore, the authors suggest that choreito may be a safe and promising therapy for the hemostasis of BKV-HC after hematopoietic stem cell transplantation.

Human Papillomavirus Vaccine Adjuvant

The human papillomavirus (HPV) E7, an oncoprotein ubiquitously expressed in the precursor lesion of cervical cancer, is a target for HPV therapeutic vaccines. A study has demonstrated that juzentaihoto and hochuekkito have adjuvant activity for oral vaccination with recombinant *Lactobacillus casei* expressing HPV-16 E7 (LacE7) in mice (Taguchi et al., 2012). Oral immunization of mice with LacE7 with mucosal adjuvant, heat-labile enterotoxin T subunit (LTB), promotes systemic E7-specific type 1 T-cell responses and a similar effect was observed with juzentaihoto or hochuekkito as an adjuvant. Oral administration of LacE7 plus either of these Japanese Kampo medicines and LTB enhances mucosal E7-specific type 1 T-cell response by approximately threefold more than after administration of LacE7 alone. Secretion of IFN-γ and IL-2 into the intestinal lumen is enhanced by juzentaihoto or hochuekkito and LTB in oral administration of LacE7. Finally, these Kampo medicines enhance the mucosal type 1 immune responses to orally immunized antigen synergistically with *Lactobacillus* and LTB. Therefore the authors suggest that juzentaihoto or hochuekkito may be an excellent adjuvant for oral *Lactobacillus*-based vaccines and may have the potential to elicit extremely high E7-specific mucosal cytotoxic immune response to HPV-associated neoplastic lesions.

Candida albicans *Infection*

C. albicans causes the majority of the opportunistic fungal infections observed in patients under treatment with immune-suppressive drugs and others, such as HIV patients. A group has suggested that several Kampo medicines might be effective as therapeutic agents against candidiasis in immunosuppressed patients. The protective effects of juzentaihoto and its ingredients against *Candida* infection were investigated using immunosuppressed mice (Abe et al., 1998, 1999). ICR mice injected with prednisolone or cyclophosphamide were orally administered 1 g/kg juzentaihoto daily and intravenously infected with a lethal dose of *C. albicans*. Juzentaihoto treatment prolonged the life span of infected mice compared to control mice. A similar protective effect was obtained by treatment with its ingredients ginseng radix, *Glycyrrhiza* radix, *A. lancea* rhizoma, or *Cnidium* rhizoma. Ninjinyoeito also had a similar effect on mice immunosuppressed with cyclophosphamide (Abe et al., 2000).

Listeria monocytogenes *Infection*

A foodborne pathogen, *L. monocytogenes* causes illness mainly in pregnant women, newborns, elderly, and immunocompromised people. Two Kampo medicines have been indicated to be effective against *L. monocytogenes* infection in mice. Shosaikoto was first described as preventing the lethal effect of *L. monocytogenes* by an intraperitoneal (ip) injection. Growth of *L. monocytogenes* in the peritoneal cavity and liver was suppressed from day 1 after the infection. The bactericidal activity of peritoneal macrophages from shosaikoto-treated mice was maintained from 1 to 3 days after ip injection of killed *L. monocytogenes*, whereas the activity of control mouse macrophages was decreased. The authors suggest that augmented accumulation of macrophages and maintenance of their bactericidal activity may be the main mechanisms of the resistance in shosaikoto-treated mice.

The effect of hochuekkito against *L. monocytogenes* infection has been reported in mouse models. Mice orally administered hochuekkito for 10 days (1 g/kg per day) were intravenously (iv) or ip infected with *L. monocytogenes*. Survival rates in mice infected iv at day 1 or infected ip at day 4 after the last administration were increased. The number of bacteria in spleen and liver was increased to kill iv-infected mice by day 5 in the nonadministered group, whereas the number of bacteria in the hochuekkito-pretreated mice was increased relatively slowly by day 3 and decreased from day 3 to day 8. A similar effect was observed in ip-infected mice. Peritoneal macrophages from hochuekkito-treated mice showed an enhanced activity to kill *L. monocytogenes* in vitro within 60 min after ingestion of bacteria. A similar effect was observed in mice undergoing restraint stress treatment and in infant mice (Yamaoka et al., 2000, 2001). In infant mice, IFN-γ-producing CD4+ T cells were increased with hochuekkito treatment independent of the deficiency in the antigen-presenting function.

Propionibacterium acnes *Infection*

P. acnes is a gram-positive commensal bacterium that causes acne on the skin. *P. acnes* releases lipase that produces fatty acids by digesting sebum, creating inflammation of the skin. Several Kampo medicines and their ingredients have been described for their inhibitory effect on the growth of bacteria. Reports have described that orengedokuto and its ingredients, Coptidis rhizoma and Phellodendri cortex (Higaki et al., 1990, 1995, 1996a,b), jumihaidokuto (Higaki et al., 2000, 2001), unseiin (Higaki and Morohashi, 2003), and keigairengyoto (Higaki et al., 1997, 2004) inhibit the growth of *P. acnes* and lipase activity. Therefore, these Kampo medicines have been used for acne.

Helicobacter pylori *Infection*

H. pylori is a gram-negative bacterium that infects the stomach and whose infection is a major cause of gastroduodenal diseases in humans. Eradication of *H. pylori* by antibiotics is a very effective treatment; however, the variable prevalence of resistant organisms has been developing (Fakheri et al., 2014). A study has investigated the antibacterial effect of hochuekkito against *H. pylori* infection in vivo and in vitro (Yan et al., 2002). The in vitro experiments demonstrate that hochuekkito inhibits the growth of antibiotic-resistant strains of *H. pylori* as well as antibiotic-sensitive strains at a dose of 2.5 mg/mL. The in vivo experiments with mice orally administered hochuekkito for 7 days before or after inoculation of *H. pylori* showed that the bacterial load in the stomach was significantly reduced in the hochuekkito group compared with the control group. Hochuekkito administration induced IFN-γ in the gastric mucosa and there were no significant differences in bacterial load between the control and the hochuekkito-treated group in IFN-γ gene-deficient mice. Therefore, the authors suggest that the antibacterial effect of hochuekkito is partly due to IFN-γ induction and its possible clinical use for treatment of *H. pylori* infection.

Vibrio cholerae *Infection*

Infection with the bacterium *V. cholerae* in the small intestine causes severe diarrheal diseases such as cholera. The causative agent of cholera is cholera toxin (CT), the virulence factor secreted by *V. cholerae*. A study has indicated that daiokanzoto inhibits CT activities such as ADP-ribosylation and Chinese hamster ovary cell elongation and identified the active compounds in this Kampo medicine (Oi et al., 2002). Among several components purified from daio extract, rhubarb galloyl-tannin, a compound characterized by a polygallate structure, is the most effective one. Synthesized gallate analogs similar to rhubarb galloyl-tannin inhibit all CT activities, including ADP-ribosylation, elongation of Chinese hamster ovary cells, and fluid accumulation in ileal loops. Therefore, the authors claim that the Kampo formulations or their gallate components might be effective adjunctive therapies with oral rehydration solution for the severe diarrhea of cholera.

Porphyromonas gingivalis *and Other Oral Microorganism Infections*

P. gingivalis is a gram-negative bacterium that is implicated in certain forms of periodontal disease. Several Kampo medicines have been reported to inhibit *P. gingivalis* growth and suggested to be effective for controlling periodontal disease. A group has tested several Kampo medicines for *P. gingivalis* growth, adherence to epithelial cells, and proteinase activity (Liao et al., 2013). Among the Kampo medicines tested, sanoshashinto has the strongest inhibitory effect, and the test identified the responsive compounds present in the Chinese rhubarb, one of the major components of sanoshashinto, to be anthraquinones such as aloe emodin and rhein. These anthraquinones also inhibit the adherence of *P. gingivalis* to oral epithelial cells and reduce its proteinase activity. The strongest antiadherence activity was observed with a Kampo medicine, mashiningan extract granules, that contains rhubarb. Therefore, the authors claim that Kampo medicines containing rhubarb and its anthraquinone derivatives may be effective for controlling periodontal disease through their capacity to inhibit *P. gingivalis* growth and virulence properties.

Certain oral microorganisms are implicated in intensifying the inflammatory process and aggravating the ulcer formation of oral mucositis (OM) in cancer patients under chemotherapy or radiotherapy. A Kampo medicine, hangeshashinto (HST), has been investigated for antimicrobial activity against several bacteria and fungi (Fukamachi et al., 2015). HST extract inhibits the growth of gram-negative bacteria, including *Fusobacterium nucleatum*, *P. gingivalis*, *Porphyromonas endodontalis*, *Prevotella intermedia*, *Prevotella melaninogenica*, *Tannerella forsythia*, *Treponema denticola*, and *Porphyromonas asaccharolytica*, and less inhibitory effects on gram-positive bacteria and the fungal strains were observed. The active ingredients in HST are identified to be baicalein, berberine, coptisine, 6-shogaol, and homogentisic acid. The authors suggest that HST may be a useful treatment for OM in patients undergoing anticancer treatment.

Streptococcus pyogenes *Infection*

S. pyogenes infection causes necrotizing fasciitis and streptococcal toxic shock syndrome. The efficacy of a Kampo medicine, hainosankyuto, for the treatment of *S. pyogenes* skin infection has been investigated in in vivo experiments using mice (Minami et al., 2011). Oral administration of hainosankyuto to infected mice for 4 consecutive days increased the survival rate and reduced the size of local skin lesions compared to control mice. Hainosankyuto attenuated the bacterial load in the blood, with increased macrophage phagocytic activity in mice, and increased the levels of IL-12 and IFN-γ and decreased the level of TNFα in the serum of *S. pyogenes*-infected mice. The authors conclude that hainosankyuto may be useful for the treatment of *S. pyogenes* infection more prophylactically than therapeutically.

References

Abe, S., Ishibashi, H., Tansho, S., Hanazawa, R., Komatsu, Y., Yamaguchi, H., 2000. Protective effect of oral administration of several traditional Kampo-medicines on lethal *Candida* infection in immunosuppressed mice. Nihon Ishinkin Gakkai Zasshi 41.

Abe, S., Tansho, S., Ishibashi, H., Akagawa, G., Komatsu, Y., Yamaguchi, H., 1999. Protection of immunosuppressed mice from lethal *Candida* infection by oral administration of a kampo medicine, hochu-ekki-to. Immunopharmacol. Immunotoxicol. 21 (2), 331–342. http://dx.doi.org/10.3109/08923979909052766.

Abe, S., Tansho, S., Ishibashi, H., Inagaki, N., Komatsu, Y., Yamaguchi, H., 1998. Protective effect of oral administration of a traditional medicine, Juzen-Taiho-To, and its components on lethal *Candida albicans* infection in immunosuppressed mice. Immunopharmacol. Immunotoxicol. 20 (3), 421–431. http://dx.doi.org/10.3109/08923979809034824.

Akbar, S.M., Yamamoto, K., Abe, M., Ninomiya, T., Tanimoto, K., Masumoto, T., Onji, M., 1999. Potent synergistic effect of sho-saiko-to, a herbal medicine, during vaccine therapy in a murine model of hepatitis B virus carrier. Eur. J. Clin. Investig. 29 (9), 786–792.

Aoki, T., Kojima, T., Kameda, N., Yoshijima, S., Ono, A., Kobayashi, Y., 1994. Anti-inflammatory effect of a traditional Chinese medicine, ren-shen-yang-rong-tang (Japanese name: ninjin-youei-to), on alveolar macrophages stimulated by RANTES or TNF-alpha. Arerugi 43 (5), 663–667.

Azzam, H.S., Goertz, C., Fritts, M., Jonas, W.B., 2007. Natural products and chronic hepatitis C virus. Liver Int. 27 (1), 17–25. http://dx.doi.org/10.1111/j.1478-3231.2006.01408.x.

Chang, J.S., Wang, K.C., Liu, H.W., Chen, M.C., Chiang, L.C., Lin, C.C., 2007. Sho-saiko-to (Xiao-Chai-Hu-Tang) and crude saikosaponins inhibit hepatitis B virus in a stable HBV-producing cell line. Am. J. Chin. Med. 35 (2), 341–351. http://dx.doi.org/10.1142/s0192415x07004862.

Chang, J.S., Yeh, C.F., Wang, K.C., Shieh, D.E., Yen, M.H., Chiang, L.C., 2013. Xiao-Qing-Long-Tang (Sho-seiryu-to) inhibited cytopathic effect of human respiratory syncytial virus in cell lines of human respiratory tract. J. Ethnopharmacol. 147 (2), 481–487. http://dx.doi.org/10.1016/j.jep.2013.03.044.

Chen, C.J., Michaelis, M., Hsu, H.K., Tsai, C.C., Yang, K.D., Wu, Y.C., Doerr, H.W., 2008. Toona sinensis Roem tender leaf extract inhibits SARS coronavirus replication. J. Ethnopharmacol. 120 (1), 108–111. http://dx.doi.org/10.1016/j.jep.2008.07.048.

Chen, X.S., Wang, G.J., Cai, X., Yu, H.Y., Hu, Y.P., 2001a. Inhibition of hepatitis B virus by oxymatrine in vivo. World J. Gastroenterol. 7 (1), 49–52.

Chen, Y., Li, J., Zeng, M., Lu, L., Qu, D., Mao, Y., Hua, J., 2001b. The inhibitory effect of oxymatrine on hepatitis C virus in vitro. Zhonghua Gan Zang Bing Za Zhi (Suppl. 9), 12–14.

Cyong, J.C., Ki, S.M., Iijima, K., Kobayashi, T., Furuya, M., 2000. Clinical and pharmacological studies on liver diseases treated with Kampo herbal medicine. Am. J. Chin. Med. 28 (3–4), 351–360. http://dx.doi.org/10.1142/s0192415x00000416.

Dan, K., Akiyoshi, H., Munakata, K., Hasegawa, H., Watanabe, K., 2013. A Kampo (traditional Japanese herbal) medicine, Hochuekkito, pretreatment in mice prevented influenza virus replication accompanied with GM-CSF expression and increase in several defensin mRNA levels. Pharmacology 91 (5–6), 314–321. http://dx.doi.org/10.1159/000350188.

Deng, G., Kurtz, R.C., Vickers, A., Lau, N., Yeung, K.S., Shia, J., Cassileth, B., 2011. A single arm phase II study of a Far-Eastern traditional herbal formulation (sho-sai-ko-to or xiao-chai-hu-tang) in chronic hepatitis C patients. J. Ethnopharmacol. 136 (1), 83–87. http://dx.doi.org/10.1016/j.jep.2011.04.008.

Dong, Y., Xi, H., Yu, Y., Wang, Q., Jiang, K., Li, L., 2002. Effects of oxymatrine on the serum levels of T helper cell 1 and 2 cytokines and the expression of the S gene in hepatitis B virus S gene transgenic mice: a study on the anti-hepatitis B virus mechanism of oxymatrine. J. Gastroenterol. Hepatol. 17 (12), 1299–1306.

Egashira, T., Takayama, F., Komatsu, Y., 2003. Changes of materials that scavenge 1,1-diphenyl-2-picrylhydrazyl radicals in plasma by per-oral administration of Kampo medicine, Ninjin-yoei-to in rats. J. Pharm. Pharmacol. 55 (3), 367–371. http://dx.doi.org/10.1211/002235702711.

Fakheri, H., Bari, Z., Aarabi, M., Malekzadeh, R., 2014. *Helicobacter pylori* eradication in West Asia: a review. World J. Gastroenterol. 20 (30), 10355–10367. http://dx.doi.org/10.3748/wjg.v20.i30.10355.

Fukamachi, H., Matsumoto, C., Omiya, Y., Arimoto, T., Morisaki, H., Kataoka, H., Kuwata, H., 2015. Effects of hangeshashinto on growth of oral microorganisms. Evid. Based Complement. Altern. Med. 2015, 512947. http://dx.doi.org/10.1155/2015/512947.

Hayashi, K., Imanishi, N., Kashiwayama, Y., Kawano, A., Terasawa, K., Shimada, Y., Ochiai, H., 2007. Inhibitory effect of cinnamaldehyde, derived from Cinnamomi cortex, on the growth of influenza A/PR/8 virus in vitro and in vivo. Antivir. Res. 74 (1), 1–8. http://dx.doi.org/10.1016/j.antiviral.2007.01.003.

Higaki, S., Hasegawa, Y., Morohashi, M., Sakamoto, K., Yamagishi, T., 1990. The influence of coptidis rhizoma to lipase activity of *Propionibacterium acnes*. Nihon Hifuka Gakkai Zasshi 100 (8), 883–886.

Higaki, S., Hasegawa, Y., Morohashi, M., Takayoshi, Y., 1995. The correlation of Kampo formulations and their ingredients on anti-bacterial activities against *Propionibacterium acnes*. J. Dermatol. 22 (1), 4–9.

Higaki, S., Kitagawa, T., Kagoura, M., Morohashi, M., Yamagishi, T., 2000. Relationship between *Propionibacterium acnes* biotypes and Jumi-haidoku-to. J. Dermatol. 27 (10), 635–638.

Higaki, S., Morimatsu, S., Morohashi, M., Yamagishi, T., Hasegawa, Y., 1997. Susceptibility of *Propionibacterium acnes*, *Staphylococcus aureus* and *Staphylococcus epidermidis* to 10 Kampo formulations. J. Int. Med. Res. 25 (6), 318–324.

Higaki, S., Morohashi, M., 2003. *Propionibacterium acnes* lipase in seborrheic dermatitis and other skin diseases and Unsei-in. Drugs Exp. Clin. Res. 29 (4), 157–159.

Higaki, S., Nakamura, M., Kitagawa, T., Morohashi, M., Yamagishi, T., 2001. Effect of lipase activities of *Propionibacterium* granulosum and *Propionibacterium acnes*. Drugs Exp. Clin. Res. 27 (5–6), 161–164.

Higaki, S., Nakamura, M., Morohashi, M., Hasegawa, Y., Yamagishi, T., 1996a. Activity of eleven kampo formulations and eight kampo crude drugs against *Propionibacterium acnes* isolated from acne patients: retrospective evaluation in 1990 and 1995. J. Dermatol. 23 (12), 871–875.

Higaki, S., Nakamura, M., Morohashi, M., Hasegawa, Y., Yamagishi, T., 1996b. Anti-lipase activity of Kampo formulations, coptidis rhizoma and its alkaloids against *Propionibacterium acnes*. J. Dermatol. 23 (5), 310–314.

Higaki, S., Nakamura, M., Morohashi, M., Yamagishi, T., 2004. *Propionibacterium acnes* biotypes and susceptibility to minocycline and Keigai-rengyo-to. Int. J. Dermatol. 43 (2), 103–107.

Hisha, H., Yamada, H., Sakurai, M.H., Kiyohara, H., Li, Y., Yu, C., Ikehara, S., 1997. Isolation and identification of hematopoietic stem cell-stimulating substances from Kampo (Japanese herbal) medicine, Juzen-taiho-to. Blood 90 (3), 1022–1030.

Hokari, R., Nagai, T., Yamada, H., 2012. In vivo anti-influenza virus activity of Japanese herbal (kampo) medicine, "shahakusan," and its possible mode of action. Evid. Based Complement. Altern. Med. 2012, 794970. http://dx.doi.org/10.1155/2012/794970.

Ikeda, K., Wu, D.Z., Ishigaki, M., Sunose, H., Takasaka, T., 1994. Inhibitory effects of sho-seiryu-to on acetylcholine-induced responses in nasal gland acinar cells. Am. J. Chin. Med. 22 (2), 191–196. http://dx.doi.org/10.1142/s0192415x94000231.

Iwagaki, H., Saito, S., 2013. Effects of a Kampo medicine on postoperative infection. Nihon Geka Gakkai Zasshi 114 (5), 241–245.

Kainuma, M., Hayashi, J., Sakai, S., Imai, K., Mantani, N., Kohta, K., Terasawa, K., 2002a. The efficacy of herbal medicine (kampo) in reducing the adverse effects of IFN-beta in chronic hepatitis C. Am. J. Chin. Med. 30 (2–3), 355–367. http://dx.doi.org/10.1142/s0192415x02000284.

Kainuma, M., Ogata, N., Kogure, T., Kohta, K., Hattori, N., Mitsuma, T., Terasawa, K., 2002b. The efficacy of a herbal medicine (Mao-to) in combination with intravenous natural interferon-beta for patients with chronic hepatitis C, genotype 1b and high viral load: a pilot study. Phytomedicine 9 (5), 365–372.

Kaji, K., Yoshida, S., Nagata, N., Yamashita, T., Mizukoshi, E., Honda, M., Kaneko, S., 2004. An open-label study of administration of EH0202, a health-food additive, to patients with chronic hepatitis C. J. Gastroenterol. 39 (9), 873–878. http://dx.doi.org/10.1007/s00535-004-1404-z.

Kakumu, S., Yoshioka, K., Wakita, T., Ishikawa, T., 1991. Effects of TJ-9 Sho-saiko-to (kampo medicine) on interferon gamma and antibody production specific for hepatitis B virus antigen in patients with type B chronic hepatitis. Int. J. Immunopharmacol. 13 (2–3), 141–146.

Kamei, T., Kumano, H., Beppu, K., Iwata, K., Masumura, S., 1998. Response of healthy individuals to ninjin-yoei-to extract—enhancement of natural killer cell activity. Am. J. Chin. Med. 26 (1), 91–95. http://dx.doi.org/10.1142/s0192415x98000129.

Kato, T., Horie, N., Matsuta, T., Naoki, U., Shimoyama, T., Kaneko, T., Sakagami, H., 2012. Anti-UV/HIV activity of Kampo medicines and constituent plant extracts. In Vivo 26 (6), 1007–1013.

Kawashima, N., Ito, Y., Sekiya, Y., Narita, A., Okuno, Y., Muramatsu, H., Kojima, S., 2015. Choreito formula for BK virus-associated hemorrhagic cystitis after allogeneic hematopoietic stem cell transplantation. Biol. Blood Marrow Transplant. 21 (2), 319–325. http://dx.doi.org/10.1016/j.bbmt.2014.10.018.

Kido, T., Mori, K., Daikuhara, H., Tsuchiya, H., Ishige, A., Sasaki, H., 2000. The protective effect of hochu-ekki-to (TJ-41), a Japanese herbal medicine, against HSV-1 infection in mitomycin C-treated mice. Anticancer Res. 20 (6a), 4109–4113.

Kubo, T., Nishimura, H., 2007. Antipyretic effect of Mao-to, a Japanese herbal medicine, for treatment of type A influenza infection in children. Phytomedicine 14 (2–3), 96–101. http://dx.doi.org/10.1016/j.phymed.2006.09.015.

Li, J., Li, C., Zeng, M., 1998. Preliminary study on therapeutic effect of oxymatrine in treating patients with chronic hepatitis C. Zhongguo Zhong Xi Yi Jie He Za Zhi 18 (4), 227–229.

Liao, J., Zhao, L., Yoshioka, M., Hinode, D., Grenier, D., 2013. Effects of Japanese traditional herbal medicines (Kampo) on growth and virulence properties of *Porphyromonas gingivalis* and viability of oral epithelial cells. Pharm. Biol. 51 (12), 1538–1544. http://dx.doi.org/10.3109/13880209.2013.801995.

Liu, J., Liu, Y., Klaassen, C.D., 1994. The effect of Chinese hepatoprotective medicines on experimental liver injury in mice. J. Ethnopharmacol. 42 (3), 183–191.

Mantani, N., Andoh, T., Kawamata, H., Terasawa, K., Ochiai, H., 1999. Inhibitory effect of Ephedrae herba, an oriental traditional medicine, on the growth of influenza A/PR/8 virus in MDCK cells. Antivir. Res. 44 (3), 193–200.

Mao, Y.M., Zeng, M.D., Lu, L.G., Wan, M.B., Li, C.Z., Chen, C.W., Zhang, H.Q., 2004. Capsule oxymatrine in treatment of hepatic fibrosis due to chronic viral hepatitis: a randomized, double blind, placebo-controlled, multicenter clinical study. World J. Gastroenterol. 10 (22), 3269–3273.

Minami, M., Ichikawa, M., Hata, N., Hasegawa, T., 2011. Protective effect of hainosankyuto, a traditional Japanese medicine, on *Streptococcus pyogenes* infection in murine model. PLoS One 6 (7), e22188. http://dx.doi.org/10.1371/journal.pone.0022188.

Mori, K., Kido, T., Daikuhara, H., Sakakibara, I., Sakata, T., Shimizu, K., Komatsu, Y., 1999. Effect of Hochu-ekki-to (TJ-41), a Japanese herbal medicine, on the survival of mice infected with influenza virus. Antivir. Res. 44 (2), 103–111.

Moscona, A., 2009. Global transmission of oseltamivir-resistant influenza. N. Engl. J. Med. 360 (10), 953–956. http://dx.doi.org/10.1056/NEJMp0900648.

Munakata, K., Takashima, K., Nishiyama, M., Asano, N., Mase, A., Hioki, K., Watanabe, K., 2012. Microarray analysis on germfree mice elucidates the primary target of a traditional Japanese medicine juzentaihoto: acceleration of IFN-alpha response via affecting the ISGF3-IRF7 signaling cascade. BMC Genom. 13, 30. http://dx.doi.org/10.1186/1471-2164-13-30.

Murayama, T., Yamaguchi, N., Iwamoto, K., Eizuru, Y., 2006. Inhibition of ganciclovir-resistant human cytomegalovirus replication by Kampo (Japanese herbal medicine). Antivir. Chem. Chemother. 17 (1), 11–16.

Nagai, T., Kataoka, E., Aoki, Y., Hokari, R., Kiyohara, H., Yamada, H., 2014. Alleviative effects of a kampo (a Japanese herbal) medicine "maoto (Ma-Huang-Tang)" on the early phase of influenza virus infection and its possible mode of action. Evid. Based Complement. Altern. Med. 2014, 187036. http://dx.doi.org/10.1155/2014/187036.

Nagai, T., Kiyohara, H., Munakata, K., Shirahata, T., Sunazuka, T., Harigaya, Y., Yamada, H., 2002. Pinellic acid from the tuber of Pinellia ternata Breitenbach as an effective oral adjuvant for nasal influenza vaccine. Int. Immunopharmacol. 2 (8), 1183–1193.

Nagai, T., Yamada, H., 1994. In vivo anti-influenza virus activity of kampo (Japanese herbal) medicine "sho-seiryu-to" and its mode of action. Int. J. Immunopharmacol. 16 (8), 605–613.

Nagai, T., Yamada, H., 1998. In vivo anti-influenza virus activity of Kampo (Japanese herbal) medicine "sho-seiryu-to"—stimulation of mucosal immune system and effect on allergic pulmonary inflammation model mice. Immunopharmacol. Immunotoxicol. 20 (2), 267–281. http://dx.doi.org/10.3109/08923979809038544.

Nagasaka, K., Kurokawa, M., Imakita, M., Terasawa, K., Shiraki, K., 1995. Efficacy of kakkon-to, a traditional herb medicine, in herpes simplex virus type 1 infection in mice. J. Med. Virol. 46 (1), 28–34.

Ohgitani, E., Kita, M., Mazda, O., Imanishi, J., 2014. Combined administration of oseltamivir and hochu-ekki-to (TJ-41) dramatically decreases the viral load in lungs of senescence-accelerated mice during influenza virus infection. Arch. Virol. 159 (2), 267–275. http://dx.doi.org/10.1007/s00705-013-1807-3.

Oi, H., Matsuura, D., Miyake, M., Ueno, M., Takai, I., Yamamoto, T., Noda, M., 2002. Identification in traditional herbal medications and confirmation by synthesis of factors that inhibit cholera toxin-induced fluid accumulation. Proc. Natl. Acad. Sci. U.S.A. 99 (5), 3042–3046. http://dx.doi.org/10.1073/pnas.052709499.

Ono, K., Nakane, H., Fukushima, M., Chermann, J.C., Barre-Sinoussi, F., 1990. Differential inhibition of the activities of reverse transcriptase and various cellular DNA polymerases by a traditional Kampo drug, sho-saiko-to. Biomed. Pharmacother. 44 (1), 13–16.

Piras, G., Makino, M., Baba, M., 1997. Sho-saiko-to, a traditional Kampo medicine, enhances the anti-HIV-1 activity of lamivudine (3TC) in vitro. Microbiol. Immunol. 41 (10), 835–839.

Saiki, I., Koizumi, K., Goto, H., Inujima, A., Namiki, T., Raimura, M., Origasa, H., 2013. The long-term effects of a kampo medicine, juzentaihoto, on maintenance of antibody titer in elderly people after influenza vaccination. Evid. Based Complement. Altern. Med. 2013, 568074. http://dx.doi.org/10.1155/2013/568074.

Shimizu, I., 2000. Sho-saiko-to: Japanese herbal medicine for protection against hepatic fibrosis and carcinoma. J. Gastroenterol. Hepatol. (Suppl. 15), D84–D90.

Smith, M.A., Chan, J., Mohammad, R.A., 2015. Ledipasvir-sofosbuvir: interferon-/ribavirin-free regimen for chronic hepatitis C virus infection. Ann. Pharmacother. 49 (3), 343–350. http://dx.doi.org/10.1177/1060028014563952.

Suzuki, M., Sasaki, K., Yoshizaki, F., Oguchi, K., Fujisawa, M., Cyong, J.C., 2005. Anti-hepatitis C virus effect of citrus unshiu peel and its active ingredient nobiletin. Am. J. Chin. Med. 33 (1), 87–94. http://dx.doi.org/10.1142/s0192415x05002680.

Taguchi, A., Kawana, K., Yokoyama, T., Adachi, K., Yamashita, A., Tomio, K., Kozuma, S., 2012. Adjuvant effect of Japanese herbal medicines on the mucosal type 1 immune responses to human papillomavirus (HPV) E7 in mice immunized orally with Lactobacillus-based therapeutic HPV vaccine in a synergistic manner. Vaccine 30 (36), 5368–5372. http://dx.doi.org/10.1016/j.vaccine.2012.06.027.

Tajiri, H., Kozaiwa, K., Ozaki, Y., Miki, K., Shimuzu, K., Okada, S., 1991. Effect of sho-saiko-to(xiao-chai-hu-tang) on HBeAg clearance in children with chronic hepatitis B virus infection and with sustained liver disease. Am. J. Chin. Med. 19 (2), 121–129. http://dx.doi.org/10.1142/s0192415x91000193.

Toriumi, Y., Kamei, T., Murata, K., Takahashi, I., Suzuki, N., Mazda, O., 2012. Utility of Maoto in an influenza season where reduced effectiveness of oseltamivir was observed – a clinical, non-randomized study in children. Forsch Komplementmed 19 (4), 179–186. http://dx.doi.org/10.1159/000341547.

Weinstock, D.M., Zuccotti, G., 2009. The evolution of influenza resistance and treatment. Jama 301 (10), 1066–1069. http://dx.doi.org/10.1001/jama.2009.324.

Wen, C.C., Shyur, L.F., Jan, J.T., Liang, P.H., Kuo, C.J., Arulselvan, P., Yang, N.S., 2011. Traditional Chinese medicine herbal extracts of *Cibotium barometz*, *Gentiana scabra*, *Dioscorea batatas*, *Cassia tora*, and *Taxillus chinensis* inhibit SARS-CoV replication. J. Tradit. Complement. Med. 1 (1), 41–50.

Yamada, H., Nagai, T., 1998. In vivo antiinfluenza virus activity of Kampo medicine Sho-seiryu-to through mucosal immune system. Methods Find Exp. Clin. Pharmacol. 20 (3), 185–192.

Yamaoka, Y., Kawakita, T., Nomoto, K., 2000. Protective effect of a traditional Japanese medicine, Bu-zhong-yi-qi-tang (Japanese name: hochu-ekki-to), on the restraint stress-induced susceptibility against *Listeria monocytogenes*. Immunopharmacology 48 (1), 35–42.

Yamaoka, Y., Kawakita, T., Nomoto, K., 2001. Protective effect of a traditional Japanese medicine Hochu-ekki-to (Chinese name: Bu-zhong-yi-qi-tang), on the susceptibility against *Listeria monocytogenes* in infant mice. Int. Immunopharmacol. 1 (9–10), 1669–1677.

Yamashiki, M., Nishimura, A., Huang, X.X., Nobori, T., Sakaguchi, S., Suzuki, H., 1999. Effects of the Japanese herbal medicine "Sho-saiko-to" (TJ-9) on interleukin-12 production in patients with HCV-positive liver cirrhosis. Dev. Immunol. 7 (1), 17–22.

Yan, X., Kita, M., Minami, M., Yamamoto, T., Kuriyama, H., Ohno, T., Imanishi, J., 2002. Antibacterial effect of Kampo herbal formulation Hochu-ekki-to (Bu-Zhong-Yi-Qi-Tang) on *Helicobacter pylori* infection in mice. Microbiol. Immunol. 46 (7), 475–482.

Yanagihara, S., Kobayashi, H., Tamiya, H., Tsuruta, D., Okano, Y., Takahashi, K., Ishii, M., 2013. Protective effect of hochuekkito, a Kampo prescription, against ultraviolet B irradiation-induced skin damage in hairless mice. J. Dermatol. 40 (3), 201–206. http://dx.doi.org/10.1111/1346-8138.12050.

Yang, W., Zeng, M., Fan, Z., Mao, Y., Song, Y., Jia, Y., Zhu, H.Y., 2002. Prophylactic and therapeutic effect of oxymatrine on D-galactosamine-induced rat liver fibrosis. Zhonghua Gan Zang Bing Za Zhi 10 (3), 193–196.

Yoshimura, A., Kuroda, K., Kawasaki, K., Yamashina, S., Maeda, T., Ohnishi, S., 1982. Infectious cell entry mechanism of influenza virus. J. Virol. 43 (1), 284–293.

CHAPTER 15

Drug Delivery Aspects of Herbal Medicines

Arunkumar Nagalingam
KMCH College of Pharmacy, Coimbatore, Tamilnadu, India

Introduction

Herbal drugs have been used since medieval times for treatment of illness in local or regional healing practices. These are naturally occurring, plant-based products with minimal or no chemical processing. In most developing countries, more than 80% of the people still rely on traditional herbal medicines to meet their health care needs. Although modern medicine exists, traditional herbal treatments have gained popularity for their historical and cultural values. Moreover, it is believed that they are safer and free from side effects compared to modern medicines. Modern research has also pointed out that many modern drug treatments suppress the symptoms of disease, leaving out the underlying problems, in contrast to natural herbal medicines, which demonstrate better results as they address the root cause of the disease more effectively (Annie, 2015).

Traditional herbal systems of medicine are gaining worldwide significance in the light of modern technological aspects. Countries like Japan, India, China, Egypt, and Pakistan and regions in Africa and the Middle East have their own forms of traditional medicine that are mostly based on plants and herbs (Table 15.1).

Herbal medicines are prepared mostly from plants by eco-friendly processes and hence they are also called "phytomedicines." The lack of scientific evidence, along with processing problems like isolation and identification of individual components and standardization of such preparations, has hindered the development of herbal products as novel formulations. Scientific research has shown that the activity of an herbal formulation is due to either a specific constituent or a blend of components. Advancements in herbal research with respect to extraction processes, isolation and identification procedures, development of bioassay techniques for efficacy testing, and standardization techniques has boosted the image of herbal medicine in the health care scenario (Mitra and Banerjee, 2012).

According to the WHO, herbal medicines are the mainstay for 75–90% people in developing countries for primary health care (Robinson and Zhang, 2011). Although herbal medicines have their own advantages there are still lacunae in the development of these drugs into palatable formulations. The lack of knowledge in regard to the physiochemical properties of the active constituents of the plants and less awareness of side effects and toxicity of

Table 15.1: Various Systems of Medicine

Country	Traditional System of Medicine
Japan	Kampo
India	Ayurveda and Siddha
China	Chinese herbal medicine
Korea	Hanbang
Pakistan	Indusynunic
Middle East	Unani
Europe	Aromatherapy, homeopathy, herbalism
United States and Australia	Western herbal medicine
Africa	Muti and Ifa

herbal drugs have made it difficult for researchers to bring out successful herbal formulations. The unsuitable molecular size and poor lipid solubility of most herbal constituents have deterred the development of herbal formulations. A multidisciplinary approach to drug delivery has to be developed to increase the scope of herbal drugs among health care professionals.

A drug delivery system is the method by which the desired quantity of a drug reaches the site of action and exerts its pharmacological action. Drug delivery systems are based on interdisciplinary approaches that combine polymer science, pharmaceutics, chemistry, and molecular biology. The chemical and pharmacological research performed since the 1990s on plants to identify the chemical compositions of extracts have suggested that the separation and purification of the various components lead to a partial or full loss of activity of the isolated/purified compound. The difficulties in isolation, identification, extraction, and standardization of herbal compounds have hindered interest of formulation scientists in developing a suitable drug delivery system for herbal drugs. But recent developments in various areas of herbal research and the latest technological innovations have laid down a pathway to developing novel drug delivery systems for herbal medicines.

Traditional Drug Delivery Systems

Herbal drugs, including Japanese Kampo medicines, are traditionally given in the form of pills, decoctions, infusions, tinctures, syrups, powders, etc. The Japanese *Pharmacopeia* has included many Kampo medicines, most of which are administered as decoctions, powders, or pills.

Examples of Kampo medicines are bai hu tang (white tiger decoction), wu pi san (five peel powder), and gui zhi fu ling wan (cinnamon twig and *Poria* pill).

Decoctions

Decoctions are normally preferred for harder herbs like roots, barks, and seeds. It is helpful to grind or crush the whole root, bark, and seeds before preparing the decoction. This is prepared by heating the required quantity of herbs with water for a period of about 30 min, until about 50% of the water is lost. The vessel must be closed during heating to prevent any essential constituents from being lost through evaporation. The extract is then removed from heat and strained using a filter, and the decoction is used either as a whole or after suitable dilution.

Examples of herbs used in decoctions are ba zhen tang (eight treasure decoction) and bai hu tang (white tiger decoction).

Infusions

Infusions are fluid preparations obtained by macerating the crude drug in water. They are prepared by moistening the crude drug, after being cut into suitable pieces, with a small quantity of water for about 15 min, and about a liter of boiling water is then added to it and heated for 5 min with continuous stirring. The fluid is then filtered after cooling and used as required.

Extracts

Extracts are prepared by concentrating extractives of crude drugs. There are two types of extracts:

1. viscous extracts
2. dry extracts

Extracts are prepared by pulverizing the crude drug to a suitable size and extracting for a particular period of time with suitable solvents by means of cold or warm extraction or by percolation. The extract is then filtered and the filtrate is concentrated or dried by a suitable method to make a millet jelly-like consistency, for the viscous type, or to make crushable solid masses, granules, or powders for the dry extracts.

Examples are *Glycyrrhiza* extract and belladonna extract.

Pills

Pills are solid spherical forms intended for oral administration. These are generally prepared by mixing the drug with additives such as diluents, binders, disintegrants, etc., and pressing it into a spherical form by a suitable method. If required these pills can be coated with a coating agent or sugar to mask the odor and taste.

Tinctures

These are liquid preparations usually prepared by extracting the crude drug with ethanol or a mixture of water and ethanol. They are prepared by maceration or percolation using coarse powders or fine cuttings of crude drugs with an appropriate solvent.

The content of the marker constituent or ethanol in tinctures prepared by either of these two methods (maceration or percolation) is specified by assaying the content using a portion of the sample and adjusting the content with a sufficient amount of percolate or solvent as required based on the result of the assay.

An example is tincture of opium.

Powders

Powders of herbal drugs are prepared by cutting the crude drugs into smaller parts, drying them completely, and pulverizing them to get the powdered drug.

Examples of powders are powdered ginseng, nux vomica extract powder, and powdered aloe.

Limitations of Traditional Drug Delivery Systems

1. There is a high chance that the herbal constituents will be destroyed in the acidic pH of the stomach.
2. Some components may be metabolized by the liver before reaching the systemic circulation and hence minimum effective concentrations cannot be achieved to produce any therapeutic effect.
3. Herbal constituents like polyphenols have good water solubility but are poorly absorbed, which limits the ability to pass the lipid membrane and hence leads to lesser bioavailability.
4. Poor patient compliance increases the chances of missing a dose when a short half-life of the drug requires frequent administration.
5. Fluctuations in blood levels may lead to overmedication or undermedication.
6. Typical drawbacks of herbal drugs, including poor lipid solubility, unsuitable molecular size, and instability, cannot be overcome by traditional drug delivery systems.

Because most of the conventional methods of herbal drug delivery systems cannot satisfy the requirements of an ideal drug delivery system, it is imperative for the formulation scientist to develop novel drug delivery systems with the requisite modifications for herbal drugs.

Ideal Drug Delivery System

An ideal drug delivery system should have the following features:

1. ensures stability of the drug in the human biological environment;
2. releases the drug at the site of action at the required time and quantity;
3. reduces fluctuation of blood levels by maintaining the drug release in a constant manner;
4. improves the palatability of the drug by masking the bitter taste and unpleasant odor of some herbal drugs;
5. improves the oral bioavailability of the drug.

Novel Drug Delivery Systems

Novel drug delivery systems (NDDSs) are advantageous in delivering herbal drugs at a predetermined rate and exhibiting site-specific action. In novel drug delivery technology, control of the distribution of the drug is achieved by incorporating the drug into a carrier system or changing the structure of the drug at the molecular level (Atmzkuri and Dathi, 2010). In phytoformulation research, nano dosage forms like liposomes, phytosomes, nanoemulsion, ethosomes, transferosomes, etc., have a number of advantages, including enhancement of solubility, stability, and bioavailability; protection from toxicity; enhancement of pharmacological activity; and protection from physical and chemical degradation (Saraf, 2010). Thus NDDSs have the potential to address various problems related to herbal medicine practice.

Liposomes

Liposomes are spherical vesicles made up of biodegradable natural or synthetic phospholipids. They usually have one or more concentric membranes. Liposomes are composed of phospholipids, which are amphipathic and are characterized by having a lipophilic tail and hydrophilic head on the same molecule (Lasic, 1993). The polar heads orient themselves toward the aqueous medium and the hydrophobic tails constitute the inner region of the membrane (Fig. 15.1) and thus form a bilayer.

This helps them to encapsulate water-soluble components in the hydrophilic compartment and lipid-soluble components in the lipid section and this property is used to alter the pharmacokinetic profile of drugs, herbs, and vitamins as well as enzymes. A number of herbal liposomal formulations have been studied, which are summarized in Table 15.2.

The unique properties of liposomes make them a potential carrier system to enhance the performance of herbal drugs by enhancing solubility, improving bioavailability, enhancing cellular uptake, altering the pharmacokinetics (Xiao and Li, 2002), and improving in vitro and in vivo stability. Liposomal delivery systems can enhance the therapeutic efficacy of a

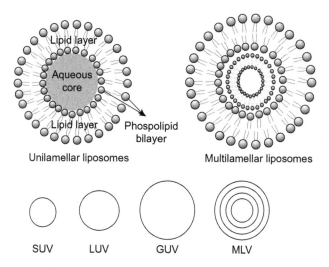

Figure 15.1

Liposomes. *GUV*, giant unilamellar vesicle; *LUV*, large unilamellar vesicle; *MLV*, multilamellar liposome vesicle; *SUV*, small unilamellar vesicle.

Table 15.2: Herbal Liposomal Formulations

Active Ingredient	Application	Use	References
Magnolol	Enhances therapeutic efficacy	Inhibiting vascular smooth muscle cell proliferation	Chen (2008)
Nux vomica	Increases stability of formulations	Antitumor, analgesic, and antiinflammatory activities	Chen et al. (2010)
Quercetin	Enhances therapeutic efficacy	Antioxidant activity	Ghosh et al. (2010)
Diospyrin	Enhancement of its antitumor effect	Anticancer activity	Hazra et al. (2005)
Artemisia arborescens	Increases antiviral activity and stability	Antiviral activity	Gortzi et al. (2008)

product by delivering it to the site of action and by maintaining the minimum effective levels for a longer period of time (Weiss and Fintelmann, 2000).

Silymarin is poorly absorbed in the gastrointestinal tract (Blumenthal et al., 2000) and hence parenteral administration shows better effect than oral administration (Carini et al., 1992). A successful liposomal dosage form of silymarin was developed for buccal delivery and was found to have better stability as well as improved bioavailability (El-Samaligy et al., 2006).

Classification of Liposomes

Liposome size can vary from very small (0.025 μm) to large (2.5 μm) vesicles. The vesicle size plays an important role in determining the circulation time of liposomes and both size and number of the bilayers affect the drug encapsulation inside the liposomes. Based on the size and the number of bilayers, liposomes are classified into two broad categories:

1. multilamellar vesicles
2. unilamellar vesicles

Unilamellar vesicles are further classified as large unilamellar vesicles and small unilamellar vesicles (Amarnath and Sharma, 1997)

Advantages of Liposomes (Himanshu et al., 2011)

Liposomes offer many distinct advantages over other forms of drug delivery:

- increased efficacy and therapeutic index;
- increased stability by encapsulation;
- nontoxic, flexible, biocompatible, and biodegradable;
- reduced toxicity of encapsulated agent.

They can trap both hydrophobic and hydrophilic compounds, avoid decomposition of entrapped components, and release the compound at the designated targets (Shehata et al., 2008).

Phytosomes

Phytosomes are also called "phytolipid delivery systems" when used for delivering herbal drugs (Gandhi et al., 2012). This is a patented technology developed by Indena to incorporate standardized plant extracts or water-soluble phytoconstituents into phospholipids to produce lipid-compatible complexes, which enhances their absorption and bioavailability (Bombardelli et al., 1989).

The phytosome approach guarantees the pharmacokinetic profile of herbal drugs without resorting to pharmacological adjuvants or structural modifications of the ingredients. The phytosome technology produces a little cell, better able to transit from a hydrophilic environment into the lipid-friendly environment of the enterocyte cell membrane and from there into the cell, finally reaching the blood. Thus it protects the valuable constituents of the herbal drug from being destroyed by gastric enzymes and gut bacteria (Murray, 2008).

Advantages (Kidd and Head, 2005)

1. Phosphatidylcholine present in the phytosome acts both as a carrier and as a hepatoprotective.
2. The bioavailability of hydrophilic phytoconstituents is increased by phytosomes, thereby increasing the efficacy of the drugs.

3. The constituents of phytosomes are safe.
4. Phytosomes are more stable compared to liposomes because of the presence of chemical bonds.
5. Phospholipids present in phytosomes add nutritional value to the product.
6. Skin permeation of phytosomes is relatively easier and hence they can be effectively used as topical preparations.
7. Phospholipids engulf/encapsulate the water-soluble phytoconstituents and thus protect them from destruction by digestive enzymes.
8. Because phosphatidylcholine is a part of the cell membrane, it nourishes the skin in addition to acting as a carrier in topical preparations.
9. Phytosome preparation methods are relatively simple.
10. As the absorption is improved by phytosomes, the dose requirement of the drug can be reduced.

Preparation of Phytosomes

The common stages of the preparation of phytosomes are charted in Fig. 15.2.

Flavonoid components are insoluble in chloroform, ether, or benzene but become extremely soluble when prepared as phytosomes. This change in the chemical and physical properties is attributed to the true stable complex formed between the phospholipid and the flavonoid (Yanyu et al., 2006). The molecular structure of phytosomes is shown in Fig. 15.3.

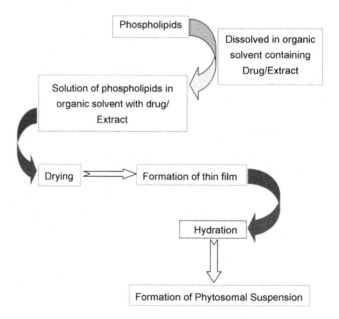

Figure 15.2
Preparation stages of phytosomes.

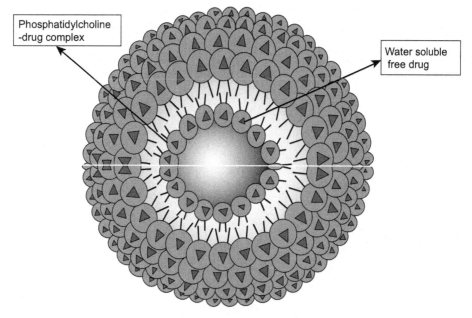

Figure 15.3
Molecular structure of a phytosome.

The success of phytosomal formulation in terms of efficacy and stability depends on various factors such as size of the phytosomes, membrane permeability, entrapment efficiency, chemical composition, and purity of the components. Hence phytosomes are generally characterized for their physical properties such as size, shape, drug entrapment, percentage drug release, chemical composition, quantity, and purity of the constituents (Jain, 2001).

Difference Between Phytosome and Liposome

The basic difference between a phytosome and a liposome is that in a phytosome, the phytoconstituent forms an integral part of the membrane by forming chemical bonds with the hydrophilic head of the phospholipid, whereas in liposomes the active herbal constituent is dissolved in the layers of the membrane and enclosed by phospholipids (Fig. 15.4) (Pandey, 2010).

Phytosomes are absorbed more than liposomes and show better bioavailability (Amin and Bhat, 2012). It was also found that phytosomes were superior to liposomes in topical formulations.

Applications of Phytosomes

Phytosome technology is most commonly used for herbal constituents that have poor absorption or poor bioavailability. This process has been widely used by researchers for many herbal extracts, including grape seed, *Ginkgo biloba*, green tea, milk thistle, ginseng, etc., and has

LIPOSOME

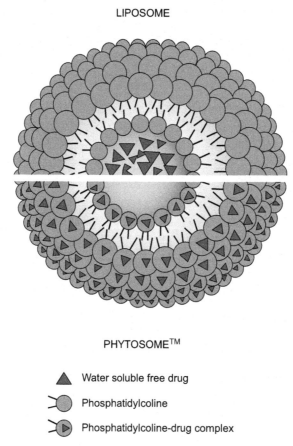

PHYTOSOME™

▲ Water soluble free drug

○ Phosphatidylcoline

○ Phosphatidylcoline-drug complex

Figure 15.4
Comparison of liposomes and phytosomes.

shown improved absorption and bioavailability in comparison with conventional extracts. This technology has been developed by Indena, an Italian company that specializes in identification, development, and production of active herbal constituents for use in pharmaceutical, nutraceutical, and cosmetic industries. Phytosome technology, a line of products, has been developed and commercialized by Indena (Table 15.3).

Phytosome formulations have the ability to cross the lipid biomembrane and reach the circulation, which results in increased absorption of active molecules when topically applied and increase in bioavailability when administered orally.

Research has shown that much work is being done to formulate herbal extracts to produce more bioavailable phytosomes. Extracts of *Aesculus hippocastanum*, saponins extracted from *Ruscus aculeatus*, Ximenoil and ximenynic acid extracted from *Santalum album*, and extracts of *Coleus forskohlii*, *Vaccinium myrtillus*, and *Serenoa repens* are being highly worked upon to improve bioavailability by formulating as phytosomes. Mukherjee et al. (2007) have

Table 15.3: Marketed Phytosome Formulations (Indena)

Brand Name	Botanical Source	Category	Activity
Bosexil	*Boswellia serrata*	Resin	Soothing, anti-photo aging
Ginkgoselect	*Ginkgo biloba*	Leaf	Antioxidant, vasokinetic
Greenselect	*Camellia sinensis*	Young leaf	Antioxidant, weight management
Ginseng Phytosome	*Panax ginseng*	Root	Tonic, skin elasticity improver
Meriva	*Curcuma longa*	Rhizome	Joint health, soothing
Silymarin Phytosome	*Silybum marianum*	Fruit	Antioxidant, liver protective
Leucoselect Phytosome	*Vitis vinifera*	Seed	Antioxidant, UV protector

regarded phytosomes as a value-added drug delivery system. A thorough study of the literature reveals that several plant extracts (crude, partially purified, or fractionated) are reported to possess various significant pharmacological or health-promoting properties. These extracts can be standardized accordingly and may be formulated as phytosomes for systematic investigation for any improved potential to be used rationally.

Transferosomes

Transferosomes are made up of phospholipids supplemented with a single-chain surfactant with a high radius of curvature, which acts as an edge activator to provide vesicle elasticity and deformability (Cevc et al., 1996). They are highly adaptable and stress-responsive complex aggregates. They overcome the skin penetration difficulty by squeezing themselves along the intercellular lipid of the stratum corneum. Transferosomes have a unique structure that is capable of entrapping hydrophilic, lipophilic, and amphiphilic drugs. They can be applicable as drug carriers for a range of small molecules, peptides, proteins, and herbal ingredients (Saraf, 2010).

Composition of Transferosomes

Transferosomes are composed of two main components (Walve et al., 2011):

1. an amphipathic ingredient (phosphatidylcholine) in which the aqueous solvents self-assemble into a lipid bilayer that closes into a simple lipid vesicle;
2. a bilayer softening component that increases lipid bilayer flexibility and permeability.

The resulting flexibility- and permeability-optimized transferosome vesicle can therefore adapt its shape easily and rapidly by adjusting the local concentration of each bilayer component and to the local stress experienced by the bilayer (Fig. 15.5).

Applications of Transferosomes

Capsaicin transferosomes were prepared by the high shear dispersion technique and the penetration of capsaicin was found to be more compared to the pure drug (Long et al., 2006).

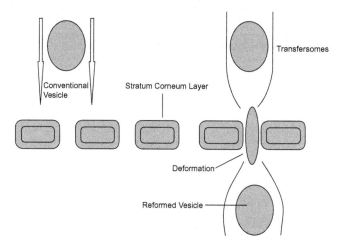

Figure 15.5
Transferosomes.

Table 15.4: Herbal Formulations of Transferosomes

Biological Source	Active Ingredient	Application	Use	References
Capsicum annuum	Capsaicin	Increase skin penetration	Treatment of rheumatism	Xiao-Ying et al. (2006)
Curcuma longa	Curcumin	Increase skin permeability	Antiinflammatory	Patel et al. (2004)
Catharanthus roseus	Vincristine	Increase permeability	Anticancer	Lu et al. (2005)
Colchicum autumnale	Colchicine	Reduction in gastrointestinal tract side effects	Treatment of gout	Singh et al. (2005)

Colchicine and curcumin transferosomes were prepared using a hand-shake method, and the formulation prevented gastrointestinal side effects associated with oral administration and provided local, sustained release and site-specific delivery of colchicine and curcumin (Singh et al., 2009). Transferosomes can penetrate the stratum corneum and supply nutrients locally to maintain their functions, resulting in maintenance of the skin. In this connection transferosomes containing capsaicin have been prepared by Xiao-Ying et al. and show better topical absorption in comparison to pure capsaicin (Xiao-Ying et al., 2006). The various herbal formulations of transferosomes are summarized in Table 15.4.

Ethosomes

Ethosomes are soft, non–invasive vesicles for the enhanced delivery of active agents. The design of topical applications is of great importance to phytomedicine for both topical and systemic drug administration. The sizes of ethosomes may vary from tens of nanometers to micrometers (Verma and Fahr, 2004).

Ethosomes are lipid-based elastic vesicles containing phospholipids, alcohol (ethanol and isopropyl alcohol) in relatively high concentrations, and water. Higher concentrations of alcohol enhance topical drug delivery and prolong the physical stability of ethosomes compared to liposomes (Dayan and Touitou, 2000).

Ethosomes may contain certain phospholipids with various chemical structures, like phosphatidylcholine, phosphatidylserine, phosphatidylethanolamine, phosphatidylglycerol, alcohol, water, and propylene glycol. This composition enables the delivery of a high concentration of active ingredients through the skin. Drug delivery can be modulated by altering the alcohol:water or alcohol–polyol:water ratio.

Mechanisms of Drug Penetration

The main advantage of ethosomes over liposomes is the increased permeation of the drug. The drug absorption probably occurs in the following two phases (Gangwar et al., 2010):

1. Ethanol effect
   Ethanol acts to enhance penetration through the skin. The mechanism of its penetration-enhancing effect is well known. Ethanol penetrates into intercellular lipids and increases the fluidity of cell membrane lipids and decreases the density of the lipid multilayer of the cell membrane.
2. Ethosome effect
   Increased cell membrane lipid fluidity caused by the ethanol of ethosomes results in increased skin permeability. So the ethosomes permeate very easily into the deep skin layers, where they are fused with skin lipids and release the drug into the deep layer of skin (Fig. 15.6).

Marketed Formulations

Novel Therapeutic Technologies, Inc., of Hebrew University has succeeded in bringing a number of products to the market based on the ethosome delivery system. Noicellex, an anticellulite formulation of ethosomes, is currently marketed in Japan. Lipoduction, another formulation currently used in the treatment of cellulite, contains pure grape seed extracts (antioxidant) and is marketed in the United States. Similarly Physonics is marketing the anticellulite gel Skin Genuity in London. Nanominox, containing minoxidil, is used as a hair tonic to promote hair growth and is marketed by Sinere (Touitou, 1996). Table 15.5 shows examples of ethosomes as a herbal drug carriers.

Transdermal Drug Delivery Systems

Transdermal drug delivery systems facilitate the passage of therapeutic quantities of drug substances through the skin and into the general circulation for their systemic effects (Shaik et al.,

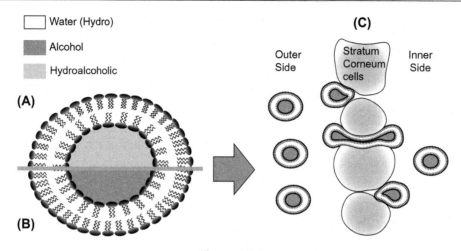

Figure 15.6
Transfer of Ethosomes across startum corneum by deformation.

Table 15.5: Ethosome Formulations of Herbal Drugs

Biological Source	Active Ingredient	Application	Use	References
Glycyrrhiza glabra	Ammonium glycyrrhizinate	Improved antiinflammatory activity and sustained release action	Treatment of dermatitis, eczema, and psoriasis	Paolinoa et al. (2005)
Cannabis sativa	Tetrahydrocannabinol	Improved patient compliance and increased skin permeation	Treatment of rheumatoid arthritis	Lodzki et al. (2003)
Tripterygium wilfordii	Triptolide	Increase in percutaneous permeability	Antiinflammatory, antitumor	Chen et al. (2004)
Sophora alopecuroides	Matrine, oxymatrine, sophoridine, sophocarpine (alkaloidal extract)	Increase in permeability	Anticancer, antiendotoxin	Zhou et al. (2010)
Curcuma longa	Curcumin	Improved bioavailability	Antiinflammatory	Maiti et al. (2007)

2011). It has been found that drugs of herbal origin can be utilized with enhanced efficacy by incorporating them into transdermal drug patches. Even herbal penetration enhancers like some terpenes are found to have enough potential to replace the conventionally available penetration enhancers like dimethyl sulfoxide, which has several disadvantages (Rathva et al., 2012). The first commercially available prescription patch, approved by the US Food and Drug Administration (FDA) in December 1979, administered scopolamine for motion sickness. The most common available transdermal drug delivery patches are the over-the-counter nicotine patches that help people quit smoking (Jatav et al., 2011). A list of marketed herbal transdermal patches is given in Table 15.6.

Table 15.6: Marketed Herbal Transdermal Patches

Brand Name	Ingredients	Use	Company
Nicoderm CQ	Nicotine	Quit smoking	GlaxoSmithKline
Transdermal SCOP	Scopolamine	Prevent motion sickness	Novartis
Forest detox foot patch	Tourmaline, chitosan, pearl stone, wood vinegar	Detoxification, increase oxygen intake	Natural pharmacy
Praan Painplast	*Angelica dahurica*, rhizoma zingerbis, Chinese *Angelica*	Pain relief	Greatline impex
Hoodia+Patch	*Hoodia gordonii*, Guaraná, *Garcinia cambogia*	Weight control	Medex scientific

Applications

The virility patch: The virility patch (RX male virility enhancement formula) is a natural herbal patch containing a variety of herbs known for promoting sexual desire and performance in men. The virility patch is an ultraconcentrated formula infused into a small, discrete dermal patch that sticks to the body. The transdermal delivery system used in these patches is approved by the FDA (Bayarski, 2010).

Transdermal slimming patch: This is entirely made of natural herbs and processed to a soft patch form with transdermal technology. It reduces the overburden of vital organs. It works 24 h—all day, all night. It eliminates hunger pangs, maintains the feeling of fullness, even when one has not eaten, and accelerates fat burning (Chaturvedi et al., 2011).

Diabetes: *Momordica charantia* is traditionally used as a medicine for diabetes. The transdermal film contains the fractionated component from an ethanolic extract of *M. charantia* fruits prepared using hydroxypropylmethylcellulose as a percentage. The release of active constituents from transdermal patches of *M. charantia* ($2\,cm^2$; $10\,mg$/patch) was found to be satisfactory (Seema, 2014).

Nanoparticles

Nanoparticles are nano- or subnano-sized structures composed of synthetic or semisynthetic polymers. Nanoparticles are colloidal systems with particles varying in size from 10 to 1000 nm. It is an effective system, as the formulation is encapsulated in it easily and can easily reach the effective site (Vyas and Khar, 2002). The drug is dissolved, entrapped, encapsulated, or attached to a nanoparticle matrix. Depending upon the method of preparation nanospheres or nanocapsules can be obtained. Nanocapsules are systems in which the drug is confined to a cavity surrounded by a unique polymer membrane, whereas nanospheres are matrix systems in which the drug is physically and uniformly dispersed. The nanoparticle system of formulation shows an advantage, as its solubility is increased and

Table 15.7: Nanoparticle Herbal Drug Delivery Systems

Biological Source	Application	Use	References
Cuscuta chinesis	Improve water solubility	Antitumor, immunostimulatory, antihepatotoxic	Yen et al. (2008)
Berberis vulgaris	Sustained drug release	Anticancer	Lin et al. (2007)
Camptotheca acuminata	Increase in solubility	Increase in bioavailability, antitumor	Xi et al. (2007)
Ginkgo biloba	Improved cerebral blood flow	Brain function activation	Shimada (2012)
Naringenin	Increase in solubility	Hepatoprotective	Yen et al. (2009)
Tripterygium wilfordii	Increase in solubility, decrease in toxicity	Antiinflammatory, antitumor	Xiong et al. (2005)
Glycyrrhiza glabra	Improve bioavailability	Antiinflammatory, antihepatotoxic	Zha et al. (2007)

the drug can reach the target site, compared to other systems. Microencapsulation of an herbal extract in nanoparticles is an effective way to protect drug or food ingredients against deterioration, volatile losses, or premature interaction with other ingredients. The advantages of the nanoparticle are that it improves the absorbency of the herbal formulation, reduces the dose of formulation, and increases its solubility (Prabhu et al., 2010). Various nanoparticle herbal formulations are summarized in Table 15.7.

Advantages of an Herbal Nanoparticle Delivery System

- A nanoparticle system delivers the herbal formulation directly to the site of action.
- Encapsulating drugs within nanoparticles can improve the solubility and pharmacokinetics of drugs.
- Nanoparticles can also provide a choice of formulations, promote transit of the drug through biological barriers, and increase bioavailability of the drug.
- They can take the drug directly to the site of action without destroying the surrounding environment.

Nanoparticles of traditional Chinese herbs (TCH) are helpful for improving their absorption and distribution in the body, and therefore enhance their efficacy. Traditional Chinese medicines, including peach seed, safflower, *Angelica* root, Szechwan lovage rhizome, *Rehmannia* root, red peony root, leech, gadfly, earthworm, and ground beetle, were mixed and prepared by drying, mincing, extracting, crushing into liquid particles with an ultrasonic wave, filtering, and nanometerizing into a nanoparticle soliquid with a nanometer collider. Nanoparticles of TCH showed significant thrombolytic effects, resulting in quick recovery from arterial embolism and diminution of thrombi. The thrombolytic effects of nanoparticles of TCHs are much intensified compared to their nonnanoparticle form. There are also some studies on integrative evaluation, pharmacokinetics, and pharmacological activity of oral prolonged-release preparations of traditional Chinese medicine (Shen et al., 2008).

Nanoemulsions

Nanoemulsions are submicrometer-sized emulsions that are under extensive investigation as drug carriers for improving the delivery of therapeutic agents. Nanoemulsions are thermodynamically stable transparent (translucent) dispersions of oil and water stabilized by an interfacial film of surfactant and cosurfactant molecules having a droplet size of less than 100 nm. A nanoemulsion, which is categorized as a multiphase colloidal dispersion, is generally characterized by its stability and clarity. Nanoemulsions are formed readily and sometimes spontaneously, generally without high energy input. In many cases a cosurfactant or cosolvent is used in addition to the surfactant, the oil phase, and the water phase (Patel and Joshi, 2012). A variety of herbal formulations have been made as emulsions for various applications (Table 15.8).

Nanoemulsions are made from surfactants approved for human consumption and common food substances that are "generally recognized as safe" by the FDA. There is an application of high shear generally obtained by a microfluidic or ultrasonic approach generally used to reduce the droplet size to nanoscale (Reza, 2011).

Solid Lipid Nanoparticles

This is a technique developed in the 1990s. These are colloidal carriers used especially for the delivery of lipophilic compounds. They are prepared by different methods—homogenization and warm microemulsion. The average mean size of solid lipid nanoparticles ranges from 50 to 1000 nm. Solid lipid nanoparticles (SLNs) are composed of a lipid matrix, which becomes solid at room temperature and also at body temperature (Pople and Singh 2006). The main features of SLNs with regard to parenteral application are excellent physical stability and protection of incorporated labile drugs from degradation. To cross the blood–brain barrier, it should be made of selected lipids and surfactants. The SLNs are prepared by different methods, such as homogenization and warm microemulsion, high-speed stirring, ultrasonication, and solvent diffusion. Lipids show compatibility with lipophilic drugs and increase the entrapment efficiency and drug loading into the SLNs (Gande, 2010). A variety of SLN herbal formulations are shown in Table 15.9.

Table 15.8: Herbal Emulsions

Herbal Ingredient	Application	Use	References
Neem oil	Reduced toxicity	Acaricidal, antifungal, antibacterial	Sun and Ouyang (2007)
Babchi oil	Improved skin permeation	Treatment of psoriasis	Ali et al. (2008)
Pilocarpine	Improved ocular retention, reduced systemic side effects	Treatment of glaucoma	Chan et al. (2007)
Triptolide	Enhanced penetration by increased hydration	Antiinflammatory	Chen et al. (2004)
Docetaxel	Improved residence time	Anticancer	Ling et al. (2007)

Table 15.9: Solid Lipid Nanoparticle Formulations of Herbal Drugs

Active Herbal Ingredient	Application of Solid Lipid Nanoparticles	Biological Activity	References
Curcumin	Increased stability	Antitumor and antioxidant	Gande (2010)
Triptolide	Enhanced penetration	Antiinflammatory	Mei et al. (2005)
Curcuminoids	Increased activity	Antitumor and antioxidant	Tiyaboonchai et al. (2007)
Garlic extract	Increased penetration	Antifungal and antidandruff	Rai et al. (2013)

Microspheres

Microspheres are spherical particles ideally of size 1–300 μm. Each particle is a matrix for the drug dispersed in the polymer and the drug is released as a first-order process. First the outer dissolution medium will diffuse the matrix, causing the entrapped drug to solubilize inside it, and then the drug is released from the system. This is one type of mechanism. In the other type the system constitutes a polymer that shows surface erosion behavior such that the surface erodes layer by layer and the release of drug occurs (Chan et al., 2010). The polymers used for the fabrication of the microspheres are biodegradable or nonbiodegradable. Various polymers have been used for fabrication of these microparticle carriers, such as albumin, gelatin, modified starch, polypropylene, dextran, polylactic acid, polylactide-co-glycolide, etc. (Burgess and Hickey, 2009). The drug release is controlled by the dissolution and degradation of the matrix. The release is effected by the size, type of matrix, polymer concentration, etc. These microparticle systems are also advantageous as they can be ingested or injected and tailored for desired release profiles.

Applications of Microspheres

Various methods, such as evaporation and ionic cross-linking techniques, have been reported (Das and Senapati, 2008) for the preparation of mucoadhesive, buoyant microspheres. These microparticle systems are advantageous as they can be ingested or injected and produce sustained release action and site-specific delivery. A number of plant ingredients have been microencapsulated for various applications (Table 15.10).

Gastroretentive floating microspheres of silymarin have been reported for sustained delivery of the drug (Garg and Gupta, 2010). Prolonged release of the drug (12 h) was achieved in simulated gastric fluid and resulted in increased drug bioavailability as well as patient compliance. Microencapsulation of zedoary turmeric oil (You et al., 2006) into microspheres via emulsion-solvent diffusion has used been used for bioavailability enhancement and sustained release application. Microspheres of turmeric oleoresin were prepared after emulsification by using a spray-drying technique. The stable emulsion product protected the resin from degradation by light, oxygen, heat, and alkaline conditions and showed increased therapeutic effect (Kshirsagar et al., 2009). Encapsulation of herbal extracts of *Piper sarmentosum* was done by

Table 15.10: Herbal Microspheres

Active Herbal Ingredient	Application of Microspheres	Biological Activity	References
Ginsenoside	Solubility and stability enhancement	Anticancer	Cheng-Bai et al. (2008)
Quercetin	Bioavailability enhancement and sustained release	Antioxidant and antiinflammatory	Natarajan et al. (2010)
Zedoary oil	Bioavailability enhancement and sustained release	Hepatoprotective	You et al. (2006)
Rutin	Cardiovascular and cerebrovas-cular targeting	Cardiovascular and cerebrovascular diseases	Xiao et al. (2008)

absorption with calcium alginate beads and it was found that there is no effect of method of encapsulation on the encapsulation efficiency, so the process can be used at industrial scale for the encapsulation of the herbal extracts. Site-specific delivery of rutin (Xiao et al., 2008) from its microspheres (rutin alginate–chitosan) was observed via targeting to cardiovascular and cerebrovascular regions. Oxidized cellulose microspheres containing camptothecin (Chao et al., 2010) were prepared by using a spray-drying process, and they have been successfully used to enhance the solubility and cytotoxicity of camptothecin.

References

Ali, J., Akhtar, N., Sultana, Y., Baboota, S., Ahuja, A., 2008. Antipsoriatic microemulsion gel formulation for topical drug delivery of babchi oil (*Psoralea corylifolia*). Methods Find. Exp. Clin. Pharmacol. 30 (4), 277–285.

Amarnath, S., Sharma, U.S., 1997. Liposomes in drug delivery: progress and limitations. Int. J. Pharm. 154, 123–140.

Amin, T., Bhat, S., 2012. A review on phytosome technology as a novel approach to improve the bioavailability of nutraceuticals. Int. J. Adv. Res. Technol. 1, 1–15.

Annie, S., 2015. Herbal medicines: keeping abreast with changing technology. Hygeia. J. D. Med. 7 (1).

Atmzkuri, L.R., Dathi, I., 2010. Current trends in herbal medicines. J. Pharm. Sci. 3 (1), 109–113.

Atram Seema, 2014. Recent development of herbal formulation—a novel drug delivery system. IAMJ 2 (6), 956.

Bayarski Y., 2010. Available from: http://www.google.com/Transdermalpatches/NDDS/Herbaldrugs.

Blumenthal, M., Goldberg, A., Brinkmann, J., 2000. Herbal Medicine. Integrative Medicine Communications, Newton.

Bombardelli, E., Curri, S.B., Della, R.L., Del, N.P., Tubaro, A., Gariboldi, P., 1989. Complexes between phospho-lipids and vegetal derivatives of biological interest. Fitoterapia 60, 1–9.

Burgess, D.J., Hickey, A.J., 2009. Microsphere technology and applications. In: Swarbrick, J. (Ed.), Enclopedia of Pharmaceutical Technology, 4. third ed. Informa Healthcare, New York, pp. 2328–2338.

Carini, R., Comoglio, A., Albano, E., Poli, G., 1992. Lipid peroxidation and irreversible damage in the rat hepatocyte model: protection by the silybin-phospholipid complex IdB 1016. Biochem. Pharmacol. 43, 2111–2115.

Cevc, G., Blume, G., Schatzlein, A., Gebauer, D., Paul, A., 1996. The skin, a pathway for systemic treatment with patches and lipid-based agent carriers. Adv. Drug Deliv. Rev. 18, 349–378.

Chan, J., Maghraby, G.M., Craig, J.P., Alany, R.G., 2007. Phase transition water in-oil microemulsions as ocular drug delivery systems: *in vitro* and *in vivo* evaluation. Int. J. Pharm. 328 (1–2), 65–71.

Chan, E.S., Yim, Z.H., Phan, S.H., Mansa, R.F., Ravindra, P., 2010. Encapsulation of herbal aqueous extract through absorption with calcium alginate hydrogel beads. Food Bioprod. Process. 88, 195–201.

Chao, P., Deshmukh, M., Kutscher, H.L., Gao, D., Rajan, S.S., Hu, P., 2010. Pulmonary targeting microparticulate camptothecin delivery system: anticancer evaluation in a rat orthotopic lung cancer model. Anticancer Drugs 21 (1), 65–76.

Chaturvedi, M., Kumar, M., Sinhal, A., Saifi, A., 2011. Recent development in novel drug delivery systems of herbal drugs. Int. J. Green Pharm. 5, 87–94.

Chen, C., 2008. Inhibiting the vascular smooth muscle cells proliferation by EPC and DPPC liposome encapsulated magnalol. J. Chin. Inst. Chem. Eng. 39, 407–411.

Chen, H., Chang, X., Weng, T., Zhao, X., Gao, Z., Yang, Y., Xu, H., Yang, X., 2004. A study of microemulsion systems for transdermal delivery of triptolide. J. Control. Release 98, 427–436.

Chen, J., Chen, Z., Wang, W., 2010. Ammonium sulphate gradient loading of brucine into liposome: effect of phospholipid composition on entrapment efficiency and physicochemical properties *in vitro*. Drug Dev. Ind. Pharm. 36, 245–253.

Cheng-Bai, Di Zhang, Xia, C., Dan, J., 2008. Preparation and characterization of biodegradedable polylactide microsphere encapsulating ginsenoside Rg3. Chem. Res. Chin. Univ. 24, 588–591.

Das, M.K., Senapati, P.C., 2008. Furosemide loaded alginate microspheres prepared by ionic cross linking technique: morphology and release characteristics. Indian J. Pharm. Sci. 70 (1), 77–84.

Dayan, N., Touitou, E., 2000. Carriers for skin delivery of trihexyphenidyl HCl, ethosomes vs. liposomes. Biomaterials 21, 1879–1885.

El-Samaligy, M.S., Afifi, N.N., Mahmoud, E.A., 2006. Increasing bioavailability of silymarin using a buccal liposomal delivery system: preparation and experimental design investigation. Int. J. Pharm. 308, 140–148.

Gande, S., 2010. Pharmacokinetic applicability of a validated liquid chromatography tandem mass spectroscopy method for orally administered curcumin loaded solid lipid nanoparticles to rats. J. Chromatogr. B Analyt. Technol. Biomed. Life Sci. 878, 3427–3431.

Gandhi, A., Dutta, A., Pal, A., Bakshi, P., 2012. Recent trends of phytosomes for delivering herbal extract with improved bioavailability. Phytojournal 1 (4), 6–14.

Gangwar, S., Singh, S., Garg, G., 2010. Ethosomes: a novel tool for drug delivery through the skin. J. Pharm. Res. 3 (4), 688–691.

Garg, R., Gupta, G.D., 2010. Gastroretentive floating microspheres of silymarin: preparation and *in vitro* evaluation. Trop. J. Pharm. Res. 9 (1), 59–66.

Ghosh, D., Ghosh, S., Sarkar, S., Ghosh, A., Das, N., Das Saha, K., 2010. Quercetin in vesicular delivery systems: evaluation in combating arsenic-induced acute liver toxicity associated gene expression in rat model. Chem. Biol. Interact. 186, 61–71.

Gortzi, O., Lalas, S., Chinou, L., 2008. Re-evaluation of bioactivity and antioxidant activity of *Myrtus communis* extract before and after encapsulation in liposome. Eur. Food Res. Technol. 226, 583–590.

Hazra, B., Kumar, B., Biswas, S., Pandey, B.N., Mishra, K.P., 2005. Enhancement of the tumour inhibitory activity, *in vivo*, of diospyrin, a plant derived quinonoid, through liposomal encapsulation. Toxicol. Lett. 157, 109–117.

Himanshu, A., Sitasharan, P., Singhai, A.K., 2011. Liposomes as drug carriers. IJPLS 2 (7), 945–951.

Jain, N.K., 2001. Controlled and Novel Drug Delivery. CBS Publisher, New Delhi.

Jatav, V.S., Saggu, J.S., Jat, R.K., Sharma, A.K., Singh, R.P., 2011. Recent advances in development of transdermal patches. Pharmacophore 2 (6), 287–297.

Kidd, P., Head, K., 2005. A review of the bioavailability and clinical efficacy of milk thistle phytosome: a silybin-phosphatidylcholine complex. Altern. Med. Rev. 10, 193–203.

Kshirsagar, A.C., Yenge, V.B., Sarkar, A., Singhal, R.S., 2009. Efficacy of pullulan in emulsification of turmeric oleoresin and its subsequent microencapsulation. Food Chem. 113, 1139–1145.

Lasic, D.D., 1993. Liposomes: From Physics to Applications. Elsevier, Amsterdam/London, New York, Tokyo.

Lin, A.H., Li, H.Y., Liu, Y.M., Qiu, X.H., 2007. Preparation and release characteristics of berberine chitosan nanoparticles *in vitro*. China Pharm. 18, 755–757.

Ling, L.I., Wang, D.K., Lin-Sui, L.I., Jia, J., Chang, D., Li, A.I., 2007. Preparation of docetaxel submicron emulsion for intravenous administration. J. Shenyang Pharm. Univ. 12, 736–739.

Lodzki, M., Godin, B., Rakou, L., Mechoulam, R., Gallily, R., Touitou, E., 2003. Cannabidiol — transdermal delivery and anti-inflammatory effect in a murine model. J. Control. Release 93 (3), 377–387.

Long, X.Y., Luo, J.B., Lin, D., Rong, H.S., Huang, W.M., 2006. Preparation and *in vitro* evaluations of topically applied capsaicin transfersomes. Zhongguo Zhong Yao Za Zhi 31 (12), 981–984.

Lu, Y., Hou, S.X., Chen, T., Sun, Y.Y., Yang, B.X., Yuan, Z.Y., 2005. Preparation of transfersomes of vincristine sulfate and study on its percutaneous penetration. Zhongguo Zhong Yao Za Zhi 30 (12), 900–903.

Maiti, K., Mukherjee, K., Gantait, A., Saha, B.P., Mukherjee, P.K., 2007. Curcumin phospholipid complex: preparation therapeutic evaluation & pharmacokinetic study in rats. Int. J. Pharm. 330 (1–2), 155–163.

Mei, Z., Li, X., Wu, Q., Hu, S., Yang, X., 2005. The research on the anti-inflammatory activity and hepatotoxicity of triptolide-loaded solid lipid nanoparticle. Pharmacol. Res. 51, 345–351.

Mitra, A., Banerjee, S., 2012. Changing landscape of herbal medicine: technology attributing renaissance. Int. J. Pharm. Pharm. Sci 4 (1), 47–52.

Mukherjee, P.K., Maiti, K., Kumar, V., 2007. Value added drug delivery systems with botanicals: approach for dosage development from natural resources. Pharma. Rev. 6, 57–60.

Murray, D., 2008. Phytosomes Increase the Absorption of Herbal Extract. [online].Available from: URL: www.doctormurray.com/articles/silybin.htm.

Natarajan, V., Madhan, B., Sehgal, P., 2010. Formulation and evaluation of quercetin polycaprolactone microsphere for the treatment of rheumatoid arthritis. J. Pharm. Sci. 100, 195–205.

Pandey, S., 2010. Phytosomes: technical revolution in phytomedicine. Int. J. PharmTech Res. 2, 627–631.

Paolinoa, D., Lucania, G., Mardente, D., Alhaique, F., Frestaa, M., 2005. Ethosomes for skin delivery of ammonium glycyrrhizinate: *in vitro* percutaneous permeation through human skin and *in vivo* anti-inflammatory activity on human volunteers. J. Control. Release 106 (1–2), 99–110.

Patel, R.P., Joshi, J.R., 2012. An overview on nanoemulsion: a novel approach. Indian J. Pharm. Sci. Res. 3 (12), 4640–4650.

Patel, R., Singh, S.K., Singh, S., Sheth, N.R., Gendle, R., 2004. Development and characterization of curcumin loaded transfersome for transdermal delivery. J. Pharm. Sci. Res. 1 (4), 71–80.

Pople, P.V., Singh, K.K., 2006. Development and evaluation of topical formulation containing solid lipid nanoparticles of vitamin A. AAPS PharmSci. Tech. 7, 91.

Prabhu, N., Gowari, K., Raj, D., 2010. Synthesis of silver phyto nanoparticles and their antibacterial activity. Digest. J. Nano. Biostructure 5, 185–189.

Rai, N., Jain, A.K., Abraham, J., 2013. Formulation and evaluation of herbal antidandruff shampoo containing garlic loaded solid lipid nanoparticles. Int. J. Pharma. Res. Rev. 2 (10), 12–24.

Rathva, S.R., Patel, N.N., Shah, V., Upadhyay, U.M., 2012. Herbal transdermal patches: a review. Int. J. Drug Discov. Herbal Res. 2 (2), 397–402.

Reza, K.H., 2011. Nanoemulsion as a novel transdermal drug delivery system. Int. J. Pharm. Sci. Res. 2 (8), 1938–1946.

Robinson, M.M., Zhang, X., 2011. Traditional Medicines: Global Situation, Issues and Challenges, third ed. The World Medicines Situation. WHO. Available from : http://www.who.int/medicines/areas/policy/world_medicines_situation/WMS_ch18_wTraditionalMed.pdf.

Saraf, A.S., 2010. Application of novel drug delivery system for herbal formulation. Fitoterapia 81, 680–689.

Shaik, H.R., Haribabu, R., Khaja Mohiddin, Vineela, J., Ravitejab, A., Pathuri, R.K., Gajavalli, S.R., Naidu, L.V., 2011. Transdermal drug delivery system—simplified medication regimen—a review. Res. J. Pharm. Biol. Chem. Sci. 2 (4), 223–238.

Shehata, T., Ogawara, K., Higaki, K., Kimura, T., 2008. Prolongation of residence time of liposome by surface-modification with mixture of hydrophilic polymers. Int. J. Pharm. 359, 272–279.

Shen, Y.J., Zhang, Z.W., Luo, X.G., Wang, X.F., Wang, H.L., 2008. Nanoparticles of traditional Chinese herbs inhibit thrombosis *in vivo*. Haematol. Heamatol. J. 93, J1457.

Shimada, S., 2012. Composition Comprising Nanoparticle Ginkgo Biloba Extract with the Effect of Brain Function Activation US 8105637 B2. , pp. 424–489.

Singh, H.P., Utreja, P., Tiwary, A.K., Jain, S., 2005. Elastic liposomal formulation for sustained delivery of colchicine: *in vitro* characterization and *in vivo* evaluation of anti-gout activity. Am. Assoc. Pharm. Sci. 11 (1), 54–64.

Singh, H.P., Utreja, P., Tiwary, A.K., Jain, S., 2009. Elastic liposomal formulation for sustained delivery of colchicine, *in vitro* characterization and *in vivo* evaluation of anti-gout activity. AAPS J. 11 (1), 54–64.

Sun, H.W., Ouyang, W.Q., 2007. The preparation of neem oil microemulsion (*Azadirachta indica*) and the comparison of acaricidal time between neem oil microemulsion and other formulation *in vitro*. J. Shanghai Jiao Tong Univ. (Agri. Sci.) 1, 60–65.

Tiyaboonchai, W., Tungpradit, W., Plianbangchang, P., 2007. Formulation and characterization of curcuminoids loaded solid lipid nanoparticles. Int. J. Pharm. 337, 299–306.

Touitou, E., 1996. Composition of Applying Active Substance to or through the Skin US Patent: 5716638.

Verma, D.D., Fahr, A., 2004. Synergistic penetration effect of ethanol and phospholipids on the topical delivery of cyclosporin A. J. Control. Release 97, 55–66.

Vyas, S.P., Khar, R.K., 2002. Targeted and Controlled Drug Delivery Novel Carrier Systems, second ed. CBS publishers and distributors, New Delhi, pp. 15–16. 346–348.

Walve, J.R., Bakliwal, S.R., Rane, B.R., Pawar, S.P., 2011. Transfersomes: a surrogated carrier for transdermal drug delivery system. Int. J. Appl. Biol. PharmaTechnol. 2 (1), 204–213.

Weiss, R., Fintelmann, V., 2000. Herbal Medicine, second ed. Thieme, Stuttgart, New York.

Xi, N., Hou, L.B., Wang, C.X., Yan, X.Q., Jiang, Q.F., Guo, D., 2007. Preparation and *in vitro* drug-release behavior of hydroxycamptothecin semisolid lipid nanoparticles. China Hosp. Pharm. J. 27, 139–142.

Xiao, Y.L., Li, B., 2002. Drug-loaded nanoparticle and TCM modernization. Chin. Trad. Herb. Drugs 33, 385–388.

Xiao, L., Zhang, Y.H., Xu, J.C., Jin, X.H., 2008. Preparation of floating rutin-alginate-chitosan microcapsule. Chin. Trad. Herb. Drugs 2, 209–212.

Xiao-Ying, L., Luo, J.B., Yan, Z.H., Rong, H.S., Huang, W.M., 2006. Preparation and *in vitro-in vivo* evaluations of topically applied capsaicin transfersomes. Yao Xue Xue Bao 41 (5), 461–466.

Xiong, F.L., Chen, H.B., Chang, X.L., Yang, Y.J., Xu, H.B., Yang, X.L., 2005. Research progress of triptolide-loaded nanoparticles delivery systems. In: Conference Proceedings IEEE Engineering in Medicine and Biology Society, 5, pp. 4966–4969.

Yanyu, X., Yunmei, S., Zhipeng, C., Quineng, P., 2006. The preparation of silybin-phospholipid complex and the study on its pharmacokinetics in rats. Int. J. Pharm 307, 77–82.

Yen, F.L., Wu, T.H., Lin, L.T., Cham, T.M., Lin, C.C., 2008. Nanoparticles formulation of *Cuscuta chinensis* prevents acetaminophen-induced hepatotoxicity in rats. Food Chem. Toxicol. 46 (5), 1771–1777.

Yen, F.L., Wu, T.H., Lin, L.T., Cham, T.M., Lin, C.C., 2009. Naringenin-Loaded nanoparticles improve the physicochemical properties and the hepatoprotective effects of naringenin in orally-administered rats with CCl_4-induced acute liver failure. Pharm. Res. 26 (4), 893–902.

You, J., Cui, F.D., Han, X., Wang, Y.S., Yang, L., Yu, Y.W., Li, O.P., 2006. Study of the preparation of sustained release microspheres containing zedoary turmeric oil by the emulsion solvent diffusion method and evaluation of the self emulsification and bioavailability of the oil. Colloids Surf. B Biointerfaces 48 (1), 35–41.

Zha, R.T., He, X.T., Du, T., Yuan, Z., 2007. Synthesis and characterization of chitosan nanoparticles modified by glycyrrhetinic acid as a liver targeting drug carrier. Chem. J. Chin. Univ. 28, 1098–1100.

Zhou, Y., Wei, Y., Liu, H., Zhang, G., Wu, X., 2010. Preparation and *in vitro* evaluation of ethosomal total alkaloids of *Sophora alopecuroides* loaded by a transmembrane pH-gradient method. Am. Assoc. Pharm. Sci. 11 (3), 1350–1358.

CHAPTER 16

Regulatory Aspects of Herbal Medicine

Alex Thomas
International Institute of Biotechnology and Toxicology, Kancheepuram, Tamilnadu, India

Introduction

Since the beginning of history, humans have been using herbs to heal their ailments. They discovered medicinal uses of herbs by observation and experimentation. The knowledge about herbs in turn led to the preparation of herbal formulations, which later gained popularity as herbal medicine. Various names were assigned to it, such as Ayurveda, Unani, Kampo, etc., with respect to its origin. Later on, methods were developed for isolating the bioactive components from the herbs and synthesizing drugs by chemical reactions.

Herbal medicines have stood the test of time for their safety, efficacy, cultural acceptability, and lesser side effects (Kamboj, 2000). People are concerned about modern drugs because of their severe side effects despite their curative properties. The commercialization of herbal medical systems and the duration and expense of the treatment resulted in compromising the quality; they did not have any specified regulatory restrictions as does modern medicine, thus they became dangerous to consume. Later on many countries came out with regulatory guidelines to control the export, import, and sale of herbal drugs within and among the countries.

Need for Regulation of Herbal Medicine

The Declaration of Alma-Ata in the year 1978 at an international conference on primary health care convened by the WHO, which called on member nations to formulate national policies, strategies, and plans to launch and sustain primary health care, encouraged the Western world to study in depth the various traditional medical systems of the world (Kumar, 2016). Today, there is an increase in the demand for botanicals worldwide, as developing countries rely heavily on plant-derived medicines for their primary health care. Developed countries impose stringent good manufacturing practices (GMP) and quality control measures on drug products derived from any manufacturing process, regardless of the primary raw material, compared to developing countries, where the relatively inexpensive process, economics, and lack of stringent product governance lead to the exploitation of traditional medicine. Major factors that hamper the full-scale application of traditional plant medicines include lack of implementation of effective quality assurance in the manufacturing process, lack of traceability in the supply chain and associated value additions, and inefficient identification of molecular species that affect the therapeutic efficacy of the final product. In other words, there lacks an assessable, causative, and prognostic relationship between the raw materials, the manufacturing process, and the final product quality. Implementation of hazard analysis and critical control points in the manufacturing process and employment of process analytical technology for ensuring minimal deviation from the manufacturing process of phytotherapeutics need to be adopted.

The general perception that herbal remedies or drugs are very safe and devoid of adverse effects is not only untrue, but also misleading. Herbs are also known to be capable of producing a wide range of undesirable or adverse reactions, some of which are capable of causing serious injuries, life-threatening conditions, and even death (Ekor, 2014).

According to reports in the literature, plants are misidentified, and potentially toxic plants are used in the manufacturing process (Chan, 1997). Toxic plants have been found in herbal medicine preparations. For example, ginseng was replaced with *Periploca sepium* in a case in which an infant was born with hirsutism following maternal ingestion of the product (Paul, 1997). Contamination of herbs with other substances such as lead, arsenic, mercury, aflatoxin, *Mycobacterium*, *Penicillium*, coliforms, *Salmonella*, *Candida*, mouse droppings, earthworms, and blister beetles has occurred. Adulteration with acetaminophen, ephedrine, indomethacin, hydrochlorothiazide, prednisone, and phenylbutazone has also been reported (Chalut, 1999).

Herbal remedies can result in indirect health risks when they delay or replace a more effective form of conventional treatment or when they compromise the efficacy of conventional medicines. The risk of an herbal remedy producing an adverse reaction depends not only on the remedy and its dosage, but also on consumer-related parameters, such as age, genetics, concomitant diseases, and concurrent use of other drugs. Another important determinant of the toxicity of herbal remedies is their quality. The risks of herbal remedies must be systematically collected, disseminated, and acted upon (De Smet, 1995).

Because of the lack of relevant and appropriate national standards, herbal knowledge is getting lost to traditional users and becoming unavailable to new users for many reasons. These reasons include failure to meet various trade registrations, import and export requirements, loss of confidence in these products due to the presence of real or perceived health risks, and increased reporting of adverse events involving the use of herbal medicines (Anonymous, 2007a).

There has been increased competition among traditional medicine practitioners, leading them to employ all tactics and strategies at their disposal. These include unethical advertising strategies such as exaggerated competence, false testimonials and claims of sources of herbs, and misinformation to lure customers to withstand the fierce competition from other service providers (Munyaradzi, 2011). With the aforementioned quandaries a meticulous regulation of herbal drugs is the need of the hour.

Regulatory Aspects of Herbal Medicine

Regulatory Status

The regulatory status of a botanical product varies from country to country, where it may be defined as a functional food, a dietary supplement, an herbal medicine, and so on (Anonymous, 2005). Factors involved in the classification of an herbal medicine include its description in a pharmacopoeia monograph, prescription status, therapeutic claim, category of ingredients or substances (scheduled, regulated, etc.), and period of usage (Anonymous, 2016a) (Tables 16.1 and 16.2).

Table 16.1: Regulatory Status of Herbal Medicine in Different Countries (Anonymous, 2005)

Prescription Medicines	Medicines that can be purchased only with a prescription
Over-the-counter medicines	Medicines that can be purchased without a prescription from a physician
Self-medication	Medicines permitted for self-medication purposes only
Dietary supplements	Substances that contain, for instance, a vitamin, a mineral, an herb or other botanical, or an amino acid. Dietary supplements may be intended to increase the total daily intake of a concentrate, metabolite, constituent, extract, or combination of these ingredients
Health foods/functional foods	Products that are presented with specific health claims and therefore regulated differently from other foods
Other	Products classified differently from the aforementioned categories

Table 16.2: Various Regulatory Agencies for Herbal Medicines

Country	Regulatory Agency
European Union	European Medicines Agency
United States	US Food and Drug Administration
United Kingdom	UK Medicines and Health Products Regulatory Agency
China	China State Food and Drug Administration
Singapore	Singapore Health Science Authority
Australia	Australia Therapeutic Goods Administration
Canada	Health Canada
Brazil	Agência Nacional de Vigilância Sanitária
India	Ministry of AYUSH
New Zealand	New Zealand Medicines and Medical Devices Safety Authority
Malaysia	National Pharmaceutical Control Bureau
Southern Africa	Southern African Development Community
Taiwan	National Laboratories of Foods and Drugs
Nigeria	Nigeria Natural Medicine Development Agency

Various countries take different legislative approaches toward herbal medicine (Anonymous, 2016a), such as:

- the same regulatory requirements for all products
- the same regulatory requirements for all products, with certain types of evidence not required for herbal/traditional medicines
- exemption from all regulatory requirements for herbal/traditional medicines
- exemption from all regulatory requirements for herbal/traditional medicines concerning registration or marketing authorization
- making herbal/traditional medicines subject to all regulatory requirements.

Quality Control

The methods of harvesting, drying, storage, transportation, and processing (for example, mode of extraction and polarity of the extracting solvent, instability of constituents, etc.) also affect herbal quality. The precise profile of constituents is likely to vary both qualitatively and quantitatively in plants with respect to inter- or intraspecies variation, environmental factors, time of harvesting, plant part used, and postharvesting factors (Kunle et al., 2012).

Several problems associated with the quality control of herbal drugs include the following (Fig. 16.1):

- Herbal drugs are usually mixtures of many constituents.
- The active principle(s) is, in most cases, unknown.
- Selective analytical methods or reference compounds may not be available commercially.
- Plant materials are chemically and naturally variable.
- Chemo-varieties and chemo-cultivars exist.
- The source and quality of the raw material are variable.

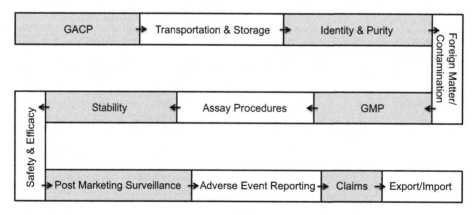

Figure 16.1

Regulatory areas to improve quality and safety of herbal medicine. *GACP*, Good Agricultural and Collection Practices; *GMP*, Good Manufacturing Practices.

Standardization

Standardization of herbal medicines is the process of prescribing a set of standards or inherent characteristics, constant parameters, and definitive qualitative and quantitative values that carry an assurance of quality, efficacy, safety, and reproducibility. It is the process of developing and agreeing upon technical standards (Anonymous, 2005). Despite the herculean task involved in the standardization of herbal medicines, measures need to be taken for its upgrade. Regulation and research to explore its potential have to be initiated in a parallel path. A proper scientific method for regulation, quality control, and standardization of herbal medicine must be developed.

Control of Starting Material

Control of starting material is a prime step in standardizing herbal medicines. Guidelines related to good agricultural and collection practices (GACP) and GMP include control of raw material, control of starting materials and intermediate substances, in-process control (standard operating procedure for processing methods), and finished product control (it should be performed with reference to the control of raw materials, starting materials, and intermediate substances). Some related aspects are discussed below.

Good Agricultural and Collection Practices

The use of fresh plants; age of the plant; part of the plant collected; period, time, and method of collection; temperature of processing; exposure to light; availability of water; availability of nutrients; drying; packing; transportation of raw material; and storage can affect the quality of the herbal material. Depending on the part of the plant used (root, stem, leaf, or fruit), the concentration of the active ingredient is likely to vary. The harvest season may also influence the concentration of the active ingredients (Chan, 1997). For example, the estimation of lipid and alkaloid content was carried out in various plant parts like leaves, bark, and wood of *Butea monosperma* during summer, monsoon, and winter for two consecutive years. The lipid concentration was observed to be highest in summer in the leaves. The alkaloid content was highest in summer in the bark and wood (Tambe et al., 2012).

Storage

The active principles may be destroyed by enzymatic processes as a result of storage for long periods from collection to marketing, resulting in a variations in composition. Wills and Stuart (2000) studied the alkamide and cichoric acid content of ground and dried *Echinacea purpurea* roots for a 60-day period. Interestingly, storage for 60 days in the dark at 5°C had no effect on the alkamide concentrations, but caused a 70% decrease in the cichoric acid concentrations. In a reverse fashion, storage of the ground roots in the light at 20°C did not decrease the cichoric acid concentrations, but decreased the alkamide concentrations by 65%.

Identity and Purity

Methods involved in identity and purity include simple chemical tests like color or precipitation and chromatographic tests, ultraviolet/visible spectroscopy, thin-layer chromatography, HPLC, GC, mass spectrometry (MS), or a combination of GC and MS, DNA finger printing, and so on.

Authentication and Reproducibility of Herbal Ingredients

Authentication of herbal ingredients can be achieved by macroscopic and microscopic comparisons with authentic material or accurate descriptions of authentic herbs, reproducibility of herbal ingredients affected by inter- or intraspecies variation, environmental factors, time of harvesting, plant part used, or postharvesting factors.

Adulteration/Substitution (Mukherjee et al., 2007)

The adulteration and substitution of herbal drugs are major problems posing a threat to the herbal drug industry and research on commercial natural products.

Types of adulteration include the following:

- adulteration with inferior commercial varieties, e.g., *Piper nigrum* adulterated by papaya seeds; adulteration by artificially manufactured substitutes, e.g., artificial invert sugar for honey;
- adulteration with exhausted drugs, e.g., clove, fennel;
- adulteration by addition of heavy metals, e.g., pieces of limestone in asafoetida, pieces of lead in opium;
- adulteration with synthetic principles, e.g., adding citral to oil of lime;
- Adulteration and substitution should be avoided by proper evaluation of raw materials, as they affect the quality/efficacy of herbal products.

Contaminants of Herbal Ingredients

Contaminants of herbal ingredients can be controlled by setting limits for parameters like ash values, foreign organic matter, microbial contamination, pesticides, fumigants, toxic metals, radioactive contaminants, and other contaminants such as endotoxins and mycotoxins.

Good Manufacturing Practices (Anonymous, 2007b)

The method of extraction, contamination with microorganisms, heavy metals, and pesticides can alter the quality, safety, and efficacy of herbal drugs. The WHO guidelines on GMP for herbal medicines include sanitation and hygiene, qualification and validation of critical instruments, handling of complaints, product recall procedures, contract production and analysis, self-inspection, personnel, training, personal hygiene, premises, equipment, materials, documentation, and good practices in production and in quality control.

Assessment of Safety and Efficacy

The phytochemistry of an herbal medicine is complex, making its evaluation of toxicity and efficacy more difficult. Moreover, if active constituents need to be analyzed, this might be an exorbitant and time-consuming operation and also it is impossible practically in the case of a mixed herbal medicine (Anonymous, 2005) (Tables 16.3–16.5).

Safety Monitoring of Herbal Medicines

Monitoring of the adverse events related to herbal medicine is very difficult to accomplish as a number of factors are contributing, which include adulteration, contamination, overdose, misuse, drug–herb interaction, allergic reactions, and so on (Anonymous, 2005).

Pharmacovigilance of Herbal Medicinal Products

The WHO international drug monitoring program, together with the WHO collaborating center in Sweden, the Uppsala Monitoring Centre (UMC), has instituted a coherent

Table 16.3: Classification of Herbal Medicines Based on Origin, Safety, and Indication (Anonymous, 2003b)

Origin	Safety	Indication
Category I: Indigenous herbal medicines historically used in a local community	Safety established by use over long time	Herbal medicine used for an **acute disease**[a]: diseases that have a rapid onset and a relatively short duration
Category II: Herbal medicines in systems, e.g., Ayurveda, Unani, etc.	Safe under specific conditions of use	Herbal medicine used for a **chronic disease**[b]: diseases that have a slow onset and last for long periods of time
Category III: Modified herbal medicines—the aforementioned types modified in some way, such as shape or form, including dose, dosage form, etc.	Herbal medicines of uncertain safety	Herbal medicine used for a **health condition**[c]: problems related to health conditions are those that, with time, could recover spontaneously
Category IV: Imported products with an herbal medicine base—all imported herbal medicines, including raw materials and products	—	—

[a]Diseases that have a rapid onset and a relatively short duration.
[b]Diseases that have a slow onset and last for long periods of time.
[c]Problems related to health conditions are those which, with time, could recover spontaneously, even without any medical intervention.

program of action for pharmacovigilance, which includes the establishment of a program for exchange of safety information, the maintenance of the global WHO database of adverse drug reaction (ADR) reports, and the provision of numerous guidelines on monitoring drug safety. National pharmacovigilance centers designated by the WHO international drug monitoring program are responsible for the collection, processing, and evaluation of case reports of suspected adverse reactions supplied by health care professionals. The WHO has described this program in two publications: *Safety Monitoring of Medicinal Products: Guidelines for Setting Up and Running a Pharmacovigilance Center* and *The Importance of Pharmacovigilance—Safety Monitoring of Medicinal Products* (Shetti et al., 2011). The UMC has taken ADR reports from over 100 countries around the world and in

Table 16.4: Minimum Requirements for Assessment of Safety of Herbal Medicines (Anonymous, 2003b)

Type	Safety Category	Safety Requirement
Indigenous herbal medicines	I	No safety data would be required for usage in local community
	II	Need to meet the usual requirements for safety of herbal medicines
	III	Considered identical to that of any new substance
Herbal medicines in systems	I	No safety data would be required
	II	No safety data would be required
	III	They have to meet the requirements for safety of "herbal medicines of uncertain safety"
Modified herbal medicines	The medicines have to meet the requirements of the safety of herbal medicines or requirements of the safety of "herbal medicines of uncertain safety," depending on the modification	
Imported/exported products with an herbal medicine base	The medicines have to meet the requirements of the safety of herbal medicines or requirements of the safety of "herbal medicines of uncertain safety," depending on the modification	

Table 16.5: Minimum Requirements for Assessment of the Efficacy of Herbal Medicines as per the Usage (Anonymous, 2003b)

Disease Category	Preclinical Data of Efficacy	Clinical Data of Efficacy	Other Data or Information Required
Acute	Needed	Control trial needed	—
Chronic	May be needed	Clinical data may or may not be needed	—
Health condition	May not be needed	May not be needed	Supported by well-established documents such as national pharmacopoeia and monographs

2010 their database contained over 4 million reports, of which approximately 21,000 included herbal or natural products (Anonymous, 2016c).

Current Scenario of Regulation

Regulation and registration of herbal medicines are different among countries. In general herbal medicines are regulated as prescription medicines or nonprescription medicines (Anonymous, 2007a). Current legal situations in different countries vary according to their legislative approaches toward herbal medicine. There exist many lacunae in the current regulation of herbal medicine. For example, people are often confused about how products are defined (e.g., herbal remedies, conventional foods, medicinal foods, or drugs). The way a product is marketed, i.e., its label and packaging, largely determine its product regulatory classification rather than its ingredients or how the consumer uses it (Chalut, 1999). National drug authorities lack general knowledge on herbal medicine and its method of evaluation, which delays updating national policies, laws, and regulation for traditional/complementary medicine, complementary/alternative medicine, and herbal medicine (Anonymous, 2005) (Fig. 16.2).

Phytomedicines are well established in some countries where they are regarded as food, which is not permitted to have medical claims (Anonymous, 2016a). A resolution on traditional medicine adopted by the 56th session of the World Health Assembly in May 2003 urged member states, where appropriate, to ensure the safety, efficacy, and quality of herbal medicines

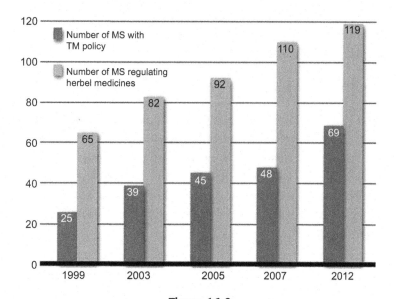

Figure 16.2

Progress of countries in regulating herbal medicine (Anonymous, 2013). *MS*, WHO member states; *TM*, traditional medicine.

by determining national standards for, or issuing monographs on, herbal raw materials and traditional medicine formulas. The WHO has developed guidelines for assessing the safety of potentially hazardous substances in herbal medicines, with particular reference to biological, chemical, and radioactive contaminants and pesticide residues (Anonymous, 2007a). Different guidelines were published by the WHO, which define the criteria for evaluating the quality, safety, and efficacy of herbal medicines, and are aimed at assisting national regulatory authorities, scientific organizations, and manufacturers (Bensoussan et al., 1998).

Regulatory Guidelines on Herbal Medicines Published by the WHO

The WHO documents and publications relating to the quality assurance of herbal medicines with regard to safety include the following:

- quality control methods for medicinal plant materials (Anonymous, 1992, 1998);
- guidelines for the assessment of herbal medicines (Anonymous, 1996a);
- quality assurance of pharmaceuticals: a compendium of guidelines and related materials, GMP, and inspection (Anonymous, 1996b);
- WHO monographs on selected medicinal plants (Anonymous, 2002);
- guide to good storage practices for pharmaceutical products (Anonymous, 2003a);
- GMP for pharmaceutical products: main principles (Anonymous, 2003c);
- WHO guidelines on GACP for medicinal plants (Anonymous, 2003c);
- good trade and distribution practices for pharmaceutical starting materials (Anonymous, 2003d);
- an international pharmacopoeia (Anonymous, 2006a, 2006b);
- guidelines on developing consumer information on the proper use of traditional, complementary, and alternative medicine (Anonymous, 2004).

International Regulatory Cooperation for Herbal Medicines

In more recent years, there has been an increased focus on regional and international collaboration on regulating medicinal products. Herbal medicines have become a specific workshop topic at meetings of the International Conference of Drug Regulatory Authorities since 1986. In the traditional medicine and complementary medicine sector, national regulatory authorities responsible for the regulation of herbal medicines have met annually since 2006 as part of the global regulatory network of the International Regulatory Cooperation for Herbal Medicines (Anonymous, 2013).

Conclusion

Herbal medicine can combat primary health care issues of a population, if dealt scientifically. The scarcity of research funds and scientific support makes it an impossible task for many developing countries. Stringent policies of regulations, market return, and freedom are also major limiting factors, which keep modern pharmaceutical companies at bay. Despite this, steps must be taken at the international level to uplift botanical medicine.

Internationally accepted monitoring authorities and guidelines have to be developed to monitor worldwide research and development in herbal medicine. A classic example of such an authority is the OECD principles of good laboratory practice (GLP). The results from GLP-certified labs are accepted internationally. This type of move will cut down the cost involved by avoiding repeated testing procedures as per the standards of different countries.

Traditional medical systems have a philosophical background that makes them more difficult to define. This puzzle can be solved only if related national authorities take steps to develop quantitative and standardized treatment methods for traditional medicines. It is applaudable that many developing countries are initiating the development of herbal monographs, making this the right time to develop international standards and monitoring systems toward their credibility (Table 16.6).

Herbs need to be classified as per their safety profiles, interactions with conventional medicines, interactions with food, adverse reactions, and efficacy. This classification can be easily achieved, if monographs are available at an internationally acceptable standard. Restrictions and bans on the use of toxic or certain herbal ingredients should be in a worldwide-accepted format (Table 16.7).

Formularies need to be developed in such a way that they can be assessed for their reliability by specific assay procedures. The development of formularies for herbal medicine can wash off many prevailing unethical and dangerous aspects. Formularies need to be accessible as a primary health care tool and strict regulations must be enacted to prevent their misuse. Currently various registration systems exist in various countries and the truth is that these registration systems have their own limitations. By promoting a single-window registration system, the status of herbal medicine can be improved. The regulatory status of herbal medicine has an important role to play in its renaissance. Well-defined criteria need to be developed, while providing status to an herbal medicine. Care is to be taken that these statuses are as per international requirements.

Research and development of any drug are an expensive process. Herbal medicines are more complex, and standardization becomes more expensive, compared to conventional medicines. Even after standardization there are still hurdles in marketing perspectives. Moreover, a worldwide cooperation is needed for the development of herbal medicine as a health care tool. Funds and sponsors need to be mobilized from national and international sectors without any business speculations.

Table 16.6: Template of an Herbal Monograph (Ana et al., 2014)

General Information	Latin Name, Synonyms, Family, Image of the Plant, Popular Names, Geographical Distribution		
Botanical authentication	Part used/organ types, macroscopic description, microscopic description, information on similar plant species that can be used as adulterants, information on voucher specimens		
Agronomic information	Biology and phenology	Sexual system, flowering time, fruiting period Form of fruit and seed dispersal	
	Production system	Information on seeds, harvesting, and processing; seed weight (by mg/1000 seeds); productivity; dormancy of seeds; longevity; and storage	
	Germination	Information on crop, description, propagation, growth and production characteristics of the soil, climatic characteristics, time of collection/harvesting, habit and regeneration, consortium, agroforestry system, breeding, and pests and diseases (occurrence, level of damage, and control)	
	Processing information	Drying, processing, expected return, packing Information on seasonal variation of markers Information about whether the management affects markers Ecological aspects	
Quality control information	**Herbal drug**	**Herbal preparation**	**Herbal medicine**
	Granulometry/particle size, organoleptic characteristics	Description, methods of production, physiochemical tests	Dosage forms, specific tests for each pharmaceutical form
	Purity requirements:		
	Microbiological tests, humidity, heavy metals, chemical residues, total ash content		
	Phytochemical analysis		
	Identification tests		
	Quantification tests (chemical constituents and concentrations):		
	Described markers or active compounds		
	Other considerations related to quality control		
Safety and efficacy information	Information on traditional use		
	Information about nonclinical and clinical assays	Nonclinical toxicology	Subchronic toxicity, chronic toxicity, genotoxicity, skin sensitization, dermal irritation, ocular irritation
		Nonclinical pharmacology	Nonclinical pharmacological assays
		Clinical trials	Phase I; phase II, including pharmacokinetics and pharmacodynamics; phase III, phase IV
	Summary of actions and indications for drug derivatives, routes of administration, daily dose, posology, period of use, contraindications, risk groups, warnings, adverse effects		
	Drug interactions	Described, potential	
	Overdose information	Description of the clinical situation, actions to be taken	
Other information	Dosage forms/formulations described in the literature, product registered in regulatory agencies, packaging and labeling information, monographs about the medicinal plant in official and unofficial documents, compendia/codices, patents applied for the plant species, curiosities		

Table 16.7: Examples of Banned and Restricted Herbal Ingredients in the United Kingdom (Anonymous, 2016b)

Botanical Source	Maximum Dose Where Permitted for Internal Use Only	Maximum Dose Where Permitted for External Use Only (%)
Adonis vernalis	100 mg (MD), 300 mg (MDD)	No dose permitted
Akebia quinata, Akebia trifoliata	Prohibited in all unlicensed medicines	Prohibited in all unlicensed medicines
Areca catechu	Can be sold only in premises that are registered pharmacies and by or under the supervision of a pharmacist	Can be sold only in premises that are registered pharmacies and by or under the supervision of a pharmacist
Artemisia cina	Same as the above	Same as the above
Brayera anthelmintica	Same as the above	Same as the above
Catha edulis	Same as the above	Same as the above
Chenopodium ambrosioides var *anthelminticum*	Same as the above	Same as the above
Claviceps purpurea	Same as the above	Same as the above
Cocculus indicus	Same as the above	Same as the above
Crotalaria berberoana	Same as the above	Same as the above
Datura stramonium, Datura inoxia	50 mg (MD), 150 mg (MDD)	Same as the above
Podophyllum resin	Can be made available only via a prescription from a registered doctor or dentist	20% or below
Schoenocaulon officinale	Same as the above	Same as the above
Senecio	Not permitted in any unlicensed medicines	Not permitted in any unlicensed medicines
Strychnos ignatii; Strychnos cuspida	Not permitted in any unlicensed medicines	Not permitted in any unlicensed medicines
Ulmus fulva, Ulmus rubra	Can be sold only in premises that are registered pharmacies and by or under the supervision of a pharmacist	Can be sold only in premises that are registered pharmacies and by or under the supervision of a pharmacist
Veratrum album	Can be made available only via a prescription from a registered doctor or dentist	Can be made available only via a prescription from a registered doctor or dentist

MD, maximum dose; *MDD*, maximum daily dose.

References

Ana, C.B., Ligia, A., Dâmaris, S., 2014. Systematic organization of medicinal plant information: a monograph template proposal. Rev. Bras. Farmacogn. 24, 80–88.

Anonymous, 1992. Quality Control Methods for Medicinal Plant Materials. World Health Organization, Geneva, pp. 1–135.

Anonymous, 1996a. Guidelines for the Assessment of Herbal Medicines WHO Technical Report Series. World Health Organization, Geneva (pp. 863; 1–185).

Anonymous, 1996b. Quality assurance of pharmaceuticals: a compendium of guidelines and related materials. In: Good Manufacturing Practices and Inspection, vol. 2. World Health Organization, Geneva, pp. 1–389.

Anonymous, 1998. Quality Control Methods for Medicinal Plant Materials. World Health Organization, Geneva, p. 122.

Anonymous, 2002. In: WHO Monographs on Selected Medicinal Plants, vol. 2. World Health Organization, Geneva, pp. 1–357.

Anonymous, 2003a. Guide to Good Storage Practices for Pharmaceutical Products. WHO Expert Committee on Specifications for Pharmaceutical Preparations (WHO Technical Report Series, No. 908) Thirty-seventh report. World Health Organization, Geneva, pp. 125–136.

Anonymous, 2003b. Guidelines for the Regulation of Herbal Medicines in the South – East Asia Region. Regional Workshop on the Regulation of Herbal Medicine. World Health Organization, Bangkok, New Delhi, pp. 1–22.

Anonymous, 2003c. WHO Guidelines on Good Agricultural and Field Collection Practices (GACP) for Medicinal Plants. World Health Organization, Geneva, pp. 1–69.

Anonymous, 2003d. Good Trade and Distribution Practices for Pharmaceutical Starting Materials (WHO Technical Report Series, No. 917). World Health Organization, Geneva, pp. 235–264. WHO expert committee on specifications for pharmaceutical preparations-thirty-eighth report.

Anonymus, 2004. Guidelines on Developing Consumer Information on Proper Use of Traditional, Complementary and Alternative Medicine. World Health Organization, Geneva, pp. 1–87.

Anonymous, 2005. National Policy on Traditional Medicine and Regulation of Herbal Medicines. World Health Organization, Geneva, pp. 1–156.

Anonymous, 2006a. In: International Pharmacopoeia, vol. 1. fourth ed. World Health Organization, Geneva.

Anonymous, 2006b. In: International Pharmacopoeia, vol. 2. fourth ed. World Health Organization, Geneva.

Anonymous, 2007a. WHO Guidelines for Assessing Quality of Herbal Medicines with Reference to Contaminants and Residues. World Health Organization, Geneva, pp. 1–89.

Anonymous, 2007b. WHO Guidelines on Good Manufacturing Practices (GMP) for Herbal Medicines. World Health Organization, Geneva, pp. 1–92.

Anonymous, 2013. WHO Traditional Medicine Strategy 2014–2023. World Health Organization, Geneva, pp. 1–70.

Anonymous, 2016a. Regulatory Situation of Herbal Medicines – a Worldwide Review. Retrieved from: http://apps.who.int/medicinedocs/pdf/whozip57e/whozip57e.pdf.

Anonymous, 2016b. https://www.gov.uk/guidance/apply-for-a-traditional-herbal-registration-thr.

Anonymous, 2016c. http://www.who-umc.org/graphics/24727.pdf.

Bensoussan, A., Talley, N.J., Hing, M., Menzies, R., Guo, Ngu, A.M., 1998. Treatment of irritable bowel syndrome with Chinese herbal medicine: a randomized controlled trial. J. Am. Med. Assoc. 280, 1585–1589.

Chalut, D., 1999. Toxicological risks of herbal remedies. Paediatr. Child Health 4, 536–538.

Chan, T.Y., 1997. Monitoring the safety of herbal medicines. Drug Saf. 17, 209–215.

De Smet, P.A., 1995. Health risks of herbal remedies. Drug Saf. 13, 81–93.

Ekor, M., 2014. The growing use of herbal medicines: issues relating to adverse reactions and challenges in monitoring safety. Front. Pharmacol. 4, 1–10.

Kamboj, V.P., 2000. Herbal medicine. Curr. Sci. 78, 35–39.

Kumar, D.S., 2016. Herbal Bioactives and Food Fortification: Extraction and Formulation. CRC Press, London, pp. 1–28.

Kunle, O.F., Egharevba, H.O., Ahmadu, P.O., 2012. Standardization of herbal medicines – a review. Int. J. Biodivers. Conserv. 4, 101–112.

Mukherjee, P.K., Venkatesh, M., Kumar, V., 2007. An overview on the development in regulation and control of medicinal and aromatic plants in the Indian system of medicine. Boletín Latinoamericano y del Caribe de Plantas Medicinales y Aromáticas 6, 129–136.

Munyaradzi, M., 2011. Ethical quandaries in spiritual healing and herbal medicine: a critical analysis of the morality of traditional medicine advertising in southern African urban societies. Pan Afr. Med. J. 10, 1–6.

Paul, A., 1997. A question of standards: herbal medicine regulations create crop controversy. Toxi-Logic 22, 41–42.

Shetti, S., Kumar, C.D., Sriwastava, N.K., Sharma, I.P., 2011. Pharmacovigilance of herbal medicines: current state and future directions. Pharmacogn. Mag. 7, 69–73.

Tambe, S.S., Deore, S., Ahire, P.P., Kadam V.B., 2012. Determination of lipid and alkaloid content in some medicinal plants of Marathwada region in Maharashtra. International Journal of Pharmaceutical Research and Bioscience 1, 195–202.

Wills, R., Stuart, D., 2000. Effect of handling and storage of alkylamides and cichoric acid in *Echinacea purpurea*. J. Sci. Food Agri. 80, 1402–1406.

Appendix

List of Kampo Medicines Manufactured by Tsumura & Co., Japan

Kampo	Ingredients	Ratio	Indications
Kakkonto (TJ-1) (7.5 g/day orally in two or three divided doses)	*Pueraria* root	4	Common cold, coryza, febrile diseases, inflammatory diseases, shoulder stiffness, neuralgia and urticaria
	Jujube	3	
	Ephedra herb	3	
	Glycyrrhiza	2	
	Cinnamon bark	2	
	Peony root	2	
	Ginger	2	
Kakkontokesankyushin'i (TJ-2) Extract (7.5 g/day orally in two or three divided doses)	*Pueraria* root	4	Nasal obstruction, emphysema, and chronic rhinitis
	Jujube	3	
	Ephedra herb	3	
	Glycyrrhiza	2	
	Cinnamon bark	2	
	Peony root	2	
	Magnolia flower	2	
	Cnidium rhizome	2	
	Ginger	1	
Otsujito (TJ-3) (7.5 g/day orally in two or three divided doses)	Japanese *Angelica* root	6	Anal fissures and hemorrhoids
	Bupleurum	5	
	Scutellaria root	3	
	Glycyrrhiza	2	
	Cimicifuga rhizome	1	
	Rhubarb	0.5	
Anchusan (TJ-5) (7.5 g/day orally in two or three divided doses)	Cinnamon bark	4	Nervous gastritis, chronic gastritis, and gastric atony
	Corydalis tuber	3	
	Oyster shell	3	
	Fennel	1.5	
	Glycyrrhiza	1	
	Amomum seed	1	
	Alpinia officinarum rhizome	0.5	

Continued

List of Kampo Medicines Manufactured by Tsumura & Co., Japan—cont'd

Kampo	Ingredients	Ratio	Indications
Jumihaidokuto (TJ-6) (7.5 g/day orally in two or three divided doses)	*Platycodon* root	3	Suppurative dermatosis or acute dermatosis, urticarial acute eczema, and tinea pedis
	Bupleurum root	3	
	Cnidium rhizome	3	
	Poria sclerotium	3	
	Quercus bark	3	
	Aralia rhizome	1.5	
	Saposhnikovia root	1.5	
	Glycyrrhiza	1	
	Schizonepeta spike	1	
	Ginger	1	
Hachimijiogan (TJ-7) (7.5 g/day orally in two or three divided doses)	*Rehmannia* root	6	Nephritis, diabetes mellitus, impotence, sciatica, low back pain, beriberi, prostatic hypertrophy, and hypertension
	Cornus fruit	3	
	Dioscorea rhizome	3	
	Alisma rhizome	3	
	Poria sclerotium	3	
	Moutan bark	2.5	
	Cinnamon bark	1	
	Powdered processed aconite root	0.5	
Daisaikoto (TJ-8) (7.5 g/day orally in two or three divided doses)	*Bupleurum* root	6	Cholelithiasis, cholecystitis, jaundice, hepatic dysfunction, hypertension, cerebral hemorrhage, urticaria, hyperchylia, acute GI catarrh, nausea, vomiting, anorexia, hemorrhoids, diabetes mellitus, neurosis, and insomnia
	Pinellia tuber	4	
	Scutellaria root	3	
	Peony root	3	
	Jujube	3	
	Immature orange	2	
	Ginger	1	
	Rhubarb	1	
Shosaikoto (TJ-9) (7.5 g/day orally in two or three divided doses) May cause intestinal pneumonia Interacts with interferon preparations	*Bupleurum* root	7	Acute febrile diseases, pneumonia, bronchitis, common cold, lymphadenitis, chronic GI disorder, insufficient postpartum recovery, and liver dysfunction due to chronic hepatitis
	Pinellia tuber	5	
	Scutellaria root	3	
	Jujube	3	
	Ginseng	3	
	Glycyrrhiza	2	
	Ginger	1	

List of Kampo Medicines Manufactured by Tsumura & Co., Japan—cont'd

Kampo	Ingredients	Ratio	Indications
Saikokeshito (TJ-10) (7.5 g/day orally in two or three divided doses)	*Bupleurum* root	5	Febrile diseases such as common cold, influenza, pneumonia, and pulmonary tuberculosis; stomach pit tension pain such as gastric ulcer, duodenal ulcer, cholelithiasis, cholecystitis; hepatic dysfunction; and pancreatitis
	Pinellia tuber	4	
	Scutellaria root	2	
	Glycyrrhiza	2	
	Cinnamon bark	2	
	Peony root	2	
	Jujube	2	
	Ginseng	2	
	Ginger	1	
Saikokaryukotsuboreito (TJ-12) (7.5 g/day orally in two or three divided doses)	*Bupleurum* root	5	Hypertension, arteriosclerosis, chronic renal disease, neurasthenia, neurotic palpitation, epilepsy, hysteria, night cry in childhood, and impotence
	Pinellia tuber	4	
	Cinnamon bark	3	
	Poria sclerotium	3	
	Scutellaria root	2.5	
	Jujube	2.5	
	Ginseng	2.5	
	Oyster shell	2.5	
	Long gu	2.5	
	Ginger	1	
Hangeshashinto (TJ-14) (7.5 g/day orally in two or three divided doses) Contraindicated in patients with aldosteronism, myopathy, and hypokalemia	*Pinellia* tuber	5	Acute or chronic GI catarrh, fermentative diarrhea, dyspepsia, gastroptosis, nervous gastritis, gastrasthenia, hangover, belching, heartburn, stomatitis, and neurosis
	Scutellaria root	2.5	
	Processed ginger	2.5	
	Glycyrrhiza	2.5	
	Jujube	2.5	
	Ginseng	2.5	
	Coptis rhizome	1	
Orengedokuto (TJ-15) (7.5 g/day orally in two or three divided doses)	*Scutellaria* root	3	Nosebleed, hypertension, insomnia, neurosis, gastritis, alcoholic hangover, climacteric disturbance and automatic imbalance syndrome peculiar to women resembling climacteric disturbance, dizziness, palpitation, eczema or dermatitis, and pruritus cutaneous
	Coptis rhizome	2	
	Gardenia fruit	2	
	Phellodendron bark	1.5	
Hangekobokuto (TJ-16) (7.5 g/day orally in two or three divided doses)	*Pinellia* tuber	6	Anxiety neurosis, nervous gastritis, hyperemesis gravidarum, coughing, hoarseness, nervous esophageal stricture, and insomnia
	Poria sclerotium	5	
	Magnolia bark	3	
	Perilla herb	2	
	Ginger	1	

Continued

Kampo	Ingredients	Ratio	Indications
Goreisan (TJ-17) (7.5 g/day orally in two or three divided doses)	*Alisma* rhizome	4	Edema, nephrosis, alcoholic hangover, acute GI catarrh, diarrhea, nausea, vomiting, dizziness, water retention in the stomach, headache, uremia, heat stroke, and diabetes mellitus
	Atractylodes lancea rhizome	3	
	Polyporus sclerotium	3	
	Poria sclerotium	3	
	Cinnamon bark	1.5	
Keishikajutsubuto (TJ-18) (7.5 g/day orally in two or three divided doses)	Cinnamon bark	4	Arthralgia and neuralgia
	Peony root	4	
	A. lancea rhizome	4	
	Jujube	4	
	Glycyrrhiza	2	
	Ginger	1	
	Powdered processed aconite root	0.5	
Shoseiryuto (TJ-19) (9 g/day orally in two or three divided doses)	*Pinellia* tuber	6	Bronchitis, bronchial asthma, rhinitis, allergic rhinitis, allergic conjuncti-vitis, and common cold
	Processed ginger	3	
	Glycyrrhiza	3	
	Cinnamon bark	3	
	Schisandra fruit	3	
	Asiasarum root	3	
	Peony root	3	
	Ephedra herb	3	
Boiogito (TJ-20) (7.5 g/day orally in two or three divided doses)	*Astragalus* root	5	Nephritis, nephrosis, nephropathy of pregnancy, hydrocele testis, obesity, arthritis, carbuncle, furuncle, myositis, edema, dermatosis, hyperhidrosis, and menstrual irregularity
	Sinomenium stem	5	
	A. lancea rhizome	3	
	Jujube	3	
	Glycyrrhiza	1.5	
	Ginger	1	
Shohangekabukuryoto (TJ-21) (7.5 g/day orally in two or three divided doses)	*Pinellia* tuber	6	Hyperemesis gravidarum (morning sickness) and vomiting associated with other diseases (acute gastroenteritis, exudative pleurisy, wet beriberi, and empyema)
	Poria sclerotium	5	
	Ginger	1.5	
Shofusan (TJ-22) (7.5 g/day orally in two or three divided doses)	*Rehmannia* root	3	Chronic dermatosis (eczema, urticaria, athlete's foot, miliaria, pruritus) with much exudation and severe itching
	Gypsum	3	
	Japanese *Angelica* root	3	
	Burdock fruit	2	
	A. lancea rhizome	2	
	Saposhnikovia root	2	
	Akebia stem	2	
	Sesame	1.5	
	Anemarrhena rhizome	1.5	
	Glycyrrhiza	1	
	Sophora root	1	
	Schizonepeta spike	1	
	Cicada slough	1	

List of Kampo Medicines Manufactured by Tsumura & Co., Japan—cont'd

Kampo	Ingredients	Ratio	Indications
Tokishakuyakusan (TJ-23) (7.5 g/day orally in two or three divided doses)	Peony root *A. lancea* rhizome *Alisma* rhizome *Poria* sclerotium *Cnidium* rhizome Japanese *Angelica* root	4 4 4 4 3 3	Anemia, malaise, climacteric disturbance (dull headache, headache, dizziness, shoulder stiffness, etc.), menstrual irregularity, dysmenorrhea, infertility, palpitation pounding, chronic nephritis, diseases during pregnancy (edema, habitual abortion, hemorrhoids, abdominal pain), beriberi, hemiplegia, and valvular diseases of the heart
Kamishoyosan (TJ-24) (7.5 g/day orally in two or three divided doses)	*Bupleurum* root Peony root *A. lancea* rhizome Japanese *Angelica* root *Poria* sclerotium *Gardenia* fruit Moutan bark *Glycyrrhiza* Ginger *Mentha* herb	3 3 3 3 3 2 2 1.5 1 1	Oversensitivity to cold, delicate constitution, menstrual irregularity, dysmenorrhea, climacteric disturbance, and automatic imbalance syndrome peculiar to women resembling climacteric disturbance
Keishibukuryogan (TJ-25) (7.5 g/day orally in two or three divided doses)	Cinnamon bark Peony root Peach kernel *Poria* sclerotium Moutan bark	3 3 3 3 3	Inflammation in the uterus and its adnexa, endometritis, menstrual irregularity, dysmenorrhea, leukorrhea, climacteric disturbance (headache, dizziness, feeling of hot flushes, shoulder stiffness, etc.), oversensitivity to cold, peritonitis, contusion, hemorrhoids, and orchitis
Keishikaryukotsuboreito (TJ-26) (7.5 g/day orally in two or three divided doses)	Cinnamon bark Peony root Jujube Oyster shell Long gu *Glycyrrhiza* Ginger	4 4 4 3 3 2 1.5	Nocturnal enuresis in childhood, neurasthenia, sexual neurasthenia, pollution, and impotence

Continued

List of Kampo Medicines Manufactured by Tsumura & Co., Japan—cont'd

Kampo	Ingredients	Ratio	Indications
Maoto (TJ-27) (7.5 g/day orally in two or three divided doses)	Apricot kernel *Ephedra* herb Cinnamon bark *Glycyrrhiza*	5 5 4 1.5	Common cold, influenza (in the initial phase), rheumatoid arthritis, asthma, nasal obstruction in suckling infants, and suckling difficulties
Eppikajyutsuto (TJ-28) (7.5 g/day orally in two or three divided doses)	Gypsum *Ephedra* herb *A. lancea* rhizome Jujube *Glycyrrhiza* Ginger	8 6 4 3 2 1	Nephritis, nephrosis, beriberi, articular rheumatism, nocturnal enuresis, and eczema
Bakumondoto (TJ-29) (7.5 g/day orally in two or three divided doses)	*Ophiopogon* tuber Brown rice *Pinellia* tuber Jujube *Glycyrrhiza* Ginseng	10 5 5 3 2 2	Coughing with a hard, obstructive sputum, bronchitis, and bronchial asthma
Shimbuto (TJ-30) (7.5 g/day orally in two or three divided doses)	*Poria* sclerotium Peony root *A. lancea* rhizome Ginger Powdered processed aconite root	4 3 3 1.5 0.5	GI disease, weak digestive system, chronic enteritis, dyspepsia, gastric atony, gastroptosis, nephrosis, peritonitis, cerebral hemorrhage, motor paralysis and anesthesia due to spinal disease, neurasthenia, hypertension, valvular diseases of heart, palpitation due to cardiac failure, hemiplegia, rheumatism, and senile pruritus
Goshuyuto (TJ-31) (7.5 g/day orally in two or three divided doses)	Jujube *Evodia* fruit Ginseng Ginger	4 3 2 1.5	Habitual migraine, habitual headache, vomiting, and cardiac beriberi
Ninjinto (TJ-32) (7.5 g/day orally in two or three divided doses)	Processed ginger *Glycyrrhiza* *A. lancea* rhizome Ginseng	3 3 3 3	Acute and chronic enterogastritis, gastric atony, gastric dilation, vomiting of pregnancy (morning sickness), and atrophic kidney
Daibotampito (TJ-33) (7.5 g/day orally in two or three divided doses)	*Benincasa* seed Peach kernel Moutan bark Rhubarb Anhydrous mirabilitum	6 4 4 2 1.8	Menstrual irregularity, dysmenorrhea, constipation, and hemorrhoid

List of Kampo Medicines Manufactured by Tsumura & Co., Japan—cont'd

Kampo	Ingredients	Ratio	Indications
Byakkokaninjinto (TJ-34) (9 g/day orally in two or three divided doses)	Gypsum	15	Thirst and hot flushes
	Anemarrhena rhizome	5	
	Glycyrrhiza	2	
	Ginseng	1.5	
	Brown rice	8	
Shigyakusan (TJ-35) (7.5 g/day orally in two or three divided doses)	*Bupleurum* root	5	Cholecystitis, cholelithiasis, gastritis, hyperacidity, gastric ulcer, nasal catarrh, bronchitis, nervousness, and hysteria
	Peony root, immature	4	
	Orange	2	
	Glycyrrhiza	1.5	
Mokuboito (TJ-36) (7.5 g/day orally in two or three divided doses)	Gypsum	10	Relief of diseases originating from the heart or kidneys, as well as edema and cardiac asthma, of those patients with a bad complexion, dyspnea with coughing, and tension and heaviness under the heart
	Sinomenium stem	4	
	Cinnamon bark	3	
	Ginseng	3	
Hangebyakujutsutemmato (TJ-37) (7.5 g/day orally in two or three divided doses)	*Citrus unshiu* peel	3	Dizziness, headache, etc., in patients with a weak GI tract and cold lower limbs
	Pinellia tuber	3	
	Atractylodes rhizome	3	
	Poria sclerotium	3	
	Gastrodia tuber	2	
	Malt	2	
	Astragalus root	1.5	
	Alisma rhizome	1.5	
	Ginseng	1.5	
	Phellodendron bark	1	
	Processed ginger	1	
	Ginger	0.5	
Tokishigyakukagoshuyushokyoto (TJ-38) (7.5 g/day orally in two or three divided doses)	Jujube	5	Chilblain, headache, lower abdominal pain, and low back pain
	Cinnamon bark	3	
	Peony root	3	
	Japanese *Angelica* root	3	
	Akebia stem	3	
	Glycyrrhiza	2	
	Evodia fruit	2	
	Asiasarum root	2	
	Ginger	1	
Ryokeijutsukanto (TJ-39) (7.5 g/day orally in two or three divided doses)	*Poria* sclerotium	6	Nervousness, neurosis, dizziness, heart pounding, shortness of breath, and headache
	Cinnamon bark	4	
	A. lancea rhizome	3	
	Glycyrrhiza	2	

Continued

List of Kampo Medicines Manufactured by Tsumura & Co., Japan—cont'd

Kampo	Ingredients	Ratio	Indications
Choreito (TJ-40) (7.5 g/day orally in two or three divided doses)	Aluminum silicate hydrate with silicon dioxide	3	Urethritis, nephritis, renal calculus, blennorrhagic inflammation, micturition pain, hematuria, edema of the lower part of the body from the waist down, feeling of residual urine, and diarrhea
	Alisma rhizome	3	
	Polyporus sclerotium	3	
	Poria sclerotium	3	
	Donkey glue	3	
Hochuekkito (TJ-41) (7.5 g/day orally in two or three divided doses)	*Astragalus* root	4	Summer emaciation, reinforcement of physical strength after illness, tuberculosis, anorexia, gastroptosis, cold, hemorrhoid, anal prolapse, uterine prolapse, impotence, hemiplegia, and hyperhidrosis
	A. lancea rhizome	4	
	Ginseng	4	
	Japanese *Angelica* root	3	
	Bupleurum root	2	
	Jujube	2	
	C. unshiu peel	2	
	Glycyrrhiza	1.5	
	Cimicifuga rhizome	1	
	Ginger	0.5	
Rikkunshito (TJ-43) (7.5 g/day orally in two or three divided doses)	*A. lancea* rhizome	4	Gastritis, gastric atony, gastroptosis, indigestion, anorexia, gastric pain, and vomiting
	Ginseng	4	
	Pinellia tuber	4	
	Poria sclerotium	4	
	Jujube	2	
	C. unshiu peel	2	
	Glycyrrhiza	1	
	Ginger	0.5	
Keishito (TJ-45) (7.5 g/day orally in two or three divided doses)	Cinnamon bark	4	Symptoms of common cold during the initial phase in patients with a declined constitution
	Peony root	4	
	Jujube	4	
	Glycyrrhiza	2	
	Ginger	1.5	
Shichimotsukokato (TJ-46) (7.5 g/day orally in two or three divided doses)	Peony root	4	Symptoms associated with hypertension (flushing, shoulder stiffness, tinnitus, and dull headache)
	Japanese *Angelica* root	4	
	Astragalus root	3	
	Rehmannia root	3	
	Cnidium rhizome	3	
	Uncaria hook	3	
	Phellodendron bark	2	
Chotosan (TJ-47) (7.5 g/day orally in two or three divided doses)	Gypsum	5	Chronic headache with hypertension in the middle aged or elderly
	Uncaria hook	3	
	C. unshiu peel	3	
	Ophiopogon tuber	3	
	Pinellia tuber	3	
	Poria sclerotium	3	
	Chrysanthemum flower	2	
	Ginseng	2	
	Saposhnikovia root	2	
	Glycyrrhiza	1	
	Ginger	1	

List of Kampo Medicines Manufactured by Tsumura & Co., Japan—cont'd

Kampo	Ingredients	Ratio	Indications
Juzentaihoto (TJ-48) (7.5 g/day orally in two or three divided doses)	*Astragalus* root	3	Declined constitution after recovery from disease, fatigue and malaise, anorexia, perspiration during sleep, cold limbs, and anemia
	Cinnamon bark	3	
	Rehmannia root	3	
	Peony root	3	
	Cnidium rhizome	3	
	A. lancea rhizome	3	
	Japanese *Angelica* root	3	
	Ginseng	3	
	Poria sclerotium	3	
	Glycyrrhiza	1.5	
Keigaitengyoto (TJ-50) (7.5 g/day orally in two or three divided doses)	*Scutellaria* root	1.5	Empyema, chronic rhinitis, chronic tonsillitis, and acne
	Phellodendron bark	1.5	
	Coptis rhizome	1.5	
	Platycodon root	1.5	
	Immature orange	1.5	
	Schizonepeta spike	1.5	
	Bupleurum root	1.5	
	Gardenia fruit	1.5	
	Rehmannia root	1.5	
	Peony root	1.5	
	Cnidium rhizome	1.5	
	Japanese *Angelica* root	1.5	
	Mentha herb	1.5	
	Angelica dahurica root	1.5	
	Saposhnikovia root	1.5	
	Forsythia fruit	1.5	
	Glycyrrhiza	1	
Junchoto (TJ-51) (7.5 g/day orally in two or three divided doses)	*Rehmannia* root	6	Constipation
	Japanese *Angelica* root	3	
	Scutellaria root	2	
	Immature orange	2	
	Apricot kernel	2	
	Magnolia bark	2	
	Rhubarb	2	
	Peach kernel	2	
	Hemp fruit	2	
	Glycyrrhiza	1.5	
Yokuininto (TJ-52) (7.5 g/day orally in two or three divided doses)	Coix seed	8	Arthralgia and myalgia
	A. lancea rhizome	4	
	Japanese *Angelica* root	4	
	Ephedra herb	4	
	Cinnamon bark	3	
	Peony root	3	
	Glycyrrhiza	2	

Continued

List of Kampo Medicines Manufactured by Tsumura & Co., Japan—cont'd

Kampo	Ingredients	Ratio	Indications
Sokeikakketsuto (TJ-53) (7.5 g/day orally in two or three divided doses)	Peony root	2.5	Arthralgia, neuralgia, low back pain, and myalgia
	Rehmannia root	2	
	Cnidium rhizome	2	
	A. lancea rhizome	2	
	Japanese *Angelica* root	2	
	Peach kernel	2	
	Poria sclerotium	2	
	Clematis root	1.5	
	Notopterygium	1.5	
	Achyranthes root	1.5	
	C. unshiu peel	1.5	
	Sinomenium stem	1.5	
	Saposhnikovia root	1.5	
	Japanese gentian	1.5	
	Glycyrrhiza	1	
	A. dahurica root	1	
	Ginger	0.5	
Yokukansan (TJ-54) (7.5 g/day orally in two or three divided doses)	*A. lancea* rhizome	4	Neurosis, insomnia, night cry in children, and peevishness in children
	Poria sclerotium	4	
	Cnidium rhizome	3	
	Uncaria hook	3	
	Japanese *Angelica* root	3	
	Bupleurum root	2	
	Glycyrrhiza	1.5	
Makyokanseikito (TJ-55) (7.5 g/day orally in two or three divided doses)	Gypsum	10	Infantile asthma and bronchial asthma
	Apricot kernel	4	
	Ephedra herb	4	
	Glycyrrhiza	2	
Gorinsan (TJ-56) (7.5 g/day orally in two or three divided doses)	*Poria* sclerotium	6	Frequent urination, micturition pain, and feeling of residual urine
	Scutellaria root	3	
	Glycyrrhiza	3	
	Rehmannia root	3	
	Plantago seed	3	
	Alisma rhizome	3	
	Japanese *Angelica* root	3	
	Akebia stem	3	
	Gardenia fruit	2	
	Peony root	2	
	Talc	3	
Unseiin (TJ-57) (7.5 g/day orally in two or three divided doses)	*Rehmannia* root	3	Menstrual irregularity, dysmenorrhea, automatic imbalance syndrome peculiar to women resembling climacteric disturbance, climacteric disturbance, and neurosis
	Peony root	3	
	Cnidium rhizome	3	
	Japanese *Angelica* root	3	
	Scutellaria root	1.5	
	Phellodendron bark	1.5	
	Coptis rhizome	1.5	
	Gardenia fruit	1.5	

List of Kampo Medicines Manufactured by Tsumura & Co., Japan—cont'd

Kampo	Ingredients	Ratio	Indications
Seijibofuto (TJ-58) (7.5 g/day orally in two or three divided doses)	*Scutellaria* root	2.5	Acne
	Platycodon root	2.5	
	Gardenia fruit	2.5	
	Cnidium rhizome	2.5	
	Glehnia root	2.5	
	A. dahurica root	2.5	
	Forsythia fruit	2.5	
	Coptis rhizome	1	
	Glycyrrhiza	1	
	Immature orange	1	
	Schizonepeta spike	1	
	Mentha herb	1	
Jizusoippo (TJ-59) (7.5 g/day orally in two or three divided doses)	*Cnidium* rhizome	3	Eczema and infantile eczema
	A. lancea rhizome	3	
	Forsythia fruit	3	
	Lonicera leaf and stem	2	
	Saposhnikovia root	2	
	Glycyrrhiza	1	
	Schizonepeta spike	1	
	Safflower	1	
	Rhubarb	0.5	
Keishikashakuyakuto (TJ-60) (7.5 g/day orally in two or three divided doses)	Peony root	6	Tenesmus alvi and abdominal pain
	Cinnamon bark	4	
	Jujube	4	
	Glycyrrhiza	2	
	Ginger	1	
Tokakujokito (TJ-61) (7.5 g/day orally in two or three divided doses)	Peach kernel	5	Menstrual irregularity, dysmenorrhea, anxiety during menstruation or following childbirth, low back pain, constipation, and accessory symptoms associated with hypertension (headache, dizziness, and shoulder stiffness)
	Cinnamon bark	4	
	Rhubarb	3	
	Glycyrrhiza	1.5	
	Anhydrous mirabilitum	0.9	
Bofutsushosan (TJ-62) (7.5 g/day orally in two or three divided doses)	Aluminum silicate hydrate with silicon dioxide	3	Accessory symptoms associated with hypertension (palpitation, shoulder stiffness, and hot flushes), obesity, swelling, and constipation
	Scutellaria root	2	
	Glycyrrhiza	2	
	Platycodon root	2	
	Gypsum	2	
	Atractylodes rhizome	2	
	Rhubarb	1.5	
	Schizonepeta spike	1.2	
	Gardenia fruit	1.2	
	Peony root	1.2	

Continued

List of Kampo Medicines Manufactured by Tsumura & Co., Japan—cont'd

Kampo	Ingredients	Ratio	Indications
	Cnidium rhizome	1.2	
	Japanese *Angelica* root	1.2	
	Mentha herb	1.2	
	Saposhnikovia root	1.2	
	Ephedra herb	1.2	
	Forsythia fruit	1.2	
	Ginger	0.3	
	Anhydrous mirabilitum	0.7	
Goshakusan (TJ-63) (7.5 g/day orally in two or three divided doses)	*A. lancea* rhizome	3	Gastroenteritis, low back pain, neuralgia, arthralgia, menalgia, headache, oversensitivity to cold, climacteric disturbance, and common cold
	C. unshiu peel	2	
	Japanese *Angelica* root	2	
	Pinellia tuber	2	
	Poria sclerotium	2	
	Glycyrrhiza	1	
	Platycodon root	1	
	Immature orange	1	
	Cinnamon bark	1	
	Magnolia bark	1	
	Peony root	1	
	Ginger	1	
	Cnidium rhizome	1	
	Jujube	1	
	A. dahurica root	1	
	Ephedra herb	1	
Shakanzoto (TJ-64) (9 g/day orally in two or three divided doses) Contraindicated in patients with aldosteronism, myopathy, and hypokalemia	*Rehmannia* root	6	Palpitation and shortness of breath in patients with a declined constitution who are easily fatigued
	Ophiopogon tuber	6	
	Cinnamon bark	3	
	Processed *Glycyrrhiza*	3	
	Jujube	3	
	Ginseng	3	
	Hemp fruit	3	
	Ginger	1	
	Donkey glue	2	
Kihito (TJ-65) (7.5 g/day orally in two or three divided doses)	*Astragalus* root	3	Anemia and insomnia
	Jujube seed	3	
	Ginseng	3	
	Atractylodes rhizome	3	
	Poria sclerotium	3	
	Longan aril	3	
	Polygala root	2	
	Jujube	2	
	Japanese *Angelica* root	2	
	Glycyrrhiza	1	
	Ginger	1	
	Saussurea root	1	

List of Kampo Medicines Manufactured by Tsumura & Co., Japan—cont'd

Kampo	Ingredients	Ratio	Indications
Jinsoin (TJ-66) (7.5 g/day orally in two or three divided doses)	*Pinellia* tuber	3	Common cold and cough
	Poria sclerotium	3	
	Pueraria root	2	
	Platycodon root	2	
	Peucedanum root	2	
	C. unshiu peel	2	
	Jujube	1.5	
	Ginseng	1.5	
	Glycyrrhiza	1	
	Immature orange	1	
	Perilla herb	1	
	Ginger	0.5	
Nyoshinsan (TJ-67) (7.5 g/day orally in two or three divided doses)	*Cyperus* rhizome	3	Neurosis before or after childbirth, menstrual irregularity, and automatic imbalance syndrome peculiar to women resembling climacteric disturbance
	Cnidium rhizome	3	
	A. lancea rhizome	3	
	Japanese *Angelica* root	2	
	Scutellaria root	2	
	Cinnamon bark	2	
	Ginseng	2	
	Areca	1	
	Coptis rhizome	1	
	Glycyrrhiza clove	1	
	Saussurea root	1	
Shakuyakukanzoto (TJ-68) (7.5 g/day orally in two or three divided doses) Contraindicated in patients with aldosteronism, myopathy, and hypokalemia	*Glycyrrhiza*	6	Pain, myalgia or arthralgia, gastric pain and abdominal pain accompanied by sudden muscle spasms
	Peony root	6	
Bukuryoin (TJ-69) (7.5 g/day orally in two or three divided doses)	*Poria* sclerotium	5	Gastritis, gastric atony, and excessive fluid retention in the stomach
	A. lancea rhizome	4	
	C. unshiu peel	3	
	Ginseng	3	
	Immature orange	1.5	
	Ginger	1	
Kososan (TJ-70) (7.5 g/day orally in two or three divided doses)	*Cyperus* rhizome	4	Symptoms in the early stage of common cold in nervous people with a weak GI tract
	Perilla herb	2	
	C. unshiu peel	2	
	Glycyrrhiza	1.5	
	Ginger	1	
Shimotsuto (TJ-71) (7.5 g/day orally in two or three divided doses)	*Rehmannia* root	3	Recovery from fatigue after childbearing or abortion, menstrual irregularity, oversensitivity to cold, chilblain, spots, and automatic imbalance syndrome peculiar to women resembling climacteric disturbance
	Peony root	3	
	Cnidium rhizome	3	
	Japanese *Angelica* root	3	

Continued

Kampo	Ingredients	Ratio	Indications
Kambakutaisoto (TJ-72) (7.5 g/day orally in two or three divided doses) Contraindicated in patients with aldosteronism, myopathy, and hypokalemia	Jujube *Glycyrrhiza* Wheat	6 5 20	Night cry and convulsion
Saikanto (TJ-73) (7.5 g/day orally in two or three divided doses)	*Bupleurum* root *Pinellia* tuber *Scutellaria* root Jujube Ginseng *Coptis* rhizome *Glycyrrhiza* Ginger *Trichosanthes* seed	5 5 3 3 2 1.5 1.5 1 3	Coughing and chest pain due to coughing
Choijokito (TJ-74) (7.5 g/day orally in two or three divided doses)	Rhubarb *Glycyrrhiza* Anhydrous mirabilitum	2 1 0.5	Constipation
Shikunshito (TJ-75) (7.5 g/day orally in two or three divided doses)	*A. lancea* rhizome Ginseng *Poria* sclerotium *Glycyrrhiza* Ginger Jujube	4 4 4 1 1 1	Weak digestive system, chronic gastritis, heavy stomach feeling, vomiting, and diarrhea
Ryutanshakanto (TJ-76) (7.5 g/day orally in two or three divided doses)	*Rehmannia* root Japanese *Angelica* root *Akebia* stem *Scutellaria* root *Plantago* seed *Alisma* rhizome *Glycyrrhiza* *Gardenia* fruit Japanese gentian	5 5 5 3 3 3 1 1 1	Micturition pain, feeling of residual urine, turbid urine, and leukorrhea
Kyukikyogaito (TJ-77) (7.5 g/day orally in two or three divided doses) Contraindicated in patients with aldosteronism, myopathy, and hypokalemia	*Rehmannia* root Peony root Japanese *Angelica* root *Artemisia* leaf *Glycyrrhiza* *Cnidium* rhizome Donkey glue	5 4 4 3 3 3 3	Hemorrhoidal bleeding
Makyoyokukanto (TJ-78) (7.5 g/day orally in two or three divided doses)	*Coix* seed *Ephedra* herb Apricot kernel *Glycyrrhiza*	10 4 3 2	Arthralgia, neuralgia, and myalgia
Heiisan (TJ-79) (7.5 g/day orally in two or three divided doses)	*A. lancea* rhizome *Magnolia* bark *C. unshiu* peel Jujube *Glycyrrhiza* Ginger	4 3 3 2 1 0.5	Acute or chronic esogastritis, gastric atony, dyspepsia, and anorexia

List of Kampo Medicines Manufactured by Tsumura & Co., Japan—cont'd

Kampo	Ingredients	Ratio	Indications
Saokoseikanto (TJ-80) (7.5 g/day orally in two or three divided doses)	*Bupleurum* root	2	Neurosis, chronic tonsillitis, and eczema
	Scutellaria root	1.5	
	Phellodendron bark	1.5	
	Coptis rhizome	1.5	
	Trichosanthes root	1.5	
	Glycyrrhiza	1.5	
	Platycodon root	1.5	
	Burdock fruit	1.5	
	Gardenia fruit	1.5	
	Rehmannia root	1.5	
	Peony root	1.5	
	Cnidium rhizome	1.5	
	Japanese *Angelica* root	1.5	
	Mentha herb	1.5	
	Forsythia fruit	1.5	
Nichinto (TJ-81) (7.5 g/day orally in two or three divided doses)	*Pinellia* tuber	5	Nausea and vomiting
	Poria sclerotium	5	
	C. unshiu peel	4	
	Glycyrrhiza	1	
	Ginger	1	
Keishininjinto (TJ-82) (7.5 g/day orally in two or three divided doses) Contraindicated in patients with aldosteronism, myopathy, and hypokalemia	Cinnamon bark	4	Headache, palpitations, chronic gastroenteritis, and gastric atony
	Glycyrrhiza	3	
	A. lancea rhizome	3	
	Ginseng	3	
	Processed ginger	2	
Yokukansankachimpihange (TJ-83) (7.5 g/day orally in two or three divided doses)	Pinellia tuber	5	Neurosis, insomnia, night cry in children, and peevishness in children
	A. lancea rhizome	4	
	Poria sclerotium	4	
	Cnidium rhizome	3	
	Uncaria hook	3	
	C. unshiu peel	3	
	Japanese *Angelica* root	3	
	Bupleurum root	2	
	Glycyrrhiza	1.5	
Daiokanzoto (TJ-84) (7.5 g/day orally in two or three divided doses)	Rhubarb	4	Constipation
	Glycyrrhiza	2	
Shimpito (TJ-85) (7.5 g/day orally in two or three divided doses)	*Ephedra* herb	5	Infantile asthma, bronchial asthma, and bronchitis
	Apricot kernel	4	
	Magnolia bark	3	
	C. unshiu peel	2.5	
	Glycyrrhiza	2	
	Bupleurum root	2	
	Perilla herb	1.5	

Continued

Kampo	Ingredients	Ratio	Indications
Tokiinshi (TJ-86) (7.5 g/day orally in two or three divided doses)	Japanese *Angelica* root	5	Chronic eczema (with little exudation) and itching
	Rehmannia root	4	
	Tribulus fruit	3	
	Peony root	3	
	Cnidium rhizome	3	
	Saposhnikovia root	3	
	Polygonum root	2	
	Astragalus root	1.5	
	Schizonepeta spike	1.5	
	Glycyrrhiza	1	
Rokumigan (TJ-87) (7.5 g/day orally in two or three divided doses)	*Rehmannia* root	5	Dysuria, frequent urination, edema, and pruritus
	Cornus fruit	3	
	Dioscorea rhizome	3	
	Alisma rhizome	3	
	Poria sclerotium	3	
	Moutan bark	3	
Nijutsuto (TJ-88) (7.5 g/day orally in two or three divided doses)	*Pinellia* tuber	4	Frozen shoulder
	A. lancea rhizome	3	
	Clematis root	2.5	
	Scutellaria root	2.5	
	Cyperus rhizome	2.5	
	C. unshiu peel	2.5	
	Atractylodes rhizome	2.5	
	Poria sclerotium	2.5	
	Glycyrrhiza	1	
	Ginger	1	
	Arisaema tuber	2.5	
	Aralia root	2.5	
Jidabokuippo (TJ-89) (7.5 g/day orally in two or three divided doses)	Cinnamon bark	3	Swelling and pain caused by contusion
	Cnidium rhizome	3	
	Nuphar rhizome	3	
	Quercus bark	3	
	Glycyrrhiza	1.5	
	Rhubarb	1	
	Clove	1	
Sehaito (TJ-90) (9 g/day orally in two or three divided doses)	Japanese *Angelica* root	3	Coughing accompanied by frequent expectoration
	Ophiopogon tuber	3	
	Poria sclerotium	3	
	Scutellaria root	2	
	Platycodon root	2	
	Apricot kernel	2	
	Gardenia fruit	2	
	Mulberry bark	2	
	Jujube	2	
	C. unshiu peel	2	
	Asparagus tuber	2	
	Fritillaria bulb	2	
	Glycyrrhiza	1	
	Schisandra fruit	1	
	Ginger	1	
	Bamboo culm	2	

List of Kampo Medicines Manufactured by Tsumura & Co., Japan—cont'd

Kampo	Ingredients	Ratio	Indications
Chikujountanto (TJ-91) (7.5 g/day orally in two or three divided doses)	*Pinellia* tuber	5	Patients with persisting fever during the convalescent phase of influenza, common cold, pneumonia, etc., or those who do not feel refreshed after the temperature has returned to normal and cannot have a good sleep, with frequent coughing or expectoration
	Bupleurum root	3	
	Ophiopogon tuber	3	
	Poria sclerotium	3	
	Platycodon root	2	
	Immature orange	2	
	Cyperus rhizome	2	
	C. unshiu peel	2	
	Coptis rhizome	1	
	Glycyrrhiza	1	
	Ginger	1	
	Ginseng	1	
	Bamboo culm	3	
Jinshihoto (TJ-92) (9 g/day orally in two or three divided doses)	*Cyperus* rhizome	3	Chronic coughing and sputum in patients with a delicate constitution
	Bupleurum root	3	
	Lycium bark	3	
	Peony root	3	
	Anemarrhena rhizome	3	
	C. unshiu peel	3	
	Japanese *Angelica* root	3	
	Ophiopogon tuber	3	
	Atractylodes rhizome	3	
	Poria sclerotium	3	
	Fritillaria bulb	2	
	Glycyrrhiza	1	
	Mentha herb	1	
Jiinkokato (TJ-93) (7.5 g/day orally in two or three divided doses)	*A. lancea* rhizome	3	Patients having a fit of coughing without sputum in a throat with little moisture
	Rehmannia root	2.5	
	Peony root	2.5	
	C. unshiu peel	2.5	
	Asparagus tuber	2.5	
	Japanese *Angelica* root	2.5	
	Ophiopogon tuber	2.5	
	Phellodendron bark	1.5	
	Glycyrrhiza	1.5	
	Anemarrhena rhizome	1.5	
Gokoto (TJ-95) (7.5 g/day orally in two or three divided doses)	Gypsum	10	Cough and bronchial asthma
	Apricot kernel	4	
	Ephedra herb	4	
	Mulberry bark	3	
	Glycyrrhiza	2	

Continued

List of Kampo Medicines Manufactured by Tsumura & Co., Japan—cont'd

Kampo	Ingredients	Ratio	Indications
Saibokuto (TJ-96) (7.5 g/day orally in two or three divided doses)	*Bupleurum* root	7	Infantile asthma, bronchial asthma, bronchitis, coughing, and anxiety neurosis
	Pinellia tuber	5	
	Poria sclerotium	5	
	Scutellaria root	3	
	Magnolia bark	3	
	Jujube	3	
	Ginseng	3	
	Glycyrrhiza	2	
	Perilla herb	2	
	Ginger	1	
Daibofuto (TJ-97) (10.5 g/day orally in two or three divided doses)	*Astragalus* root	3	Articular rheumatism of the lower limbs, chronic arthritis, and gout
	Rehmannia root	3	
	Peony root	3	
	A. lancea rhizome	3	
	Japanese *Angelica* root	3	
	Eucommia bark	3	
	Saposhnikovia root	3	
	Cnidium rhizome	2	
	Glycyrrhiza	1.5	
	Notopterygium	1.5	
	Achyranthes root	1.5	
	Jujube	1.5	
	Ginseng	1.5	
	Processed ginger	1	
	Powdered processed aconite root	1	
Ogikenchuto (TJ-98) (18 g/day orally in two or three divided doses)	Peony root	6	Delicate constitution, weakness during convalescence, and night sweats
	Astragalus root	4	
	Cinnamon bark	4	
	Jujube	4	
	Glycyrrhiza	2	
	Ginger	1	
Shokenchuto (TJ-99) (15 g/day orally in two or three divided doses)	Peony root	6	Delicate constitution in childhood, fatigue and malaise, nervousness, chronic gastroenteritis, nocturnal enuresis in children, and night cry
	Cinnamon bark	4	
	Jujube	4	
	Glycyrrhiza	2	
	Ginger	1	
Daikenchuto (TJ-100) (15 g/day orally in two or three divided doses)	Processed ginger	5	Abdominal cold feeling and pain accompanied by abdominal flatulence
	Ginseng	3	
	Zanthoxylum fruit	2	
Shomakakkonto (TJ-101) (7.5 g/day orally in two or three divided doses)	*Pueraria* root	5	Common cold during the initial phase and dermatitis
	Peony root	3	
	Cimicifuga rhizome	2	
	Glycyrrhiza	1.5	
	Ginger	0.5	

List of Kampo Medicines Manufactured by Tsumura & Co., Japan—cont'd

Kampo	Ingredients	Ratio	Indications
Tokito (TJ-102) (7.5 g/day orally in two or three divided doses)	Japanese *Angelica* root	5	Patients who have a feeling of coldness in the back and feeling of enlarged abdomen or abdominal pain
	Pinellia tuber	5	
	Cinnamon bark	3	
	Magnolia bark	3	
	Peony root	3	
	Ginseng	3	
	Astragalus root	1.5	
	Processed ginger	1.5	
	Zanthoxylum fruit	1.5	
	Glycyrrhiza	1	
Sansoninto (TJ-103) (7.5 g/day orally in two or three divided doses)	Jujube seed	10	Patients who suffer from physical and mental fatigue and weakness and cannot sleep well
	Poria sclerotium	5	
	Cnidium rhizome	3	
	Anemarrhena rhizome	3	
	Glycyrrhiza	1	
Shin'iseihaito (TJ-104) (7.5 g/day orally in two or three divided doses)	Gypsum	5	Nasal obstruction, chronic rhinitis, and empyema
	Ophiopogon tuber	5	
	Scutellaria root	3	
	Gardenia fruit	3	
	Anemarrhena rhizome	3	
	Lilium bulb	3	
	Magnolia flower	2	
	Loquat leaf	2	
	Cimicifuga rhizome	1	
Tsudosan (TJ-105) (7.5 g/day orally in two or three divided doses)	Immature orange	3	Menstrual irregularity, menalgia, climacteric disturbance, low back pain, constipation, bruise (contusion), and symptoms associated with hypertension (headache, dizziness, and shoulder stiffness)
	Rhubarb	3	
	Japanese *Angelica* root	3	
	Glycyrrhiza	2	
	Safflower	2	
	Magnolia bark	2	
	Sappan wood	2	
	C. unshiu peel	2	
	Akebia stem	2	
	Anhydrous mirabilitum	1.8	
Unkeito (TJ-106) (7.5 g/day orally in two or three divided doses)	*Ophiopogon* tuber	4	Menstrual irregularity, dysmenorrhea, leukorrhea, climacteric disturbance, insomnia, neurosis, eczema, cold feeling in the lower limbs and waist, and chilblain
	Pinellia tuber	4	
	Japanese *Angelica* root	3	
	Glycyrrhiza	2	
	Cinnamon bark	2	
	Peony root	2	
	Cnidium rhizome	2	
	Ginseng	2	
	Moutan bark	2	
	Evodia fruit	1	
	Ginger	1	
	Gelatin	2	

Continued

List of Kampo Medicines Manufactured by Tsumura & Co., Japan—cont'd

Kampo	Ingredients	Ratio	Indications
Goshajinkigan (TJ-107) (7.5 g/day orally in two or three divided doses)	*Rehmannia* root	5	Leg pain, low back pain, numbness, blurred vision in old patients, pruritus, dysuria, frequent urination, and edema
	Achyranthes root	3	
	Cornus fruit	3	
	Dioscorea rhizome	3	
	Plantago seed	3	
	Alisma rhizome	3	
	Poria sclerotium	3	
	Moutan bark	3	
	Cinnamon bark	1	
	Powdered processed aconite root	1	
Ninjin'yoeito (TJ-108) (7.5 g/day orally in two or three divided doses)	*Rehmannia* root	4	Declined constitution after recovery from disease, fatigue and malaise, anorexia, perspiration during sleep, cold limbs, and anemia
	Japanese *Angelica* root	4	
	Atractylodes rhizome	4	
	Poria sclerotium	4	
	Ginseng	3	
	Cinnamon bark	2.5	
	Polygala root	2	
	Peony root	2	
	C. unshiu peel	2	
	Astragalus root	1.5	
	Glycyrrhiza	1	
	Schisandra fruit	1	
Shosaikotokakikyosekko (TJ-109) (7.5 g/day orally in two or three divided doses)	Gypsum	10	Tonsillitis and peritonsillitis
	Bupleurum root	7	
	Pinellia tuber	5	
	Scutellaria root	3	
	Platycodon root	3	
	Jujube	3	
	Ginseng	3	
	Glycyrrhiza	2	
	Ginger	1	
Rikkosan (TJ-110) (7.5 g/day orally in two or three divided doses)	*Asiasarum* root	2	Pain after tooth extraction and toothache
	Cimicifuga rhizome	2	
	Saposhnikovia root	2	
	Glycyrrhiza	1.5	
	Japanese gentian	1	
Seishirenshiin (TJ-111) (7.5 g/day orally in two or three divided doses)	*Ophiopogon* tuber	4	Feeling of residual urine, pollakiuria, and micturition pain
	Poria sclerotium	4	
	Nelumbo seed	4	
	Scutellaria root	3	
	Plantago seed	3	
	Ginseng	3	
	Astragalus root	2	
	Lycium bark	2	
	Glycyrrhiza	1.5	

List of Kampo Medicines Manufactured by Tsumura & Co., Japan—cont'd

Kampo	Ingredients	Ratio	Indications
Choreitogoshimotsuto (TJ-112) (7.5 g/day orally in two or three divided doses)	Aluminum silicate hydrate with silicon dioxide	3	Difficulty in micturition, micturition pain, feeling of residual urine, and frequent urination
	Rehmannia root	3	
	Peony root	3	
	Cnidium rhizome	3	
	Alisma RHIZOME	3	
	Polyporus sclerotium	3	
	Japanese *Angelica* root	3	
	Poria sclerotium	3	
	Donkey glue	3	
Sano'shashinto (TJ-113) (7.5 g/day orally in two or three divided doses)	*Scutellaria* root	3	Symptoms associated with hypertension (flushing, shoulder stiffness, tinnitus, dull headache, insomnia, and anxiety), nosebleed, hemorrhoidal bleeding, constipation, climacteric disturbance, and automatic imbalance syndrome peculiar to women resembling climacteric disturbance
	Coptis rhizome	3	
	Rhubarb	3	
Saireito (TJ-114) (9 g/day orally in two or three divided doses)	*Bupleurum* root	7	Watery diarrhea, acute gastroenteritis, sunstroke, and edema
	Alisma rhizome	5	
	Pinellia tuber	5	
	Scutellaria root	3	
	A. lancea rhizome	3	
	Jujube	3	
	Polyporus sclerotium	3	
	Ginseng	3	
	Poria sclerotium	3	
	Glycyrrhiza	2	
	Cinnamon bark	2	
	Ginger	1	
Ireito (TJ-115) (7.5 g/day orally in two or three divided doses)	*Magnolia* bark	2.5	Food poisoning, heat stroke, cold abdomen, acute gastroenteritis, and abdominal pain
	A. lancea rhizome	2.5	
	Alisma rhizome	2.5	
	Polyporus sclerotium	2.5	
	C. unshiu peel	2.5	
	Atractylodes rhizome	2.5	
	Poria sclerotium	2.5	
	Cinnamon bark	2	
	Ginger	1.5	
	Jujube	1.5	
	Glycyrrhiza	1	

Continued

List of Kampo Medicines Manufactured by Tsumura & Co., Japan—cont'd

Kampo	Ingredients	Ratio	Indications
Bukuryoingohangekobokuto (TJ-116) (7.5 g/day orally in two or three divided doses)	*Pinellia* tuber *Poria* sclerotium *A. lancea* rhizome *Magnolia* bark *C. unshiu* peel Ginseng *Perilla* herb Immature orange Ginger	6 5 4 3 3 3 2 1.5 1	Anxiety neurosis, nervous gastritis, hyperemesis gravidarum, water brash, and gastritis
Inchingoreisan (TJ-117) (7.5 g/day orally in two or three divided doses)	*Alisma* rhizome *A. lancea* rhizome *Polyporus* sclerotium *Poria* sclerotium *Artemisia capillaris* flower Cinnamon bark	6 4.5 4.5 4.5 4 2.5	Vomiting, urticaria, hangover nausea, and swelling
Ryokyojutsukanto (TJ-118) (7.5 g/day orally in two or three divided doses)	*Poria* sclerotium Processed ginger *Atractylodes* rhizome *Glycyrrhiza*	6 3 3 2	Low back pain, cold low back, and nocturnal enuresis
Ryokankyomishingeninto (TJ-119) (7.5 g/day orally in two or three divided doses)	Apricot kernel *Pinellia* tuber *Poria* sclerotium *Schisandra* fruit Processed ginger *Glycyrrhiza* *Asiasarum* root	4 4 4 3 2 2 2	Bronchitis, bronchial asthma, cardiac weakness, and kidney disease
Orento (TJ-120) (7.5 g/day orally in two or three divided doses) Contraindicated in patients with aldosteronism, myopathy, and hypokalemia	*Pinellia* tuber *Coptis* rhizome Processed ginger *Glycyrrhiza* Cinnamon bark Jujube Ginseng	6 3 3 3 3 3 3	Acute gastritis, hangover, and stomatitis
Sammotsuogonto (TJ-121) (7.5 g/day orally in two or three divided doses)	*Rehmannia* root *Scutellaria* root *Sophora* root	6 3 3	Hot flushes in the limbs
Hainosankyuto (TJ-122) (7.5 g/day orally in two or three divided doses) Contraindicated in patients with aldosteronism, myopathy, and hypokalemia	*Platycodon* root *Glycyrrhiza* Immature orange Peony root Jujube Ginger	4 3 3 3 3 1	Purulence with a reddened, swollen, and painful lesion; carbuncle; furuncle; facial furuncle; and other furunculosis
Tokikenchuto (TJ-123) (7.5 g/day orally in two or three divided doses)	Peony root Cinnamon bark Jujube Japanese *Angelica* root *Glycyrrhiza* Ginger	5 4 4 4 2 1	Menalgia, lower abdominal pain, hemorrhoids, and pain of proctoptosis

List of Kampo Medicines Manufactured by Tsumura & Co., Japan—cont'd

Kampo	Ingredients	Ratio	Indications
Senkyuchachosan (TJ-124) (7.5 g/day orally in two or three divided doses)	*Cyperus* rhizome *Cnidium* rhizome *Notopterygium* *Schizonepeta* spike *Mentha* herb *A. dahurica* root *Saposhnikovia* root *Glycyrrhiza* Green tea leaf	4 3 2 2 2 2 2 1.5 1.5	Common cold, automatic imbalance syndrome peculiar to women resembling climacteric disturbance, and headache
Keishibukuryogankayokuinin (TJ-125) (7.5 g/day orally in two or three divided doses)	*Coix* seed Cinnamon bark Peony root Peach kernel *Poria* sclerotium Moutan bark	10 4 4 4 4 4	Menstrual irregularity, automatic imbalance syndrome peculiar to women resembling climacteric disturbance, acne, spots, and roughness of the hands and feet
Mshiningan (TJ-126) (7.5 g/day orally in two or three divided doses)	Hemp fruit Rhubarb Immature orange Apricot kernel *Magnolia* bark Peony root	5 4 2 2 2 2	Constipation
Maobushisaishinto (TJ-127) (7.5 g/day orally in two or three divided doses)	*Ephedra* herb *Asiasarum* root Powdered processed aconite root	4 3 1	Common cold and bronchitis
Keihito (TJ-128) (7.5 g/day orally in two or three divided doses)	*A. lancea* rhizome *Poria* sclerotium *Dioscorea* rhizome Ginseng *Nelumbo* seed *Crataegus* fruit *Alisma* rhizome *C. unshiu* peel *Glycyrrhiza*	4 4 3 3 3 2 2 2 1	Weak digestive system, chronic gastroenteritis, dyspepsia, and diarrhea
Daijokito (TJ-133) (7.5 g/day orally in two or three divided doses)	*Magnolia* bark Immature orange Rhubarb Anhydrous mirabilitum	5 3 2 1.3	Chronic constipation, acute constipation, hypertension, neurosis, and food poisoning
Keishikashakuyakudaioto (TJ-134) (7.5 g/day orally in two or three divided doses)	Peony root Cinnamon bark Jujube *Glycyrrhiza* Rhubarb Ginger	6 4 4 2 2 1	Acute enterocolitis, large intestinal catarrh, habitual constipation, fecal impaction, and tenesmus alvi
Inchinkoto (TJ-135) (7.5 g/day orally in two or three divided doses)	*A. capillaris* flower *Gardenia* fruit Rhubarb	4 3 1	Jaundice, hepatic cirrhosis, nephrosis, urticaria, and stomatitis

Continued

List of Kampo Medicines Manufactured by Tsumura & Co., Japan—cont'd

Kampo	Ingredients	Ratio	Indications
Seishoekkito (TJ-136) (7.5 g/day orally in two or three divided doses)	*A. lancea* rhizome	3.5	Heat stroke, anorexia, diarrhea, and general malaise due to heat and emaciation in summer
	Ginseng	3.5	
	Ophiopogon tuber	3.5	
	Astragalus root	3	
	C. unshiu peel	3	
	Japanese *Angelica* root	3	
	Phellodendron bark	1	
	Glycyrrhiza	1	
	Schisandra fruit	1	
Kamikihito (TJ-137) (7.5 g/day orally in two or three divided doses)	*Astragalus* root	3	Anemia, insomnia, mental anxiety, and neurosis
	Bupleurum root	3	
	Jujube seed	3	
	A. lancea rhizome	3	
	Ginseng	3	
	Poria sclerotium	3	
	Longan aril	3	
	Polygala root	2	
	Gardenia fruit	2	
	Jujube	2	
	Japanese *Angelica* root	2	
	Glycyrrhiza	1	
	Ginger	1	
	Saussurea root	1	
Kikyoto (TJ-138) (7.5 g/day orally in two or three divided doses) Contraindicated in patients with aldosteronism, myopathy, and hypokalemia	*Glycyrrhiza*	3	Tonsillitis and peritonsillitis
	Platycodon root	2	

All the information in this table was collected from the individual Kampo pamphlets provided by Tsumura & Co. Ltd., Tokyo, Japan. *GI*, gastrointestinal.

Index

'*Note*: Page numbers followed by "f" indicate figures and "t" indicate tables.'